Aging, Health, and Behavior

Aging, Health, and Behavior

edited by
Marcia G. Ory
Ronald P. Abeles
Paula Darby Lipman

SAGE PUBLICATIONS
The International Professional Publishers
Newbury Park   London   New Delhi

For information address:

SAGE Publications, Inc.
2455 Teller Road
Newbury Park, California 91320

SAGE Publications Ltd.
London EC2A 4PU
United Kingdom

SAGE Publications India Pvt. Ltd.
M-32 Market
Greater Kailash I
New Delhi 110 048 India

Printed in the United States of America

Library of Congress Cataloging-in-Publication Data

Main entry under title:

Aging, health, and behavior / edited by Marcia G. Ory, Ronald P.
   Abeles, Paula Darby Lipman.
       p.   cm.
   Includes bibliographical references and index.
   ISBN 0-8039-4342-3 (cloth.) – ISBN 0-8039-4343-1 (pbk.)
   1. Aged–Health and hygiene. 2. Health behavior. I. Ory, Marcia
G. II. Abeles, Ronald P., 1944-   . III. Lipman, Paula Darby.
   [DNLM: 1. Aging–psychology. 2. Health Behavior. 3. Health
Promotion. 4. Health Services for the Aged. 5. Social Environment.
WT 104 A26753]
RA564.8.H392   1991
618.97–dc20
DNLM/DLC
for Library of Congress   91-18529
                                                                  CIP

92 93 94 15 14 13 12 11 10 9 8 7 6 5 4 3 2

Sage Production Editor: Astrid Virding

Contents

Foreword

MATILDA WHITE RILEY

The chapters in this volume reflect a decade of progress within the emerging area of research on health and behavior, and they point to an agenda for the future. Because their special focus is on aging, they infuse into the earlier static treatments of health and behavior the special dimension of time—with its reference to process and change. Thus a unique feature of both the past progress and the future agenda is the dynamic perspective. Two major projects provide much of the background for these chapters and their special perspective, one early in the decade and one in mid-decade. In both, the National Institute on Aging (NIA) was closely involved.

A report by the Institute of Medicine (IOM) laid the groundwork for the broad area addressed in these chapters and elaborated some of the conceptual and methodological complexities with which they contend. That report, published in 1982, was titled *Health and Behavior: Frontiers of Research in the Biobehavioral Sciences* (Hamburg, Elliott, & Parron). Based on several years of work by more than 400 behavioral and biomedical scientists, and drawing on formulations by the newly established Academy for Behavioral Medicine Research (Weiss, Herd, & Fox, 1981), this report confronted the discovery that the heaviest burdens of illness in the United States are related to individual behaviors and life-styles. The several conferences and studies involved in the project examined the varied linkages between health and behavior and demonstrated the importance for health promotion and disease prevention of understanding these linkages. Emphasizing that human behavior can be observed "systematically, reliably, and reproducibly," and setting out an array of unprecedented scientific opportunities, the report concluded that "underlying causes will be identified with more certainty when the intimate interplay between genetics and environmental factors and the rich variability of individuals and societies are taken into account" (Hamburg, Elliott, & Parron, 1982, p. 4).

The report also made clear that the very complexity of the field presents its own difficulties. Pursuit of scientific opportunities requires spanning the range of sciences from anthropology, sociology, and psychology to neuroanatomy, psychneuroendocrinology, and behavioral genetics. It also requires a broadly integrative approach that blends basic, applied, and clinical aspects of all these behavioral, social, and biomedical sciences.

Nevertheless, the approach to research on health and behavior as understood at that time was not dynamic. Despite the seminal contributions of the report, its concern with the "rich variability of individuals and societies" took little account of the fact that both individuals and societies are continually moving and changing over time. To be sure, one of the six conferences contributing to the report was devoted to "health, behavior, and aging" and explicated the processes of aging and cohort flow as a "new paradigm" for understanding the health-behavior linkages (Riley, 1981). But the essential relevance of such a dynamic paradigm was lost in the overall report. The mistaken notion that individuals, as well as their social environments, are fixed in time remained obstinate. A case in point is the related report of the IOM's Committee on Stress and Health, also published in 1982 (Elliott & Eisdorfer, 1982). This committee delved deeply into the relationships among four elements: environmental stressors, their antecedents, the consequent health outcomes, and the causal connections among them. Yet, as members of that committee, Beatrix Hamburg and I had practically no success in convincing the other members that these elements not only influence each other over time and within a changing environment but also are closely intertwined with the social, psychological, and biological processes of aging. In another instance, an edited volume in social psychology (Abeles, 1987), itself a linkage field, found practically no recognition of a dynamic life-course perspective.

Several years later, a second major project explicitly incorporated aging as a process-oriented or dynamic force into research on health and behavior. This project, which began with a conference, was published in 1987 under the title *Perspectives in Behavioral Medicine: The Aging Dimension* (Riley, Matarazzo, & Baum). The project was jointly sponsored by the Academy for Behavioral Medicine Research (ABMR) and the NIA—a joint sponsorship that is noteworthy because it juxtaposed ABMR's broad integration between biomedical and social-behavioral knowledge with the NIA's involvement with the dynamic dimension of this knowledge. Contributors, who focused on selected areas (cognitive, neurological, immunological, physiological), not only continued (as in the IOM project) to investigate the interplay between health and behavior but also examined this interplay in a new light, as involving human beings who are growing older over time.

The opening chapter of that book enunciated guiding principles for research on aging, as follows:

> Aging is multifaceted, consisting of social and psychological as well as biological processes;
>
> Aging is not entirely fixed for all time, but varies with social structure and social change;
>
> And, as a corollary, because aging is not immutable, it is subject to a degree of social and behavioral as well as biomedical modification and intervention. (Riley, 1987, p. 2)

Already, in 1987, it was acknowledged that these principles may seem more self-evident to the social and behavioral scientists than to the biomedical scientists:

> While [the former] emphasize the conditions of social and cultural variability and change in aging, the biomedical scientists are more likely to emphasize the species-specific universals in the aging process. Yet, members of the human species do not grow old in laboratories. And universal aging processes must be gleaned, not from studies of any single cohort, but from many cohorts under the most widely varying social and temporal conditions. (Riley, 1987, p. 2)

In elucidating and specifying these global principles, the goal of the project on the aging dimension of health and behavior was "to share multidisciplinary understandings of what is known, take inventory of what is currently under study, and outline research agendas for the future in this increasingly integrated area" (Riley, 1987, p. 2). This ABMR-NIA project took the early steps toward that goal.

Only recently, however, have signal advances toward the goal been set in motion—advances that are abundantly illustrated in the current volume *Aging, Health, and Behavior*. Two interrelated components of the dynamic perspective, as announced in the ABMR-NIA project (see also Riley, Abeles, & Teitelbaum, 1982), are now useful in considering how far the field has come and what further directions lie ahead:

> *a life-course perspective*, which examines biomedical and psychosocial processes as they continually influence each other from birth to death; and
>
> *a cohort perspective*, which examines how these multifaceted aging processes respond to social change, so that cohorts of people who are growing old today age differently from cohorts who grew old in the past and from those who will grow old in the future. (Riley, 1987, p. 3)

Much of the material in this volume demonstrates for the field of health and behavior the growing power of the life-course perspective (see Abeles & Riley, 1976-1977). From this perspective, the task is to take into account all the diverse strands of the aging processes, which include

> *biological* aging processes (neural, immunological, endocrine, and other physiological changes);
>
> *cognitive and biopsychological* aging processes (change or constancy in intellectual or sensori-motor functioning);
>
> *attitudinal and motivational* aging processes (change or constancy in self-esteem, personal control, coping, maintaining a sense of personal identity); and
>
> *social* aging processes (not only reactions to "events" but also growing older within particular roles, actively shaping these roles, relating to and interacting with significant other people). (Riley, 1987, p. 7)

Throughout the ensuing chapters are numerous examples of how these strands, themselves changing with age, interact with one another as a person grows older and also of how change in any one strand creates feedback loops in the others.

Of course, many discussions of health and behavior in this volume focus not on aging as a process but on age differences and current interactions between older people and younger people at a given period of time. This focus typically requires cross-sectional, rather than longitudinal, analyses. At the same time, few scientists today make the mistake of interpreting these cross-sectional age differences as describing aging as a process. Now informed by the life-course perspective, they rarely fall into the trap of the "life-course fallacy." Indeed, they go far toward expunging the persistent residues of this fallacy, which—because, in cross section, old people tend to be less advantaged than young people—have so long perpetuated the doctrine of inevitable and universal aging decline.

While recent work in health and behavior has progressed rapidly in the use of the life-course perspective, the cohort perspective by contrast is still little developed, is obfuscated by much conceptual and methodological confusion, and thus offers wide opportunities for future progress. The variability of the aging process, and the conditions under which the process is mutable and subject to intervention, can be probed not only by tracing the lives of individuals who are growing old today but also by comparing different cohorts of individuals who—because they are born, grow up, and grow old under differing historical and future social conditions—grow old in very different ways.

Insofar as this volume typifies the literature in the field as a whole, there is still too little scrutiny of the interconnections between historical trends or long-term policies and the differing interactions between health and behavior in successive cohorts. And there is still too little recognition of the special power of cohort analyses for improving forecasts, in that many facts are already known about the earlier lives of cohort members now alive who will be the old people of the future.

Nevertheless, experience with the "baby boom" cohorts means that scientific and even popular awareness of the cohort perspective is now emerging. This awareness serves as a guard against the fallacy of "cohort centrism"—that is, erroneously defining aging in general as we ourselves have experienced it in our own particular cohorts. The numerous dramatic evidences that cohort differences exist show emphatically that old age as it is today, or will be in the coming years, cannot be understood by relying on existing studies of people who were old in the recent past. In this sense, and quite apart from disease, social and behavioral scientists are beginning to recognize that the expression *normal aging* can be misleading, that what seems "normal" may mean merely "cohort centric."

In sum, the chapters in this volume build firmly on the work on health, behavior, and aging that has been accumulating in the past decade, and they look ahead to potentially more fruitful avenues in the coming decade. Speaking for the NIA, I take great satisfaction in the significant contributions by the scientific staff of the Social and Behavioral Research program to these developments, past and future. All members of this staff have continually encouraged research in this area. And, in particular, the NIA has held the lead in the all-NIH Working Group on Health and Behavior, which provided major sponsorship for the IOM project of 1982 and has continued throughout the decade to coordinate relevant work in all the NIH institutes (and, on occasion, in all the agencies of the Public Health Service). Moreover, it was the NIA that took the initiative in organizing and implementing the ABMR-NIA project of 1987, which established aging as a basic dimension of health and behavior.

I wish to express special appreciation for the ongoing contributions of Marcia Ory and Ronald Abeles: the former for her skillful management of the program in psychosocial geriatric research at the NIA, and the latter for his splendid implementation of the NIH and NIA initiatives in the broad area of health and behavior research. It is fitting that these two scholars, together with a more recent colleague, bring much of this work to fruition in this volume. My own efforts here have been, and will continue to be, greatly enlarged by those of the editors.

REFERENCES

Abeles, R. P. (Ed.). (1987). *Life-span perspectives and social psychology.* Hillsdale, NJ: Lawrence Erlbaum.

Abeles, R. P., & Riley, M. W. (1976-1977). A life-course perspective on the later years of life: Some implications for research. *Social Science Research Council annual report* (pp. 1-16). New York: Social Science Research Council.

Elliott, G. R., & Eisdorfer, C. (Eds.). (1982). *Stress and human health: Analysis and implications of research.* New York: Springer.

Hamburg, D. A., Elliott, G. R., & Parron, D. L. (1982). *Health and behavior: Frontiers of research in the biobehavioral sciences* (Institute of Medicine Publication 82-010). Washington, DC: National Academy Press.

Riley, M. W. (1981). Health behavior of older people: Toward a new paradigm. In D. L. Parron, F. Solomon, & J. Rodin (Eds.), *Health, behavior and aging.* Washington, DC: National Academy Press.

Riley, M. W. (1987). Aging, health, and social change: An overview. In M. W. Riley, J. D. Matarazzo, & A. Baum (Eds.), *Perspectives in behavioral medicine: The aging dimension* (pp. 1-14). Hillsdale, NJ: Lawrence Erlbaum.

Riley, M. W., Abeles, R. P., & Teitelbaum, M. S. (Eds.). (1982). *Aging from birth to death: Vol. 2. Sociotemporal perspectives.* Boulder, CO: Westview.

Riley, M. W., Matarazzo, J. D., & Baum, A. (Eds.). (1987). *Perspectives in behavioral medicine: The aging dimension.* Hillsdale, NJ: Lawrence Erlbaum.

Weiss, S. M., Herd, J. A., & Fox, B. H. (Eds.). (1981). *Perspectives on behavioral medicine.* New York: Academic Press.

Acknowledgments

We gratefully acknowledge the help of many people in the preparation of this book. It is the outgrowth of many of the NIA's activities on aging, health, and behavior, including our research program on psychosocial geriatrics research and participation in the NIH Working Group on Health and Behavior. Valuable research/editorial assistance was provided by Sharon Ardison, Lydia Schlinder, and Diane Zablotsky. We especially thank Claudette Grubelich and Michelle Blanco for their assistance in preparation of this manuscript and Nhi Chau and Tung Nguyen for their supportive role.

The principles of aging research outlined in Chapter 1 are drawn primarily from the seminal work of Matilda White Riley, who contributed valuable comments and editorial suggestions for the introduction. We also thank the contributors to the volume and the anonymous reviewers for each chapter.

1

Introduction: An Overview of Research on Aging, Health, and Behavior

MARCIA G. ORY

RONALD PETER ABELES

PAULA DARBY LIPMAN

Two interrelated revolutionary trends during the twentieth century are giving rise to a new orientation toward both health and aging. At the beginning of this century, acute, infectious conditions were the major causes of death. By the closing decade of this century, the conquest of these conditions by modern medicine and public health policy has ironically given rise to a *revolution in chronic illness and disability*, where, for the first time in human history, conditions such as heart disease, cancer, and stroke are the leading causes of morbidity and mortality. These chronic illnesses are often slow in developing, are long lasting, and are not readily treated by methods based upon a germ theory of illness. This transition from acute to chronic conditions has resulted in a shift away from the search for a single infectious germ and its corresponding "magic bullet" cure. Instead, emphasis is increasingly placed upon understanding the complex interactions among environmental, social, behavioral, and biological factors.

At the same time, industrialized countries have been experiencing a virtual *revolution in aging* (Abeles & Riley, 1987; Havlik et al., 1987; Torrey, Kinsella, & Tauber, 1987; U.S. Senate, 1989). With the triumph over the lethal, acute diseases of childhood during the first half of the twentieth century, ever greater proportions of each successive birth

AUTHORS' NOTE: The authors of this chapter are employees of the federal government; therefore, the text of this chapter cannot be copyrighted and is in the public domain.

1

cohort have survived to old age. The U.S. Bureau of the Census estimates that, among babies born in 1980, 77% could look forward to reaching age 65, as compared with about 41% in 1900 (National Center for Health Statistics, 1985; U.S. Bureau of the Census, 1984). Moreover, during the second half of this century, similar improvements in the mortality experiences of older people have become evident. For example, the proportion of 65-year-olds in 1980 who could expect to reach age 85 was more than twice the 1900 proportion (Rosenwaike, 1985).

Not only are people living longer, but older people compose a greater proportion of the population than ever before. Improvements in mortality at both younger and older ages have combined with declines in birth rates to produce a dramatic reshaping of the population "pyramid." While older people constituted 4% of the U.S. population in 1900, they now represent about 12% (U.S. Bureau of the Census, 1988). Moreover, the size of this population is projected to increase significantly through 2030, when there will be approximately 66 million people over age 65, representing 22% of the American people (U.S. Senate, 1989).

An appreciation of this "revolution in aging"—increasing longevity and an increasing population of older people—has stimulated the expansion of the scientific study of aging as a multidisciplinary endeavor. Although a significant and growing amount of research has been devoted separately to psychosocial aspects of health and aging, relatively little attention has been focused on their confluence. The purpose of this volume is to encourage understanding of the interactions among aging and psychosocial factors as they influence health and effective functioning. This initial chapter provides an overview of basic concepts in health and behavior research, discusses social and behavioral principles of aging research, and introduces the reader to *psychosocial geriatrics research*, an emerging field of inquiry that examines the relationship of age to health and behavior. Individual chapters are briefly highlighted and future research needs identified.

BEHAVIORAL MEDICINE:
HEALTH AND BEHAVIOR RESEARCH

More than a decade ago, the 1979 U.S. Surgeon General's Report *Healthy People* (U.S. Department of Health, Education and Welfare, 1979) directed the national spotlight at the relationship between health and behavior by documenting the extent to which life-styles contributed to the burden of chronic illness in the United States and other industrialized countries. Since then, health professionals and the public alike have become increasingly aware of the critical role of behaviors and life-styles in promoting health and preventing disease and disability (Berkman & Breslow, 1983; Hamburg, Elliot, & Parron, 1982; Kasl, 1986; Riley & Bond, 1983; U.S. Department of Health and Human Services, 1990; U.S. Department of Health, Education and Welfare, 1980). The scientific study of the interactions between health and behavior has been spurred by the establishment of *behavioral medicine*, an interdisciplinary field that integrates knowledge in the biomedical and behavioral sciences as applied to the prevention, diagnosis, treatment, and rehabilitation of disease (Schneiderman & Tapp, 1985; Schwartz & Weiss, 1979; Weiss, Herd, & Fox, 1981).

Mechanisms Linking Health and Behavior

Quite apart from research on aging, a growing body of research focuses on factors affecting behavior and the mechanisms through which behaviors are translated step by step into health outcomes (Berkman, 1989; Cohen, 1988; Hamburg et al., 1982; McQueen & Siegrist, 1983). Such studies can be characterized by a progressive specification of all pathways involved. For example, as will be detailed in the individual chapters in this volume, there are increased efforts toward understanding direct and indirect social and behavioral processes, intervening physiological pathways, and various stages in the onset and course of disease processes and outcomes. The fact that social and behavioral conditions are associated with a wide range of outcomes, not a single disease entity, suggests that several pathways lead from social and behavioral factors to illness and/or that certain factors act to increase general susceptibility to disease (Berkman, 1989; Cassel, 1976).

A schema for viewing the relations between health and behavior has been developed over the years by the National Institutes of Health's Working Group on Health and Behavior, especially in this Group's Annual Reports. As diagrammed in Figure 1.1, the schema represents a simplified pathway leading from health-related behaviors to health outcomes through intervening physiological or psychosocial variables. Included in this schema (Abeles, 1988) are two types of *health attitudes and behaviors* and one type of *intervening mechanism* linking behavior to physical illness:

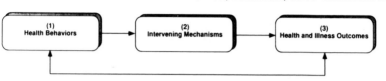

Figure 1.1. Health and Behavior Linkages: A Simplified Schema

- **habits and life-styles,** such as smoking, heavy drinking, exercise, diet, hygienic practices, and social activity and participation in social networks;
- **reactions to illness** by the patient, his or her family, health care providers, social organizations, and so on (e.g., denying or minimizing the significance of symptoms, delaying medical care, and failing to prescribe or comply with treatment and rehabilitation regimens); and
- **alterations of tissue functioning** through the central nervous system, hormone production, or physiological responses to psychosocial stimuli (e.g., stress).

While this simplified schema is useful for some purposes, more complex schemata are obviously needed to depict the dynamic interactions between health and behavior, and we have developed a new schema in Figure 1.2. This second schema incorporates several important facets: (a) the influence of exogenous social and environmental factors on health-related behaviors and intervening variables (Box 1); (b) the separation of health attitudes from health behaviors (Box 2), psychosocial from physiological mediators (Boxes 3 and 4), and biological effects from health/disease outcomes (Boxes 5 and 6); (c) attention to interactions between physical and mental health (Box 6); and (d) recognition of reciprocal relationships (e.g., one's state of health can influence health-related behaviors or intervening processes). With respect to Box 6, it is important to note that quality of life, while related to physical health and functioning, does not always depend directly on health factors. Some older people are able to achieve a high quality of life despite poor health and vice versa. Many of the individual chapters in this volume present detailed conceptual frameworks that focus on particular aspects of such a schema as this.

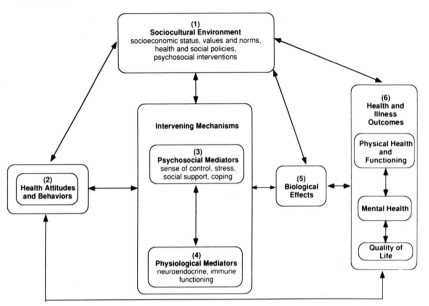

Figure 1.2. Health and Behavior Linkages: An Expanded Schema

Categories of Research on Health and Behavior

In closing this brief exposition of basic concepts in research on health and behavior, it may be useful to indicate the breadth of topics encompassed by research on health and behavior, given that various chapters in this volume are illustrative of these kinds of research. Current investigations can be classified into the following categories, which were also developed by the NIH Working Group on Health and Behavior (Abeles, 1990):

Identification and distribution of psychosocial risk factors. This includes research on correlations between (a) particular behavioral, social, and cultural factors and (b) various aspects of health and functioning. Such research also considers the spectrum and prevalence of such factors in different population groups.

Development, maintenance, and change of health-related behaviors. This category encompasses research on particular health-related behaviors, such as smoking or sedentary life-style, and the antecedent factors establishing, maintaining, and altering these behaviors. Here the research goal is to understand the mechanisms by which behaviors correlated with negative health and functioning outcomes could be prevented or changed and how behaviors correlated with positive outcomes could be supported.

Basic biobehavioral mechanisms. Research in this area addresses the mechanisms or processes through which behavior influences, and is influenced by, health and illness. The emphasis is on identifying the physiological processes that explicate the correlations identified by psychosocial risk-factor analyses (e.g., the effects of stress on health through changes in immune functioning).

Behavioral and social interventions to prevent and treat illness or to promote health. Research in this category develops and evaluates behavioral and social interventions (e.g., clinical trials, field experiments) guided by the research supported under the prior categories.

Effects of health upon behavior. The focus of these kinds of studies is on how physical health and health care treatments of illness influence mental, emotional, or behavioral states. Included are also studies of the interplay between physical health and mental disorders.

SOCIAL AND BEHAVIORAL
PRINCIPLES OF RESEARCH ON AGING

Research on aging, health, and behavior requires an understanding of some of the basic principles of aging and its related social processes. Popular assumptions about older people and the aging process are often ill informed, based more on misconceptions than on scientific knowledge. A substantial body of research exists now, elucidating how social and behavioral factors, interacting with biological factors, influence health and functioning in the middle and later years. Riley and her colleagues (Abeles, 1987; Abeles & Riley, 1976-1977; Ory, 1988; Ory & Bond, 1989; Riley, 1985; Riley & Bond, 1983; Riley, Foner, & Waring, 1988; Riley, Matarazzo, & Baum, 1987) have postulated several related principles of aging as a guide for analyzing and designing research on aging, and many of these principles are echoed throughout this book.

The Heterogeneity of the Older Population

Despite the stereotypic view that most older persons are ill or dependent on others for their care, there is great variability in the health and functioning of older people. Indeed, research often reveals greater variability on functional indicators among older than among younger adults (Maddox, 1987; Rowe, 1985; Rowe & Kahn, 1987). The oft-quoted statistic that 80% of older persons have at least one chronic disease or disability obscures the fact that most older persons live independently in the community and can manage their health care on a daily basis without extensive medical intervention or social services (Havlik et al., 1987; U.S. Senate, 1989). The range of functioning among even the oldest-old population is just beginning to be recognized (Suzman & Riley, 1985; Suzman, Willis, & Manton, 1990).

Some recent reports emphasize the health and relative wealth of the older population (Committee on Population, 1987; Palmer, Smeeding, & Torrey, 1988). While a more favorable impression of the health or income status of older people counters the characteristically negative stereotypes of the past, a view of later life that is overly optimistic may lead to policies detrimental to the health or social needs of especially vulnerable subgroups of the older population (e.g., the oldest old, the rural elderly, those with limited education and incomes, minority and ethnic populations) who are still in need of support and service (Binstock, 1983, 1985; Commonwealth Fund Commission, 1989).

Aging as a Life-Course Process

Aging is best understood within a life-course perspective. Persons do not suddenly become old at age 65; aging reflects an accumulation of a lifetime of interacting social, behavioral, and biomedical processes. Genetics may predispose an individual to certain diseases or conditions that are translated by biological mechanisms into morbidities and mortality, but research shows that length and quality of life are also highly dependent on health-related attitudes and behaviors, life-style factors, and social environments.

Similarly, people's attitudes about their health, their responses to illness symptoms, and their use of health care have been shaped throughout their lives. For example, an older person's previous experiences with the health care system and health care providers affect later health care attitudes and behaviors (Haug & Ory, 1987; Ory & Bond, 1989).

Aging and the Social Context

Aging is influenced by, and also influences, the social context in which people grow older. This is apparent in the heterogeneous aging patterns of people in different ethnic, geographic, or socioeconomic subcultures. It is also apparent in the differing aging patterns of people living in different historical periods. Cohorts of people born in different eras age in different ways because of the particular social circumstances, health behaviors, medical care, and other sociocultural factors operative at the time. Because society changes over time, people in different cohorts will inevitably age in different ways (the "principle of cohort differences"). It is often inappropriate to attribute presumed age-related differences in health attitudes, behaviors, other social characteristics, and their biological sequelae, to the aging process, because most of the existing research is cross-sectional and cannot separate change over the life course from changes in the social context. The erroneous interpretation of cross-sectional age differences as aging processes is known as the "life-course fallacy" (Riley, 1985; Riley et al., 1988).

The Potential for Intervention

The observation that variations in social conditions affect the aging process underscores that this process is malleable and hence responsive to some degree of human intervention and control. Research is challenging previous notions about inevitable declines in older people's cognitive functioning and is testing the limits of abilities and performance (Kliegl & Baltes, 1987). Behavioral or social interventions have been shown to postpone or compensate for aging-related changes in cognitive and other functional domains. Such research has demonstrated late-life improvements in intellectual functioning under certain conditions (e.g., if life situations are challenging, if people continue to use their skills, and if the social environment provides incentives and opportunities for learning; Baltes & Willis, 1982; Riley & Riley, 1989; Schaie, 1983).

Examples of successful behavioral interventions can be found in a wide variety of domains. For example, a longitudinal research project is establishing that relatively brief and simple interventions can improve cognitive functioning among community-living older people to that of 14 years prior. Another series of studies demonstrates that undesirable behaviors (e.g., wandering) of progressively deteriorating Alzheimer's disease patients can be eliminated, or at least attenuated, by teaching caregivers behavioral management skills or redesigning the physical environment (Gallagher, Lovett, & Zeiss,

1989). Still other studies show that, despite common assumptions to the contrary, urinary incontinence can often be cured or managed by older persons, their families, or health care providers through behavioral interventions (National Institutes of Health, 1988).

THE RELATION OF AGE TO HEALTH AND BEHAVIOR

Psychosocial Geriatrics Research

In living longer, individuals accumulate a host of life-styles and behaviors that can facilitate or impede the development and course of many chronic illnesses and conditions throughout the life course. Despite this obvious fact, specific studies of older people—or of how aging processes affect or are affected by interacting health and psychosocial processes—are rare (Riley, Matarazzo, & Baum, 1987; Schroots, Birren, & Svanborg, 1988; Siegler, 1989; Siegler & Costa, 1985; Wolinsky, 1990). Fortunately, an emerging field of inquiry, *psychosocial geriatrics research*, is beginning to examine the dynamic interactions among health, behavior, and aging processes (National Institute on Aging, 1989; National Institutes of Health, 1983a, 1983b). Drawing on several related disciplines, such as medical sociology, health psychology, medical anthropology, and psychosocial epidemiology, this area of study adds an explicit aging perspective to the already established field of behavioral medicine.

Psychosocial geriatrics research addresses the origins, correlates, and malleability of health-related attitudes and behaviors of older people and their caregivers. It is particularly concerned with beliefs about the nature of the aging process and how older people perceive, interpret, or act upon symptoms of illness. It seeks to understand how particular behaviors and attitudes influence the health of people as they age; how health attitudes and behaviors interact with physiological and psychosocial aging processes to influence health and functioning; and how social conditions affect the development, maintenance, and potential modification of these attitudes and behaviors. While *behavioral geriatrics research* might be the preferred term because of its easy association with behavioral medicine, the term psychosocial geriatrics research will be used in this volume to emphasize the contributions of both psychological and social factors.

Conceptual Model

As illustrated in Figure 1.3, we hypothesize several possible pathways through which age influences the relationship between health and behavior (see the Foreword in this volume; Green & Gottlieb, 1989). The relationship between age and biological effects and related health outcomes is well documented (Box 1 to Box 5). Age-related factors can also affect the sociocultural environment and people's health attitudes and behaviors (Box 1 to Box 2 and to Box 3) as well as each of the hypothesized psychosocial and physiological mediators (Box 1 to Box 4 through Box 2 and/or 3).

Societal aging. This term refers to the relative proportion of different age groups in a given society. Until the twentieth century, societies were relatively young, with larger numbers of infants and children than of adults and older people. However, falling infant mortality rates and birthrates, combined with greater longevity, have resulted in the unprecedented situation where infants and children are becoming minorities in modern industrialized countries. Such societal aging influences the sociocultural environment in which people live by shaping the structure of groups and social systems. Norms about health behavior and expectations regarding health are different for individuals who grow old under differing historical and social conditions.

Age differences in health behaviors and attitudes. From the perspective of the aging of individuals, older people are believed to hold different health attitudes and engage in different health behaviors from those of younger persons, although it is not always clear whether this represents an aging or a cohort effect.

Reductions in resources and capabilities. It has also been hypothesized that the relationship between health and behavior is intensified in old age because the physical and social circumstances of old age may diminish psychosocial resources and adaptive abilities (e.g., sense of control, social support, coping strategies) while increasing vulnerability to physiological responses (e.g., immune or neuroendocrine effects) to stressful situations (Rodin, 1986). The individual chapters in this volume will discuss these hypotheses further and provide evidence for the variety of ways that age-related factors interact with health and behavior.

Changing risk factors with aging. Aging can also influence the relationship between health and behavior by changing one's profile of risk factors. Recent research from the well-known Alameda County study is demonstrating the health consequences of recommended

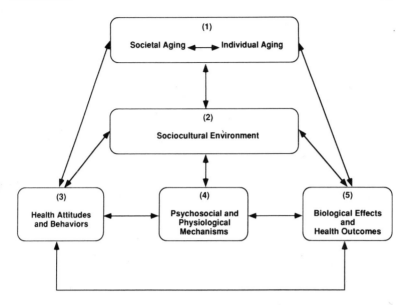

Figure 1.3. Schema of Aging, Health, and Behavior Linkages

health practices and life-style factors such as smoking, physical activity, and social integration even for older people (Kaplan & Haan, 1989; Kaplan, Seeman, Cohen, Knudsen, & Guralnik, 1987).

Nevertheless, our understanding of the relationship between health and behavior in old age is complicated by the subtle ways in which aging processes influence the existence or potency of risk factors. For example, the relationship between psychosocial variables and health outcomes may be different for younger versus older populations. Research from the Alameda County study indicates that marital status may not be a significant predictor of mortality risk among older women, for whom widowhood is more or less normative (Kaplan et al., 1987). Additionally, there is much debate about whether some behaviors shown to be risk factors for illness among younger persons are equally as potent as health predictors for older persons. And, even when epidemiological linkages are found between risk factors and health outcomes, it is not widely demonstrated that eliminating or reducing the risk factor will improve health and function in older people (Branch & Jette, 1984; Evans, 1984; Kane, Kane, & Arnold, 1985; Kannel & Gordon, 1980; Kasl & Berkman, 1981).

Both substantive and methodological explanations have been given (see especially Berkman, 1989; Evans, 1984) for the changing risk factor patterns with aging. Diseases of old age are often multi-causal, and it may simply be harder to isolate any one specific risk factor from a multitude of interacting physical, social, or behavioral causes that have accumulated over a lifetime. Moreover, true measures of risk factors may be harder to obtain, because intraindividual variance increases on most measures with aging.

Finally, there may be critical periods of exposure. Vulnerability may change with aging, or the most susceptible persons may have died before reaching old age. While preventive health habits cannot be banked toward future health (the benefits often cease when the behavior is stopped), there is some suggestion that the adoption of healthy life-styles (e.g., increased physical activity) can appreciably improve functioning—even in very old people (Fries, Green, & Levine, 1989; Kaplan & Haan, 1989).

A major research challenge is to improve our knowledge about the mutability of risk factors and about how different mechanisms may work at different ages to reduce or eliminate undesirable risk factors. There is also a need to understand how changes in risk factors at different points in an individual's life affect morbidity and mortality.

ORGANIZATION OF THE BOOK

Following this introduction, this volume is organized into four major parts addressing various aspects of the interrelationships among aging, health, and behavior as previously illustrated by the boxes of interacting variables depicted in Figure 1.3. Each of the major sections focuses on one or more sets of variables.

Part I: Health and Illness Behaviors

The first part examines specific aspects of health and illness behaviors among older persons (see Figure 1.3, Box 3), including social and cultural factors associated with a wide range of health-related self-care behaviors; an examination of the linkages between self-, informal, and formal care behaviors; and a microanalysis of how the social structure of institutions affects the behaviors of patients and staff (see also Box 2).

A major concern in this part, and throughout the entire volume, is the role of age as a determinant of health-related behaviors and as a mediator of the relationship between health and behavior. Health and illness behaviors do not exist in a vacuum; they are affected by social and cultural factors and, in turn, affect the health and functioning of people throughout their lives. The chapter by Dean examines different approaches to the study of health-related behaviors, considers methodological and conceptual issues, and presents empirical findings from a series of self-care studies conducted over the last decade in Denmark.

Going beyond most previous studies, which have failed to conceptualize and analyze both direct and indirect influences on health-related behaviors, Dean examines how the response to illness is shaped by complex interactions among social situational and attitudinal variables that affect symptom evaluation and the utilization of professional medical care. Previous inconsistencies regarding the influence of age on self-care practices become clearer as the complexities of interacting aging processes are explored. While independent age effects are small, age exerts considerable indirect effects through the social, psychological, and situational variables that directly shape behavior and health, indicating the importance of examining interrelationships among many moderate and small influences in understanding the influence of age on behavior and health.

The chapter by DeFriese and Woomert provides a conceptual framework for understanding self-care, informal care, and formal health care and for examining the interactions among these different types of care. The relative balance among self-care and informal and formal care depends in large part on the health and functional status of the older person and the existence of informal social networks. Yet, even when older people's health care needs are great and formal health care/social services are available, rarely does formal care substitute for various services provided informally by family and friends.

This thoughtful review reveals a lack of scientific evidence to support many popular assumptions about the benefits of various types of health care. The failure of many large-scale health services/social services programs to demonstrate measurable improvements in older people's health underscores the importance of the appropriate conceptualization and measurement of the structure, processes, and outcomes of such care as well as the interactions among different types of self-care, informal care, and formal care. Too often studies have been inadequately designed or analyzed and the real impact remains unknown.

The chapter by Baltes and Wahl examines the effect of social relational variables on health-related behaviors. Complementing the broad overview of health-related practices and care provided by Dean and DeFriese and Woomert, this chapter offers a microanalysis of resident-staff interaction to understand behavior frequently exhibited by patients in long-term care settings. The impact of the environment on the aging individual is hypothesized to be particularly strong given the biological vulnerabilities associated with aging. This chapter presents an alternative view to the generally negative impression of the behavioral and social world of institutionalized elderly. Rather than expressing "learned helplessness," dependent actions in nursing home settings are seen to represent a complementary interaction pattern that allows older people to exert personal control over the environment. Viewed in this adaptive context, these dependent actions elicit supportive responses from the social environment and thus allow some degree of self-regulation.

Part II: Biopsychosocial Mechanisms Linking Health and Behavior

The second part presents different theoretical frameworks for understanding the linkages between health and behavior in an aging population (see Figure 1.3, Boxes 3 and 4). Separate chapters address how older people perceive and respond to illness symptoms; how they cope with chronic illness and disability, particularly Alzheimer's disease; how personality attributes such as sense of personal control affect health in old age; and the psychobiological linkages between stress and illness.

The chapter by Leventhal, Leventhal, and Schaefer focuses on psychological and cognitive processes used by individuals in the face of perceived or actual threats to health. Viewing the individual as an active problem solver, these investigators ask how age affects the process of perceiving and responding to illness symptoms and how individuals cope with both the health threat itself and the emotional and psychological reactions to it.

Examining age differences in health and illness behavior in both healthy people and patients undergoing medical treatment, Leventhal and colleagues conclude that older people appear to be more vigilant in responding to health threats than are middle-aged and young adults. Older people's tendency toward vigilant coping and rapid seeking of care must be seen in the context of other findings, which suggest that older people are more likely than their younger counterparts to attribute symptoms (especially those that are mild or have slow onset) to aging rather than illness—and also that such attributions slow the vigilant coping response typically seen in older persons. Attention to the dynamic process of understanding and responding to perceived threats to health, and how this process varies with age, can provide useful guidelines for the development of health-promotion programs and tools.

The nature, determinants, and consequences of coping behaviors are explored further in the chapter by Kiyak and Borson. The modes of coping employed in response to chronic illness may have considerable effects on both psychological and physical adaptation. How age affects coping responses to stress has not been adequately researched. For the most part, however, the specific illness or disability appears to be more important than the patient's age per se. Cognitively impaired older people may show deficits in adequacy and scope of their coping responses, but otherwise effective coping can be expected throughout the life span. Future research will need to explore how older people cope with chronic or multiple disabilities/diseases and determine the benefit of teaching older people and their caregivers specific coping strategies.

Enhanced personal control has been linked to positive health outcomes for persons of all ages. Exploring the hypothesis that the relationship between control and health may strengthen with age, the chapter by Rodin and Timko suggests that aging presents challenges to the older person's actual and perceived control, in terms of social and personal events that diminish older people's sense of control over their lives as well as biologically driven changes that increase vulnerability to stressors and feelings of loss of control over their bodies. While age per se does not directly relate to control expectancies, it may indirectly influence the relationship between levels of control and healthy psychological and physical functioning by affecting mediating mechanisms such as behavioral/cognitive processes and/or physiological responses. Age-related events not only can affect one's sense of control but can also modify the consequences of lack of control on health outcomes in old age. For example, losses in predictability and control are associated with neuroendocrine arousal and depressed immune response. Because physiological changes in the endocrine and immune systems accompany aging, older people may be more biologically susceptible to the negative effects of stressful events that attack their sense of control.

Adopting a synthesizing biopsychosocial approach, the chapter by Vogt seeks to clarify existing literature relating social and psychological factors to aging, health, and illness. Inconsistencies in reported relationships can be explained, in part, by lack of specificity in conceptualization and measurement of predictors, mediators, and/or outcomes. Vogt focuses on the mechanisms linking stress and illness and asks how social and psychological factors interact with biological processes to affect specific health outcomes at different points in the life course.

Several conceptual models have been developed for relating social and psychological factors to declines in health. Previous attempts to link social and psychological factors to disease outcomes may have been hampered by the lack of a clear conceptual framework for hypothesizing biologically realistic pathways between specific psychosocial factors and disease outcomes. To alleviate this problem, Vogt recommends the use of a three-category disease classification model organized in terms of stress-related illness outcomes: (a) diseases thought to be related to chronic hyperarousal (primarily cardiovascular conditions); (b) diseases thought to be related to hyperreactivity of the pituitary-adrenal axis and that require a healthy immune resistance (infections, cancers); and (c) diseases of hyperimmunity.

Part III: Social and Behavioral Interventions

The third part focuses on social and behavioral interventions in middle and later life. Building on an understanding of social and behavioral influences on health outcomes, the third part of this volume addresses conceptual and methodological issues involved in designing and evaluating health-promotion/disease-prevention interventions for older people. (See Figure 1.3, interactions among Boxes 2, 3, and 5.)

The chapter by Rakowski focuses particularly on preventive health habits and the promotion of life-style changes as well as their application to community-based interventions. Several factors influence the impact and interpretation of health-promotion/disease-prevention programs. Although most programs seek evidence of success at the physiological level, and/or reduced mortality and morbidity, programs geared to older people must consider several other issues. For example, the positive physiological correlates of changes in behavioral risk factors (diet, smoking, and so on) may not be as apparent or measurable with older participants. Likewise, preexisting medical conditions may complicate assessment of benefits of behavioral change. Realistic outcome indicators for older people, particularly the oldest old, should include quality of life, efforts at behavioral change, and improvements in functional health.

Future research is needed to address several important issues. Although there are clearly several different dimensions to personal health, research has not yet identified statistically significant clusters of health practices. Health-promotional programs usually target single behaviors such as specific dietary changes, seat belt use, or smoking cessation. Factors that are naturally associated with health-related practices also need to be distinguished from factors that promote behavioral change. Research in this area is becoming increasingly more sophisticated. The challenge is to specify health practices beneficial to older people as well as the criteria for evaluating the success of interventions across the complete range of the later years.

In contrast to the individually oriented health-promotion programs reviewed by Rakowski, the chapter by Levi focuses on health-related interventions targeted at social systems. A theoretical systems model (which includes many of the process variables discussed elsewhere in this volume) is proposed for understanding the interactive processes among the physical and social environment, the individual's health-related attitudes and behaviors, and associated levels of health and well-being. Intersectoral cooperation, interdisciplinary approaches to intervention and evaluation, and participatory interaction among policy planners and the research and lay communities are all important components of this system's approach.

The last part of this chapter is devoted to examples of experimental intervention in social systems. These studies, conducted primarily in Sweden, focus on manipulations of behavioral and social factors aimed at enhancing physical and psychological well-being. Additional research is needed to examine the effectiveness of social interventions at different points in the life course and the relationship of such timing to the achievement of desired health-promotion/disability-prevention goals.

Part IV: Implications for Public Policy

The final part addresses how public policies affect and are affected by health care needs and societal conditions in an aging society (see Figure 1.2, Boxes 1 and 2). A major theme throughout this volume is that the health status of populations is determined not just by genes, biology, and life-style but also by one's position in the social stratification systems of age, race, sex, income, and other social forces that affect the experience of illness and health. The chapter by Estes and Rundall explores several important social structures and social characteristics that play a role in defining health and health-related behavior among older people. Research into the causes of health and disease in populations must incorporate the relationships among social characteristics and health and their influence on the development of public policies surrounding health and health care.

To address the needs of the aging population of tomorrow, major changes in social structural factors are needed. Social policy and perceptions of older people, along with trends in health, functioning, and quality of life, will shape the health policy of the future. A public policy that integrates health care and social services across the full spectrum of health and illness needs will do much to contribute to the health and well-being of persons of all ages and social situations.

The last chapter, by Manton and Suzman, focuses on the forecasting of health services and manpower needs of aging populations. Such forecasts are based on assumptions, echoed throughout this volume, that the health and functioning of older people are largely a result of the life-course accumulation of risk factors, not an immutable consequence of biological aging. The forecasting of health services and manpower needs of the elderly is extremely important for allocating future resources to improve the health, health care, and quality of life of older people. Forecasting and modeling techniques are becoming increasingly mathematically sophisticated and biosocially realistic, as indicated by the material presented in this chapter. Nevertheless, current projections are subject to some degree of error due to our current inabilities to forecast with certainty the health and functioning of future cohorts of older people, the types of health services they will require in the future, and changes in public policies regarding the delivery and financing of health care services.

A CALL FOR FUTURE RESEARCH

The chapters in this volume examine the nature, determinants, and consequences of various health-related behaviors and patterns of care. Theoretical models of psychosocial and physiological linkages between health and behavior are proposed and the interacting influence of age as a biopsychosocial process and/or structural feature of society is explored. Key issues in designing and evaluating interventions for enhancing health and effective functioning across the life course are discussed. We see the important role of individual behaviors, societal conditions, and public policies for determining the health of older people today and in the future.

Substantial conceptual and methodological advances have been made in the years since the publication of *Healthy People* (U.S. Department of Health, Education and Welfare, 1979). Yet the complexities involved in examining the dynamic interactions among aging, health, and behavior cannot be underestimated. Continued efforts are needed to specify further the predictors and modifiers of health behaviors throughout life, the mechanisms linking particular behaviors to specific health outcomes at different points in the life course, and the reciprocal effects of health on behavior as they accumulate over a lifetime.

While there is general recognition of the complex interactions among physical illnesses, mental disorders, and health care behaviors in old age, most of the research cited in this book, nevertheless, focuses on the physical dimension of older people's health and functioning. More research is needed to examine how mental and physical health operate together to influence the need for and use of health care. This is especially important in later life, when mental disorders may present differently and may be harder to diagnose and treat.

We know surprisingly little about the dynamics of aging, health, and behavior within subgroups of the older population—the oldest old, racial and ethnic minorities, and rural older people. Additional study is certainly warranted in these areas. Furthermore, while this volume does draw on both U.S. and European experiences, more attention to research in other countries with different social and cultural systems would also be useful for furthering our understanding of what happens as people grow older in particular social contexts.

Recognizing the omission of some topics (as noted above), this volume presents a wide range of basic and applied research on aging, health, and behavior. Understanding both the pathways linking health and behavior and the interacting influence of age is important for identifying factors influencing the health and quality of life of older people. Such research on health and behavior can direct individual and community-level psychosocial interventions for promoting health and effective functioning in the later years.

REFERENCES

Abeles, R. P. (Ed.). (1987). Introduction. In R. P. Abeles (Ed.), *Life-span perspectives and social psychology* (pp. 1-16). Hillsdale, NJ: Lawrence Erlbaum.

Abeles, R. P. (1988). *Health and behavior research initiatives by the National Institutes of Health, FY 1989.* Unpublished report prepared for the Department of Health and Human Services and submitted to the Senate Committee on Appropriations for the Departments of Labor, Health and Human Services, and Education, and Related Agencies.

Abeles, R. P. (1990, February). *Health and behavior research initiatives by the National Institutes of Health.* Unpublished report prepared for the Department of Health and Human Services and submitted to the Senate Committee on Appropriations for the Departments of Labor, Health and Human Services, and Education, and Related Agencies.

Abeles, R. P., & Riley, M. W. (1976-1977). A life-course perspective on the later years of life: Some implications for research. In *Social Science Research Council annual report* (pp. 1-16). New York: Social Science Research Council.

Abeles, R. P., & Riley, M. W. (1987). Longevity, social structure and cognitive aging. In C. Schooler & K. W. Schaie (Eds.), *Cognitive functioning and social structure over the Life course* (pp. 161-175). Norwood, NJ: Ablex.

Baltes, P. B., & Willis, S. (1982). Enhancement (plasticity) of intellectual functioning in old age: Penn State's Adult Development and Enrichment Project (ADEPT). In F. L. M. Craik & S. E. Trehub (Eds.), *Aging and cognitive process* (pp. 353-389). New York: Plenum.

Berkman, L. (1989). Maintenance of health, prevention of disease, a psychosocial perspective. In National Center for Health Statistics, *Health of an aging America: Issues on data for policy analysis* (pp. 39-55; Vital and Health Statistics. Series 4, No. 25. DHHS Pub. No. [PHS] 89-1488). Washington, DC: Government Printing Office.

Berkman, L., & Breslow, L. (1983). *Health and ways of living: The Alameda County study.* New York: Oxford University Press.

Binstock, R. H. (1983). The aging as scapegoat. *The Gerontologist, 23,* 136-143.

Binstock, R. H. (1985). *Aging 2000: Our health care destiny.* New York: Springer-Verlag.

Branch, L. G., & Jette, A. M. (1984). Personal health practices and mortality among the elderly. *American Journal of Public Health, 74,* 1126-1129.

Cassel, J. (1976). The contributions of the social environment to host resistance. *American Journal of Epidemiology, 104*(2), 1072-1123.

Cohen, S. (1988). Psychosocial models of the role of social support in the etiology of physical disease. *Health Psychology, 7*(3), 269-297.

Committee on Population, Commission on Behavioral and Social Sciences and Education, and National Research Council. (1987). *Demographic change and the well-being of children and the elderly: Proceedings of a workshop.* Washington, DC: National Academy Press.

Commonwealth Fund Commission on Elderly People Living Alone. (1989). *Old, alone and poor: A plan for reducing poverty among elderly people living alone.* Baltimore, MD: Commonwealth Fund.

Evans, J. G. (1984). Prevention of age-associated loss of autonomy: Epidemiological approaches. *Journal of Chronic Diseases, 37,* 353-363.

Fries, J., Green, L., & Levine. S. (1989, March 4). Health promotion and compression of morbidity. *The Lancet,* pp. 481-483.

Gallagher, D., Lovett, S., & Zeiss, A. (1989). Interventions with caregivers of frail elderly persons. In M. G. Ory & K. Bond (Eds.), *Aging and health care: Social science and policy perspectives* (pp. 145-166). London: Routledge.

Green, L. W., & Gottlieb, N. H. (1989). Health promotion for the aging population: Approaches to extending active life expectancy. In J. R. Hogress (Ed.), *Health care for an aging society* (pp. 139-154). New York: Churchill Livingstone.

Hamburg, D. A., Elliott, G. R., & Parron, D. L. (1982). *Health and behavior frontiers of research in the biobehavioral sciences* (Institute of Medicine Publication 82-010). Washington, DC: National Academy Press.

Haug, M. R., & Ory, M. (1987). Issues in elderly patient- provider interactions. *Research on Aging, 9,* 3-44.

Havlik, R. J., Liu, B. M., Kovar, M. G., et al. (1987, June). Health statistics on older persons, United States, 1986. In *Vital and Health Statistics* (series 3, no. 25. DHHS pub. no [PHS] 871409, National Center for Health Statistics, Public Health Service). Washington, DC: Government Printing Office.

Kane, R. L., Kane, R., & Arnold, A. (1985). Prevention in the elderly: Risk factors. *Health Services Research, 19,* 945-1006.

Kannel, W. B., & Gordon, T. (1980). Cardiovascular risk factors in the aged: The Framingham study. In S. Haynes & M. Feinleib (Eds.), *Second Conference on the Epidemiology of Aging* (NIH Publication No. 80-969). Bethesda, MD: National Institutes of Health.

Kaplan, G. A., & Haan, M. N. (1989). Is there a role for prevention among the elderly? Epidemiological evidence from the Alameda County study. In M. G. Ory & K. Bond (Eds.), *Aging and health care: Social science and policy perspectives* (pp. 27-51). London: Routledge.

Kaplan, G. A., Seeman, T. E., Cohen, R. D., Knudsen, L. P., & Guralnik, J. M. (1987). Mortality among the elderly in the Alameda County study: Behavioral and demographic risk factors. *American Journal of Public Health, 77,* 307-312.

Kasl, S. (1986). The detection and modification of psychosocial and behavioral risk factors. In L. Aiken & D. Mechanic (Eds.), *Applications of social science to clinical medicine and health policy.* New Brunswick, NJ: Rutgers University Press.

Kasl, S., & Berkman, L. F. (1981). Some psychosocial influences on the health status of the elderly: The perspective of social epidemiology. In J. L. McGaugh & S. B. Kiesler (Eds.), *Aging, biology and behavior* (pp. 345-385). New York: Academic Press.

Kliegl, R., & Baltes, P. (1987). Theory-guided analysis of mechanisms of development and aging through testing the limits and research on expertise. In C. Schooler & K. Warner Schaie (Eds.), *Cognitive functioning and social structure over the life course* (pp. 98-119). Norwood, NJ: Ablex.

Maddox, G. L. (1987). Aging differently. *The Gerontologist, 27,* 557-564.

McQueen, D. V., & Siegrist, J. (1983). Social factors in the etiology of chronic diseases: An overview. *Social Science and Medicine, 16,* 353-367.

National Center for Health Statistics. (1985). *Vital Statistics of the United States, 1982* (Vol. 2, Sec. 6, Life Tables; DHHS Publication No. PHS 85-1104). Washington, DC: Government Printing Office.

National Institute on Aging. (1989). *Behavioral and social research program annual report.* Unpublished document.

National Institutes of Health. (1983a). Health and effective functioning in the middle and later years. *Guide for Grants and Contracts, 12*(6), 10-15.

National Institutes of Health. (1983b). Health behaviors and aging: Behavioral geriatrics research. *Guide for Grants and Contracts, 12*(11), 24-27.

National Institutes of Health. (1988). *Urinary incontinence in adults* (Consensus Development Conference statement). Bethesda, MD: Author.

Office of the Surgeon General. (1988). *Surgeon General's Workshop: Health promotion and aging: Proceedings of a workshop.* Washington, DC: Government Printing Office.

Ory, M. (1988). Considerations in the development of age-sensitive indicators for assessing health promotion. *Health Promotion, 3*(2), 139-150.

Ory, M., & Bond, K. (Eds.). (1989). Health care for an aging society. In *Aging on health care: Social science and policy perspectives.* London: Routledge.

Palmer, J. L., Smeeding, T., & Torrey, B. B. (1988). *The vulnerable.* Washington, DC: Urban Institute Press.

Riley, M. W. (1985). Age strata in social systems. In R. H. Binstock & E. Shanas (Eds.), *Handbook of aging and the social sciences* (pp. 369-411). New York: Van Nostrand Reinhold.

Riley, M. W. (1987). Aging, health and social change: An overview. In M. W. Riley, J. D. Matarazzo, & A. Baum (Eds.), *Perspectives in behavioral medicine: The aging dimension* (pp. 12-14). Hillsdale, NJ: Lawrence Erlbaum.

Riley, M. W., & Bond, K. (1983). Beyond ageism: Postponing the onset of disability. In M. W. Riley, B. B. Hess, & K. Bond (Eds.), *Aging in society: Selected reviews of recent research.* Hillsdale, NJ: Lawrence Erlbaum.

Riley, M. W., Foner, A., & Waring, J. (1988). A sociology of age. In N. J. Smelser & R. Burt (Eds.), *Handbook of sociology.* Newbury Park, CA: Sage.

Riley, M. W., Matarazzo, J. D., & Baum, A. (Eds.). (1987). *Perspectives in behavioral medicine: The aging dimension.* Hillsdale, NJ: Lawrence Erlbaum.

Riley, M. W., & Riley, J. W., Jr. (Eds.). (1989). The quality of aging: Strategies for interventions. *The Annals of the American Academy of Political and Social Science, 503,* 9-147.

Rodin, J. (1986). Aging and health: Effects of the sense of control. *Science, 233,* 1271-1276.

Rosenwaike, I. (1985). *The extreme aged in America: A portrait of an expanding population.* Westport, CT: Greenwood.

Rowe, J. W. (1985). Health care of the elderly. *The New England Journal of Medicine, 312,* 827-835.

Rowe, J. W., & Kahn, R. L. (1987). Human aging: Usual and successful. *Science, 237,* 143-149.

Schaie, K. W. (Ed.). (1983). *Longitudinal studies of adult psychological development.* New York: Guilford.

Schneiderman, N., & Tapp, J. T. (1985). *Behavioral medicine: The biopsychosocial approach.* Hillsdale, NJ: Lawrence Erlbaum.

Schroots, J. (1988). Current perspectives on aging, health and behavior. In J. Schroots, J. Birren, & A. Svanborg (Eds.), *Health and aging: Perspectives and prospects* (pp. 3-24). New York: Springer.

Schroots, J., Birren, J., & Svanborg, A. (Eds.). (1988). *Health and aging: Perspectives and prospects.* New York: Springer.

Schwartz, G. E., & Weiss, S. M. (1979). *Proceedings of the Yale Conference on Behavioral Medicine.* Washington, DC: Government Printing Office.

Siegler, I. (1989). Developmental health psychology. In M. Storandt & G. R. Vanden Bos (Eds.), *Continuity and change in the adult years.* Washington, DC: American Psychological Association.

Siegler, I., & Costa, P. (1985). Health-behavior relationships. In J. Bissen & K. W. Schale (Eds.), *Handbook of the psychology of aging* (2nd ed.). New York: Van Nostrand Reinhold.

Suzman, R., & Riley, M. W. (Eds.). (1985). The oldest old. *Milbank Memorial Fund Quarterly: Health and Society, 63*, 177-451.

Suzman, R., Willis, D., & Manton, K. (1990). *The oldest old.* London: Oxford University Press.

Torrey, B., Kinsella, K., & Tauber, C. (Eds.). (1987). *An aging world.* Washington, DC: Bureau of Census, Department of Commerce.

U.S. Bureau of the Census. (1984). Demographic and socioeconomic aspects of aging in the United States. In *Current Population Reports* (Series P-23, No. 138). Washington, DC: Government Printing Office.

U.S. Bureau of the Census. (1988, March). Current population estimates, by age, sex, and race: 1980-1987. In *Current Population Reports* (Series P-25, No. 1020). Washington, DC: Government Printing Office.

U.S. Department of Health and Human Services. (1990). *Promoting health/preventing disease: Year 2000 objectives for the nation.* Washington, DC: Government Printing Office.

U.S. Department of Health, Education and Welfare. (1979). *Healthy people: The surgeon general's report on health promotion and disease prevention* (Public Health Service). Washington, DC: Government Printing Office.

U.S. Department of Health, Education and Welfare, Public Health Service. (1980). *Healthy people 2000: National health promotion and disease prevention objectives for the nation.* Washington, DC: Government Printing Office.

U.S. Senate, Special Committee on Aging. (1989). *Aging America: Trends and projections.* Washington, DC: Government Printing Office.

Weiss, S. M., Herd, J. A., & Fox, B. A. (Eds.). (1981). *Perspectives on behavioral medicine.* New York: Academic Press.

Wolinsky, F. (1990). *Health and health behavior among elderly Americans: An age-stratification perspective.* Detroit: Wayne State Press.

PART I

Self-, Informal, and Formal Health Care Behaviors

2

Health-Related Behavior: Concepts and Methods

KATHRYN DEAN

Early concepts of biological aging were influenced by a pathological model based on notions of inevitable decline (Brocklehurst, 1978; Riley, Hess, & Bond, 1983). Widespread misconceptions about the aging process stemmed from research comparing age groups from cross-national samples of populations. Yet many of these studies were actually assessing the effects of different combinations of social, psychosocial, and behavioral variables in the various age strata. Such misinterpretations of earlier research are slowly being supplanted with research findings documenting the extent to which aging is a complex process affected by multiple influences that may vary sharply for different cohorts of people moving through time (Riley, 1987).

While researchers in the field no longer consider aging immutable (Maddox & Campbell, 1985; Riley & Bond, 1985), little is known about the complex biological, behavioral, and social interactions and processes that determine the way people age. The mechanisms behind the relationships remain uncharted. Few research investigations have been directed toward assessing the relative and interactive influences of different behaviors. Likewise, the direct effects on health of social and psychosocial variables and the indirect effects operating through behaviors generally are not understood.

HEALTH-RELATED BEHAVIORS

The examination of health-related behaviors has drawn on several research traditions. Epidemiological research focuses on relationships between behavioral risk factors and morbidity or mortality.

Social science research approaches investigate the cultural meanings of illness and behavior, processes shaping health and illness behavior, and factors predicting the utilization of health care. The lines between these different research traditions are blurring as behavioral or psychosocial research studies increasingly incorporate concepts and methodologies from various approaches.

Epidemiological Risk-Factor Approaches

Epidemiological studies have linked the behavioral practices of individuals with morbidity and mortality (Abdellah & Moore, 1988; Hamburg, Elliott, & Parran, 1982; U.S. Department of Health, Education and Welfare, 1979). Behavioral influences have for the most part been conceptualized as risk factors for specific diseases rather than in terms of general health, well-being, or functioning. An exception is the comprehensive work of the Human Population Laboratory of the California Department of Health Services, which, through its studies of general health and functional capacity, greatly accelerated the assimilation of behavioral research into the sociomedical sciences. In 1972, Belloc and Breslow reported findings that associated seven "health practices" with an index of physical health in an adult population. Each of the practices (hours of sleep, physical exercise, alcohol consumption, cigarette smoking, obesity, eating between meals, and eating breakfast regularly) was associated with high scores on an index used to measure health status. Subsequent follow-up investigations with the original respondents found significant relationships between health practices and age-standardized mortality rates traced over a five-year period (Belloc, 1973).

Wiley and Camacho (1980) reinterviewed a subsample of the original respondents nine years after the first interview data were obtained. Findings from this follow-up confirmed initial analyses linking life-style factors to health outcomes. Especially relevant to this chapter are recently completed analyses that show that behavior and behavioral change affect health status well into the sixth and seventh decades of life. Long-term follow-up from the Alameda County study reveals that health behaviors and social conditions are not fixed over the life course but can change, and changes influence subsequent mortality risks, even for those 70 and older (Kaplan & Haan, 1989).

European researchers have also documented similar kinds of findings in their prospective community studies. For example, in Denmark, a great deal of information about relationships between behavior and disease has been obtained from more than 20 years of study in Glostrup (Hansen, 1977). Specific behavioral habits, especially smoking and alcohol consumption, have been linked with specific diseases or abnormalities (Agner, 1985; Grandjean, Olesen, & Hollnagel, 1981; Hagerup and Larsen, 1971; Ibsen et al., 1981; Melgaard, Sælan, & Hedegaard, 1986). Such findings are consistent with results from prevalence studies, case control studies, and various types of longitudinal investigations from other European studies (Fraser, 1986, chaps. 7, 8, 12, 13; Reid et al., 1976; Rose et al., 1977; Rosengren, Wilhelmsen, & Wedel, 1988). Most recently, cohort differences in social situational variables have become a subject of research interest in these studies. Thus investigations of the effects of cohort changes in social and psychosocial variables on health and functional ability will soon be possible.

In recognition of the influence of specific behaviors on the onset and course of major chronic diseases, a number of applied health-promotion and disease-prevention programs based on epidemiological risk-factor models were initiated in the 1970s. Early clinical applications focused on high-risk individuals with elevated levels of serum cholesterol and/or blood pressure. In addition to clinical studies, communitywide prevention research and demonstration projects were undertaken. The origins of these public health projects have been traced to community projects and studies coordinated by the World Health Organization (WHO) Cardiovascular Unit in the 1960s (Blackburn, 1983). The first major community project in primary cardiovascular disease prevention was the North Karelia Project in Finland (Puska, Juomilehti, & Salonem, 1981). Three major community projects conducted under the auspices of the National Institutes of Health in the United States are located in California (Farquhar, Moccaby, & Soloman, 1984), Minnesota (Blackburn et al., 1984), and Rhode Island (Lasates et al., 1984).

These community intervention projects concentrate on specific behaviors of individuals and examine the effectiveness of educational approaches for encouraging recommended attitudinal and behavioral change. Such interventions are based on a behavioral model of health that assumes that educating individuals to change or avoid certain behaviors, or never to practice them, will protect their health and improve the general health of postindustrial populations. These community projects move from a narrow focus on individuals at high risk to a concern with primary prevention in general populations. They address multiple behavioral risks or life-style factors in contrast to single-risk-factor campaigns. Through such large-scale community studies, "life-style" research has become firmly established in the health field in a remarkably short period of time. Only in 1972 did *Index Medicus* begin listing articles under the heading "lifestyle"; by 1985, the number of references indexed annually under the term had tripled (Coreil, Levin, & Jaco, 1985).

Nevertheless, a problem with applying the traditional epidemiological risk-factor approach to the concept of life-style is that little attention has been focused on modeling the underlying cultural and social influences. Rather, a quite separate research tradition has developed around the subject of social causes of illness (Badura, 1983; Cohen & Syme, 1985; Townsend & Davidson, 1982), leading to a fragmentation in research efforts. Moreover, conceptualizing health problems in terms of discrete risk ignores the complex social and behavioral processes involved in the maintenance or deterioration of health. A related problem is that health behaviors are often identified as causal risk factors even though the behaviors generally are neither independent of social factors (Hollnagel, Madsen, & Larsen, 1982; Rose & Marmot, 1981) nor sufficient to explain disease patterns in society (Badura, 1983; Kaplan, 1984; Kaplan & Haan, 1986; Marmot, Rose, Shipley, & Hamilton, 1978). For example, while smoking is a major behavioral risk factor for cardiovascular or malignant diseases, smoking behavior cannot be understood when separated from the social and cultural context in which it occurs.

Although epidemiological approaches have expanded our knowledge of the factors involved in many specific diseases, with few exceptions (e.g., Pearlin et al., 1981) little attention has been given to methodological designs and statistical procedures directly concerned with understanding multiple causation and ways in which different levels of influence interrelate to affect general health and well-being. Focusing on modeling of macro-level and micro-level influences on health and functioning can expand our understanding of healthy aging. More specifically, such approaches could begin to disentangle the effects of chronic diseases and accumulated multiple pathologies from biological aging processes.

Social Science Approaches

Social science approaches draw upon several related disciplines such as medical anthropology, medical sociology, and health psychology. In contrast to the epidemiological tradition, which focuses on the distribution of disease and death in the population, social science approaches to the study of health-related behavior have generally focused on behavioral variables as the consequence of social and cultural factors. A rich body of anthropological literature examines cultural meanings of illness. Most of these studies have been conducted in non-Western societies or among traditional ethnic groups within Western societies. Additionally, much of the work of medical anthropologists has focused on processes of care seeking in folk healing and professional sectors, neglecting self-care and care obtained from family and community networks (Chrisman & Kleinman, 1983). Nevertheless, this body of literature has clearly documented that, in all groups, people monitor their health in terms of cultural concepts and standards of normality (Fabrega, 1973; Kleinman, 1980). The very recognition of symptoms as well as behavioral responses are grounded in the cultural context and in social learning (Helman, 1978; Zborowski, 1958; Zola, 1966).

There are two research traditions within medical sociology. An extensive body of behavioral research has been organized around the concepts of health behavior and illness behavior (Antonovsky, 1972; Kasl & Cobb, 1966; Mechanic, 1972, 1978; Rosenstock, 1974; Rosenstock & Kirscht, 1979; Suchman, 1967). This research tradition, which also includes the perspective of health psychologists, is characterized by process studies that examine the influence of factors such as social networks, health beliefs, psychological distress and other social influences on health-related decision making, the use of medical services, and compliance with medical advice. Research investigations in this vein have generated a wealth of information on care seeking, with special attention to the influence of social and psychosocial variables on the utilization of health care services.

Another research tradition within medical sociology examines the use of professional services by means of large-scale population survey studies and multivariate research methodologies (Wan, 1989). In this approach to the study of health care utilization (probably the dominant approach in medical sociology today), psychosocial variables have been found to make little or no independent contribution to utilization behavior when controlling for other factors (Andersen, Kravits, & Anderson, 1975; Berkanovic, Telesky, & Reeder, 1981; Kohn & White, 1976; Mossey, Havens, & Wolinsky, 1989; Wolinsky, 1978). Large-scale survey investigations repeatedly show that illness variables (such as perceived seriousness of or worry over symptoms, perceived health status, or disability days) account for most of the variation in the use of medical services. The findings of the population surveys suggest that it is "need," rather than social, psychosocial, or economic variables, that determines illness behavior. These results are inconsistent with the earlier evidence from smaller-scale studies demonstrating the importance of social and cultural factors in influencing health behaviors. Only modest amounts of the variation in use of professional services have ever been explained by any of the multivariate models of health care use (Wan, 1989).

Dynamics of Health-Related Behaviors

One explanation for the apparent contradiction in these research traditions is that the dynamic processes that govern health-related behavior cannot be studied in the statistical models often used to analyze the data. Concern for health, health-protective patterns of behavior, attention to pain, and perceptions regarding the seriousness of symptoms are not simply indicators of health status. They involve a dynamic process of interpretation and behavior. People with identical symptoms respond differently depending on what is happening in daily life at the time, and on situational factors creating options and constraints, just as healthy people with similar knowledge and beliefs act differently to maintain their health (Dean, 1984; Mechanic, 1979; Shanas & Maddox, 1985).

A major problem with previously discussed large-scale population survey studies is their conceptualization and analysis of variables representing the illness experience. Perceptions of illness may be proxy measures summing the effects of many other variables. Indeed, they may themselves be outcome variables shaped by social and psychosocial factors. The effects of the underlying factors may be hidden when proximate influences are defined as independent variables and analyzed simultaneously with more distal influences in single-equation regression models. For example, disability days, often used to represent a measure of need, are most likely affected by the tendency to assume sick role behavior as well as options in the social and medical environment (e.g., available social supports or professional care). When such variables are included in single-equation regression models, they "soak up" or hide the influence of other variables. Complex interactions and processes cannot be identified in the regression procedures typically used in such studies.

Discussing the apparent contradictions in the literature on the utilization of health care services, Mechanic concluded:

The results of these multivariate studies can be attributed in part to gross measurement of subtle processes of response by summary measures that are not specific enough to capture important variations among respondents. Moreover, the variance attributed to "illness" in multivariate models that have only a very general theoretical rationale often masks the effects of important psychosocial processes. What are called "illness" and "need" in these studies are usually summary measures of illness behavior that incorporate psychological and attitudinal components and are correlated at a zero-order level with many relevant psychosocial measures. The introduction of the global illness measures in a regression equation simultaneous with other social and behavioral measures will often reduce the betas of such variables correlated with it to insignificance. From a theoretical standpoint, however, one should have a model that posits the interrelationships between the global illness behavior measures and other psychosocial factors. (Mechanic, 1983, pp. 602-603)

Need for Further Conceptualization and Analysis

The separate epidemiological and social science approaches described above have tended to focus narrowly on the association of specific health behaviors with disease outcomes or on the prediction of the use of health services. While our knowledge of health-related behavior has increased over the last 20 years, different approaches are now needed to advance our understanding further. Both the conceptualization and the modeling of variables need careful consideration. This includes the range of behavior studied and the modeling of antecedent and intervening influences. For example, the range of health-related behaviors has seldom been a focus for research, although a few health diary studies have explored the range of responses to illness and factors associated with alternative responses (Alpert, Kosa, & Haggerty, 1967; Brody, Klebon, & Moles, 1983; Rakowski, Julius, Hickey, Verbrugge, & Holter, 1988; Verbrugge & Ascione, 1987). There is also a need to explore how behaviors cluster and to use multivariate analytic techniques in new ways to study in greater depth the influence of social situational variables. If certain life-styles are associated with negative health outcomes, we must not only discover which behaviors cluster in more and less healthy ways of living but also why the behaviors are deleterious and what factors create and maintain them (Dean, 1984).

RESEARCH ON SELF-CARE

The concept of self-care began to emerge in the mid-1970s as more studies documented the role of individual behavioral practices in health and the extent to which illness is cared for without recourse to medical care. In spite of the volume of evidence linking personal behavior and health protection, some early references, explicitly or implicitly, referred to self-care only in terms of response to illness. In some instances, the concept not only was limited to symptom responses but also sharply contrasted with seeking professional help. However, because most medical contacts are preceded and followed by self-treatments, and because consultation cannot occur without symptom evaluation and decision making by the lay individual, the continuum of care and the self-care aspects of decisions to seek help could not be ignored (Dean, 1981, 1986c).

Definition and Integration of the Concept

From the onset, self-care was defined broadly in conceptual discussions and literature overviews (Dean, 1981; Harberden & Lafaille, 1978; Levin, 1977; Levin, Katz, & Holst, 1976; Williamson & Danaher, 1978). Self-care is now widely conceptualized as the range of health and illness behavior undertaken by individuals on behalf of their own health. Personal decision making and interaction with professional providers are included as important aspects of self-care behavior (Dean, 1986b, 1989; WHO, 1983).

In an integrated approach to health-related behavior, each person's behavior is a continuum organized by the perceptions, decisions, and options available to that individual. Regardless of the type or level of professional services used, the forces that shape care decisions (to do nothing, to actively promote health, to self-treat, to seek care from another, and to follow advice) operate through the individual, who assimilates the influences and determines the care. Components of self-care (health-maintenance behavior, self-treatment, care seeking, and so on) can be studied separately or as part of the continuum of health-related behavior. The nature of professional consultation is determined by complex processes and is placed in its appropriate perspective as a component of the continuum of care. This conceptualization, appropriate for understanding the range of care in all countries, is especially relevant where chronic diseases and injuries are the major threats to health. Self-care in the face of chronic illness may be the most relevant aspect of the subject with regard to aging populations.

Recognition of the vital role of self-care is reflected in the rapid integration of the concept in the health field. In an investigation of self-care programs in America, it was estimated that 60% of health service organizations operate one or more self-care educational programs (DeFriese, Woomert, Guild, Steckler, & Konrad, 1989). The widespread acceptance of a broad self-care concept was illustrated in the range of subjects taught. Of the programs, 94% offered instruction directed toward health maintenance while 59% dealt with diagnosis and symptom assessment of common illnesses, chronic diseases, or injuries; 63% of the educational programs taught the prevention of further deterioration or spread of already existing conditions. Advocacy skills were addressed in nearly half of the programs. Prevention of iatrogenic illness was discussed in over a quarter of the programs.

Nature and Determinants of Self-Care

Relatively little is known about the range and determinants of health-maintenance behaviors. It is known that routine habits that are potentially harmful to health differ in subgroups of the population. Gender differences in dangerous self-care practices are well documented. Men's higher lifetime use of alcohol and tobacco along with male driving behavior are among major differences (Langlie, 1977; Verbrugge, 1985). There is evidence that women more often obtain preventive physical examinations, brush teeth, and have a greater intake of vitamins, while men have higher levels of physical activity, especially strenuous exercise. Statistical interactions between heavy drinking and heavy smoking among men in contrast to women suggest an important gender difference in life-style behavior, and there is some evidence that women may, on the average, live healthier life-styles (Dean, 1989b).

The available evidence discerns no consistent relationships between age and different health-maintenance behaviors. Likewise, although some studies find social class differences in health-related habits (e.g., positive relationships for alcohol intake and exercise with social class, and inverse relationships between smoking and social class), the evidence is not consistent and at this time remains inconclusive.

U.S. and European research on illness-related self-care in adult populations shows that the vast majority of symptoms are not brought to the attention of the medical care system but are treated by individuals and their lay networks. In one of the few studies of self-care responses to illness in the United States, perceptions about health and numbers of symptom episodes were independently associated with the reported tendency to care for symptoms without seeking medical advice among persons over 45 years of age (Haug, Wykle, & Namazi, 1989). For symptoms considered serious, lower faith in medical care was also related to the tendency for self-treatment. The attitudinal, behavioral, and psychological distress variables included in the study were generally not independently associated with self-care behavior. The psychological distress variable, however, was related to the number of symptoms reported, which, in turn, influenced self-care behavioral responses.

Another U.S. study examined behavioral responses to daily symptoms in a community sample of persons 62 to 94 years of age (Rakowski et al., 1988). Major findings included a tendency for women to respond more actively to symptoms than men, an association between pain/discomfort and increased use of medicines, and a tendency for persons expressing satisfaction with their income level to be more likely to seek professional help for symptoms.

Most self-care studies have focused on specific health behaviors or practices. For example, medication behavior has been studied in numerous investigations (Bush & Rabin, 1976; Dean, 1981; Dunnell & Cartwright, 1972; Fryklöf & Westerling, 1983; White et al., 1967). While the results are not always consistent, most studies find that the use of medicines, especially prescription medicines, increases with age and is more prevalent among women (Ory, 1987-1988). Older people, who tend to have multiple chronic conditions, frequently take multiple drugs simultaneously, a situation referred to as *polypharmacy*. Additionally, they often take psychotropic drugs in combination with other prescription medications (Brown Eve, 1986; Cartwright & Anderson, 1981; Christopher, Bellinger, Shepherd, Ramsey, & Crooks, 1978; Hemminki & Heikkila, 1975; Scott, Stansfield, & Williams, 1982).

Extensive self-medication is involved in the use of prescription drugs. Alterations in the use of medically prescribed drugs, a form of self-medication, range from not taking the prescribed medicine to changing the dosage, duration, or time of its use (Graham-Smith,

1975; McEwen, 1979). The most common response to illness symptoms in one large U.S. self-care study was to take a previously prescribed medication (Haug et al., 1989). The extent to which self-medication is a result of lay judgment regarding side effects or ineffectiveness of drugs, in contrast to errors involving taking more or less medication than the amount prescribed, is unknown.

Although not extensively studied, the bulk of self-treatment involves behaviors other than medicine taking (Dean, 1986b, 1986c; Dean, Holst, & Wagner, 1983). Some of the most frequent types of self-treatment involve dietary practices and forms of rest and relaxation. Home remedies involve many types of procedures and preparations. Avoidance behaviors are also frequent; these range from avoiding particular movements or practices to staying away from or reducing stressful situations. Social forms of care (Freer, 1980) and appropriately engaging in sick role behavior (Berkman, 1975) may be especially beneficial forms of self-care.

Appropriateness of Self-Care

A major clinical issue is the extent to which self-care treatments are appropriate. From the limited amount of research information available on self-treatment before medical consultations, it appears that lay practices are predominantly appropriate and safe. Home medical guides may not be kept up to date (Elliot-Binns, 1973), but it appears that treatment behaviors are seldom dangerous (Anderson, Buck, Danaher, & Fry, 1977). In Denmark, Pedersen (1976) concluded that self-treatment had been relevant in 90% of the cases he studied and somewhat helpful nearly two-thirds of the time. In an investigation of self-care behavior in the Norwegian population, persons practicing self-treatment were found to have shorter episodes of illness (Grimsmo, 1984). General practitioners evaluating the effectiveness of self-medication in Britain found 75% of the medication behavior adequate and only 5% potentially harmful (Williamson & Danaher, 1980).

The streams of research cited above illustrate the extensive range and importance of self-care behaviors. Very little is known, however, about the development or maintenance of self-care behaviors over the life course, the ways in which such behaviors cluster, or the psychosocial factors shaping patterns of behaviors and life-styles.

STUDIES OF SELF-CARE BEHAVIOR IN DENMARK

In contrast to many self-care studies using varying conceptualizations and methodologies, a series of coordinated studies have been conducted over the past decade in Denmark. This set of studies will be described in some detail to illustrate the cumulative nature of self-care research. Reflecting a social situational perspective, a goal of these studies is to gain understanding of the interrelationships among social, psychosocial, and behavioral variables. As a Western industrialized country with a capitalistic economy, relative cultural unity, and a highly developed social welfare system, Denmark provides both important similarities to and differences from the United States that make the study of self-care behavior highly informative (Anderson, 1975; Haro, 1975; Holst & Wagner, 1975).

Review of Two Early Studies

In the first study, self-care responses to six common illness conditions (colds, influenza, skin rash, lumbar pain, depression, and chest pain) were studied in a random sample of more than 1,400 adult Danes representative of the age, sex, and marital status distribution of the population (Dean et al., 1983). A wide range of self-treatment responses (predominantly alterations in activity level or routine behavior, use of some type of mechanical aid, or changes in the amount or type of fluid intake) were reported for the common conditions. Four types of behaviors were common to the six conditions: nonmedication self-treatment, use of medication, physician consultation, and decision to take no action in response to the onset of symptoms.

Of the variables included in this study, age, sex, perceived health status, and a reliant attitude toward physicians with regard to nonmedical problems were the most important variables related to the four types of self-care behavior. However, the relationships between these variables and self-care behaviors were not always simple and direct. Interactions among the categories of "independent" variables often accounted for the variation in self-care responses to common illnesses. For example, although age, sex, and the tendency to discuss nonmedical problems with physicians did not separately influence the nonmedication self-treatments, their complex interaction did. Thus, in this early study, older people, especially older women, more often practiced ameliorative-type responses to illness. At the same time, women relied on physicians more than men with regard to confiding and discussing nonmedical problems.

Similarly, the influence of age on medication behavior and physician consultation for common illness was not simple. Both tendency to seek counsel for nonmedical problems from physicians and perceived health status were related to taking medicines and contacting doctors for common symptoms. At the same time, older persons who relied on physicians for counsel on nonmedical problems more often had a poor perception of their own health than those who did not rely on physicians for such matters. Moreover, more women than men reported both discussing nonmedical problems with their doctors and having poor health.

To elaborate on the findings of the first survey, a follow-up investigation was designed to study more systematically the influence of social, psychosocial, and situational variables on self-care responses to all reported illness episodes for a period of six months. Findings from this second investigation point to factors behind the links usually found between age and illness behaviors. The only direct, clearly independent relationships between age and self-care responses to illness were modest age correlations with bed rest and professional consultation. Age was, however, related to several social, situational, and attitudinal variables, some of which directly influenced self-care responses to illness. For example, in contrast to younger people, older people more often lived alone, reported fewer contacts with friends in the prior month, and were less satisfied with their social support. Older people were also more likely to engage in different types of stress-reduction behaviors, feel that their health was due to chance, and have greater faith in the capability of medical science to protect health. This second investigation partially supported the hypothesis that perceived seriousness of symptoms serves as an intervening variable through which social, structural, and attitudinal variables shape self-care behavioral responses to illness.

Age as a Variable Shaping Self-Care Behavior

Distinct age-related patterns of self-care, identified in our prior work (Dean, 1986b; Dean et al., 1983), are consistent with findings of other investigators. We find older age related to greater use of medications, ameliorative care rather than behavior directed toward the source of symptoms, more frequent professional consultation, and less active and preventive coping behavior.

Self-care responses to illness, however, are shaped by complex interactions among social situational, attitudinal, and health variables rather than age per se. Such personal and situational variables affect symptom perceptions, which, in turn, are related to medical care utilization. Thus episodes perceived to be serious are more likely to result in medical contacts than those believed to be less serious. For example, our early research (Dean, 1986b) showed that episodes of illness were more often experienced as serious among people who (a) were divorced or widowed, (b) considered themselves in relatively poor health, (c) responded to feeling stressed by taking medicine or trying to forget their problems, (d) were older, (e) expressed strong faith in the capacity of medical science to preserve or restore health, or (f) expressed strong faith in the benefit of pharmaceuticals.

At first glance, it appears that the effects of age, operating through perceptions of illness, exerted less influence on self-care responses than did marital status, perceived health status, and the ways people cope with stress. This impression is not entirely correct, however. While age in itself does not cause these differences, these factors are themselves directly associated with age. That is, age exerted both small direct and considerable indirect effects on perceptions regarding the seriousness of illness episodes. Thus it appears that factors that have little or nothing to do with chronological age per se, but arise from social, structural, and cultural influences that often combine in the personal life situations of old people, shape self-care behaviors.

These social, structural, and cultural influences operate to shape older people's health-related behavior and attitudes. Research suggests that older people often assume a passive and pessimistic approach to their own health and well-being; for example, older age has been associated with beliefs that good health is a matter of chance (Cicirelli, 1980; Dean, 1984). In addition, negative stereotypes of aging, acceptance of disabilities as inevitable, and palliative care could preclude preventive or corrective treatment, both in the form of self-care and in the form of professional treatment. A negative approach to aging probably reduces attempts to create positive environments, control stress, expand functional capacity, and seek social interaction. Further research on age differences in self-care behavior may help determine how social and psychological variables, often associated with age, exert influence on health and functional capacity.

Review of Third Danish Study

In our most recent research, we have given priority to identifying influences that arise from situations more common to old age and those due directly to old age. It is impossible in a cross-sectional study to separate effects of age from period effects and cohort effects. Therefore, our goal was to examine age differences in statistical modeling focusing on intervening influences and any direct effects of age that might exist after the control of all other variables in the model.

Methodology and statistical analysis. In 1982, interviews were conducted with a random sample of 465 persons over 45 years of age from a Danish community of urban, suburban, and rural residences. The sample is representative of the age, sex, and marital status distributions of the study population. Three forms of self-care behavior were examined: routine habits, conscious health maintenance behavior, and symptom care. Self-care responses to illness included (a) no action taken, (b) nutritional treatment, (c) "home remedy" (nondietary), (d) medication, (e) bed rest, and (f) decision to seek professional advice. For each illness episode, a self-care response sheet was completed to collect information on whether or not one or more of the six types of behavioral responses occurred and on the nature of the particular practice (i.e., which food or medicine was used or which type of professional was contacted).

Three measures of attitudes toward health and medical care were examined in this study: faith in medical care, internal health locus of control, and confidence in one's own ability to make decisions regarding health. Measures of social network, social support, and stressful problems/events were used to study the influence of social situational variables on the three components of self-care behavior. Income, type of occupation, and employment status were also assessed to obtain measures of socioeconomic status.

A major goal of the analysis in this investigation was to elaborate the direct and indirect statistical effects of age on self-care behavior. Contrary to the usual focus on independent statistical relationships, our major interest was in examining age as an antecedent variable to identify social and psychosocial variables and interrelationships among variables that shape behaviors that affect health over time. Statistically independent effects of age on behavior were of less concern. Because the data to be analyzed were cross-sectional, causal relationships could not be directly assessed. The specific intent of this analysis was to identify interactions among variables and potential chains of influence. To achieve this goal, statistical methods were needed that could elaborate interrelationships among many complex variables and test levels of influence among the variables.

The large number of quantitative and discrete variables indicated that multivariate techniques for analyzing contingency tables would be the most appropriate statistical methods for the analysis of the data. The statistical procedures used are based on mathematical graph models for the analysis of multiway contingency tables (Kreiner, 1987; Wermuth & Lauritzen, 1983). Of the available methods for analyzing survey data, the graphic models are best suited to address the research questions posed in the investigation as well as in terms of the nature of the data to be analyzed. Variables were included in the investigation because of their known or hypothesized influence on health-related behavior. Generally, the variables were neither continuous nor normally distributed. While the data set is mixed, the variables are mostly discrete, either categorical or ordinal, and skewed in their distributions. The graphic models can determine the structure of the data and do so without building on assumptions that are generally violated in health and social survey data.

An a priori decision was made to conduct separate analyses for men and women. This decision was based on the consistent sex differences found in our earlier studies of self-care behavior (Dean, 1986b; Dean et al., 1983) and in multiple investigations of health-related behavior in different settings (Dean, 1981; Langlie, 1977; Verbrugge, 1985). It was felt that gender effects could not be fully elaborated in the combined data, so they were assessed separately.

Because the limits of causal modeling with cross-sectional data are clearly recognized, to avoid ad hoc manipulations of the data, it was important to conduct the analyses on the basis of a theoretically determined recursive structure for levels of influence among variables. Figure 2.1 shows this model. In this structure, age is considered an antecedent variable that, at any point in time, represents for individuals the accumulated effects of social, psychosocial, and behavioral influences as well as the effects of social and economic conditions in a given community. The variables in each box interrelate among themselves and also affect the parallel and subsequent levels of influence. As complex as the statistical model is, the reality consists of far more complicated processes and interactions.

Research findings. Surprisingly few age differences in self-care behavior were found (see Table 2.1). The modest negative correlations between age and tobacco consumption represent the only statistically independent age differences. It is not possible to determine whether or not these differences in tobacco consumption represent responses to already existing diseases. This question must be explored in detailed analyses of the smoking and morbidity variables and in a prospective study of the effects of behavior on morbidity and mortality.

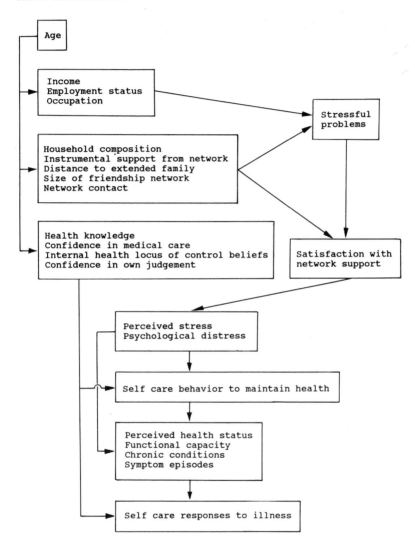

Figure 2.1. Analytic Model for Hypothesized Levels of Influence Among Variables Affecting Self-Care Behavior

The negative relationships between age and both routine physical exercise and dental examination were indirect relationships arising from age differences in income. Both routine physical exercise and dental examinations occurred more frequently among persons living

Table 2.1

Statistical Associations for Age and Self-Care Behaviors Among Persons over 45 Years of Age in a Danish Community

	Men (N = 211)		Women (N = 253)	
	γ^*	p	γ^*	p
Health-related behavior:				
tobacco consumption[a]	−.17	.014	−.20	.003
alcohol consumption	−.14	.016	.03	.350
physical activity	−.22	−.002	−.33	.000
health-promoting behavior	.15	.074	−.02	.404
avoidance behavior	.03	.396	−.05	.321
dental exam[b]	−.40	.000	−.47	.000
blood pressure measurement	.15	.083	.02	.408
breast exam	—	—	−.24	.017
Illness responses	(899 episodes)		(1345 episodes)	
bed rest	−.04	.457	−.03	.443
dietary change	.01	.483	.28	.103
liquid intake	.42	.083	−.13	.225
home remedy	−.20	.187	−.21	.073
medication	.21	.055	.00	.495
professional contact	.15	.191	.15	.097

a. This row denotes an independent statistical relationship.
b. This row denotes an indirect statistical relationship.
* Gamma correlations with associated p values calculated by Exact tests (kreiner, 1987).

in families with high incomes while older people more often had lower incomes.

The modest increase in professional contacts for both sexes and use of medications by men were also indirect relationships arising from older people's more often living in situations that led to more frequent professional consultation. The relative lack of statistically independent age differences in medical contacts and use of medicine in this study, compared with many other investigations, may result from the nurse interviewers' having obtained more information on the chronic conditions and symptoms of older respondents than usually is reported in interviews. The inclusion of such detailed health variables in this analysis may have resulted in smaller age differences in use of care in comparison with the well-reported age differences in morbidity.

The medication findings reported here do not take account of multiple medication use in responses to illness episodes; instead, the analysis reported here examined the relative proportion of medication responses to illness episodes rather than the volume of medicine taking. Therefore, the correlations in Table 2.1 do not represent possible age differences in the total amount of drugs consumed. The frequently reported tendency for women to take medicine for illness more often than men was not found, although women did report relatively more symptoms. Women reported an average of 5.3 illness episodes for the two-month study period compared with the male average of 4.3 episodes. However, at the same time, the female group was somewhat older: 15% of the women were over 75 years of age compared with 11% of the men.

Figures 2.2 and 2.3 summarize the interrelationships among the age, social, psychological, behavioral, and health variables for men and women, respectively. While there are some similarities in the interrelationships among specific variables for the two sexes, dissimilarities are more prevalent and are especially striking in relation to the variables related to self-care behavior.[1]

Interpretation of findings. The serious limitations inherent in trying to draw any conclusions from cross-sectional data on factors influencing behavior cannot be overlooked. Yet, by moving away from static analytic models that concentrate on relative weights and implied relative causation, it is possible to analyze cross-sectional data in process designs with more flexible and valid analytic techniques. Before the advent of widespread computer analysis of survey data, more careful attention was directed toward modeling antecedent, intervening, and other types of relationships into analyses. Gradually, what the computer could readily do replaced conceptual modeling in many investigations. Variables that themselves are shaped/ influenced by other variables in the model often are included as parallel factors in analytic procedures that cannot identify or account for the interrelationships. Large correlations and betas are often the focus of attention regardless of methodological and conceptual limitations inherent in the use of some procedures and regardless of how much of the variation in the outcome measure of interest is explained. Because causation is complex and gradual, it is perhaps the opposite emphasis that is needed—understanding the interrelationships

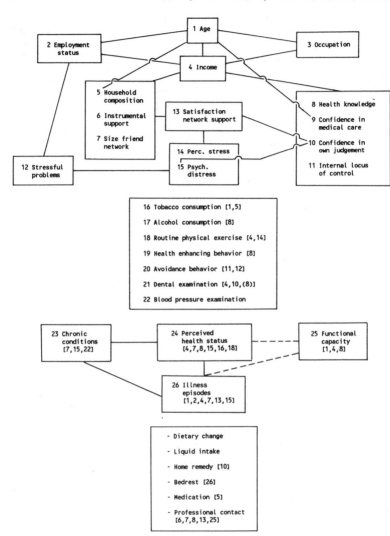

Figure 2.2. Levels of Influence Among Variables Affecting Self-Care Behavior Among Men over 45 Years of Age in a Danish County

NOTE: Lines between age, social, and psychological variables refer to statistically independent direct relationships between variables. When the line connects with a box, the influence is independently related to all variables in the box. Each variable is preceded by a variable number for identification purposes. The variables exerting direct independent statistical influence on self-care behavior and health variables are listed in brackets after each behavioral or health variable. Variables exerting meaningful indirect influences are shown in parentheses.

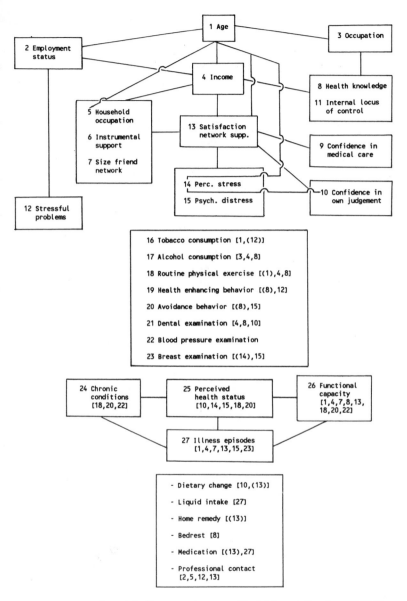

Figure 2.3. Levels of Influence Among Variables Affecting Self-Care Behavior Among Women over 45 Years of Age in a Danish County

NOTE: Lines between age, social, and psychological variables refer to statistically independent direct relationships between variables. When the line connects with a box, the influence is independently related to all variables in the box. Each variable is preceded by a variable number for identification purposes. The variables exerting direct independent statistical influence on self-care behavior and health variables are listed in brackets after each behavioral or health variable. Variables exerting meaningful indirect influences are shown in parentheses.

among the many moderate and small influences. Rather than discounting small and moderate independent effects, perhaps large correlations should be examined to assess their conceptual and analytic validity.

While it is not possible to assess causation in cross-sectional data, it can be useful to test logically modeled relationships on the basis of theoretical or substantive considerations. It is immediately helpful to know whether self-care behavior arises from health beliefs, psychological distress, or social situational influences. The study of interrelations among these levels of influences also provides useful information for the design of longitudinal investigations of health behavior.

The findings of this last investigation suggest possible pathways through which social, psychosocial, and behavioral influences may influence health and aging. It is significant to find that it is not health beliefs or self-confidence in matters related to health that shape self-care but social situational variables.

Neither confidence in the ability of medical care to preserve health nor (with one exception) belief in personal control over health was related to self-care. The measure of knowledge regarding ways to prevent cancer and cardiovascular disease was related to health-protective practices among both men and women and to professional contacts among men. It appears that health-specific knowledge regarding beneficial effects does increase particular behaviors while more generalized beliefs are less important. It is relevant to note in this regard that confidence in the ability of medical care to protect health and the knowledge measure were inversely related. The locus of health control variable did affect the male health-related avoidance behavior. This finding supports other evidence that the locus of control health perspective may be more important in altering health-damaging behaviors than as a generalized behavioral influence (Dean, 1984).

The self-confidence in health decisions measure apparently reflects personal self-confidence in some way. Because the items in this measure include sometimes disagreeing with one's doctor and sometimes following one's own opinion rather than medical advice, it clearly reflects the self-care aspects of compliance behavior. The inverse relationship with dental visits was consistent with this interpretation. It is interesting that there was a strong positive relationship between the self-confidence variable and confidence in medical care.

The dominance of the social situation, especially satisfaction with social support in determining professional care seeking (irrespective of age, measures of health, or health beliefs), points once again to the importance of the social network. Satisfaction with network support influenced medical care seeking independent of the type or amount of illness. Equally interesting to note is that it was not stressful life events that led directly to illness episodes and perceived health status but psychological distress. Psychological distress was shaped by some combination of stressful change in the life situation, network support, and self-confidence among men. For women, support from the network appears to be a dominant aspect of psychological distress. Neither stressful problems nor self-confidence in health matters was related to the distress variable among women. The absence of support in and of itself constituted a major stressor for women. At the same time, women less often than men reported satisfactory support and help from the personal network.

For men, psychological distress is shaped via another route of situational influences. The relationship between employment status and reported stressful problems in the life situation, independent of income, network, and support influences, points to the stressful nature of retirement in and of itself for men. The extent to which network support and personal coping can moderate psychological distress arising from retirement and resulting in symptoms of illness needs to be explored in these and other data.

Clearly, the disentanglement of the contributions of social network and personal functioning to perceived support and stress reduction is an area in need of careful research study. Both for understanding the processes that maintain or damage health and for developing appropriate and cost-effective professional services, information is needed on the extent to which social network influences on health are either the direct result of stress reactions arising from nonsupportive networks, and/or arise from stress-buffering mechanisms, and/or operate through the personal functioning and self-care behavior of individuals who become ill. In this investigation, the influence of network and support variables on illness episodes independent of chronic conditions and functional capacity supports the findings of many other investigations showing that nonsupportive networks are directly damaging to health. Buffering effects of the network and interrelationships with personal functioning are yet to be explored in subanalyses, but findings from our earlier work clearly supported buffering effects as well (Dean, 1986a).

The findings do not indicate that social support affects health maintenance behavior as studied in this investigation. Living alone was related to greater male tobacco consumption, but otherwise it was health knowledge, income, occupation, and stressful situations, either acute or chronic, that appeared to influence these widely studied behaviors. One may question the extent to which the behaviors studied here represent the range of behavioral influences through which social network may affect health over time. One thing is clear, however; we must begin to address the many unanswered questions to understand processes of health maintenance and healthy aging.

SUMMARY AND CONCLUSIONS

Age is one of the strongest predictors of health and the use of medical services (Ory & Bond, 1989). Correlations between age and health variables reflect a multitude of interacting biological, behavioral, and social factors. The dynamic linkages among these classes of variables are slowly becoming the focus of researchers.

In investigations of self-care behavior in Denmark, age is conceptualized as an antecedent variable, which, at any point in time, collects the accumulated influence of multiple social, psychosocial, and behavioral influences. The results of our investigations suggest that independent effects of age are small. Rather, age is statistically related to social and psychosocial variables that directly influence behavior and health and thus should perhaps be considered in more technical terms as a summary collector of causal influences. The task then is to disentangle the summary effects and identify the combinations of factors that lead to the preservation or breakdown of health.

The findings of our studies may be affected by national and cultural conditions specific to Denmark. However, it is interesting to note in this regard that the limited information available for the United States suggests some important parallels. Haug and colleagues (1989), studying a general population sample of persons over 45 years of age, also found that health maintenance is unrelated to illness-related self-care. It appears that quite different influences shape these forms of behavior. In both settings, attitudes and beliefs exerted much less influence on behavior than did situational variables. Likewise, in both investigations, psychological distress (while exerting little direct influence on behavior) was an important factor related to the health status measures. The findings suggest the relevance of the Danish studies for U.S. research as well as the importance of cross-national investigations for purposes of replicating the findings and clarifying the cultural and social structural influences affecting the aging process.

NOTE

1. A detailed analysis of the findings can be obtained from the author.

REFERENCES

Abdellah, F., & Moore, S. (Eds.). (1988). *Surgeon General's workshop: Health promotion and aging*. Washington, DC: U.S. Public Health Service.

Agner, E. (1985). Smoking and health in old age: A ten year follow-up study. *Acta Medica Scandinavica, 218*, 311.

Alpert, J., Kosa, J., & Haggerty, R. (1967). A month of illness and health care among low income families. *Public Health Reports, 820*, 705.

Andersen, R., Kravits, J., & Anderson, O. (1975). *Equity in health services.* Cambridge, MA: Ballinger.

Anderson, J., Buck, C., Danaher, K., & Fry, J. (1977). Users and non-users of doctors: Implications for self-care. *Journal of the Royal College of General Practitioners, 27*, 155.

Anderson, O. (1975). What can the U.S. learn from Scandinavia? *Scandinavian Review, 63*, 5.

Antonovsky, A. (1972). A model to explain visits to the doctor, with specific reference to the case of Israel. *Journal of Health and Social Behavior, 13*, 446.

Badura, B. (1983). Social epidemiology in theory and practice. *European Monographs in Health Education Research, 5*, 27.

Belloc, N. (1973). Relationship of health practices and mortality. *Preventive Medicine, 2*, 67-81.

Berkanovic, E., Telesky, C., & Reeder, S. (1981). Structural and social psychological factors in the decision to seek medical care for symptoms. *Medical Care, 19*, 693.

Berkman, P. (1975). Survival and a modicum of indulgence in the sick role. *Medical Care, 13*, 85.

Blackburn, H. (1983). Research and demonstration projects in community cardiovascular disease prevention. *Journal of Public Health Policy, 4*, 398-421.

Blackburn, H., et al. (1984). The Minnesota Heart Health program: A research and demonstration project in cardiovascular disease prevention. In S. Weiss (Ed.), *Settings for health promotion in behavioral health*. Silver Spring, MD: John Wiley.

Brocklehurst, J. (1978). Aging and health. In D. Hobmon (Ed.), *The social challenge of ageing*. London: Croom Helm.

Brody, E., Klebon, M., & Moles, E. (1983). What older people do about their day to day mental and physical health symptoms. *Journal of the American Geriatric Society, 31*, 489.

Brown Eve, S. (1986). Self medication among older adults in the United States. In K. Dean, T. Hickey, & B. Holstein (Eds.), *Self-care and health in old age*. London: Croom Helm.

Bush, P. J., & Rabin, D. L. (1976). "Who's using nonprescribed medicines?" *Medical Care, 14*, 1014-1023.

Cartwright, A., & Anderson, R. (1981). *General practice revisited*. London: Tavistock.

Chrisman, N., & Kleinman, A. (1983). Popular health care, social networks and cultural meanings: The orientation of medical anthropology. In D. Mechanic (Ed.), *Handbook of health, health care and the professions*. New York: Free Press.

Christopher, L. J., Bellinger, B. R., Shepherd, A. M. M., Ramsey, A., & Crooks, G. (1978). Drug prescribing patterns in the elderly: A cross-sectional study of in-patients. *Age & Aging, 7*, 74-82.

Cicirelli, V. (1980). Relationship of family background variables to locus of control in the elderly. *Journal of Gerontology, 35*, 108.

Cohen, S., & Syme, L. (1985). Issues in the study and application of social support. In S. Cohen & L. Syme (Eds.), *Social support and health*. New York: Academic Press.

Cohen, S., & Syme, L. (Eds.). (1985). *Social support and health*. New York: Academic Press.

Coreil, J., Levin, G., & Jaco, G. (1985). Life style: An emerging concept in the sociomedical sciences. *Culture, Medicine and Psychiatry, 9*, 423-437.

Dean, K. (1981). Self-care responses to illness: A selected review. *Social Science and Medicine, 15A*, 673.

Dean, K. (1984). Influence of health beliefs on lifestyles: What do we know? *European Monographs in Health Education Research, 6*, 127-151.

Dean, K. (1986a). Social support and health: Pathways of influence. *Health Promotion, 1*, 133.

Dean, K. (1986b). Self care: Implications for aging. In K. Dean, T. Hickey, & B. Holstein (Eds.), *Self care and health in old age*. London: Croom Helm.

Dean, K. (1986c). Lay care in illness. *Social Science and Medicine, 22*, 275.

Dean, K. (1989a). Conceptual, theoretical and methodological issues in self-care research. *Social Science and Medicine, 29*, 117.

Dean, K. (1989b). Self care behavioral elements of lifestyles: Gender, attitudes and the social situation. *Social Science and Medicine, 29*, 137.

Dean, K., Holst, E., & Wagner, M. (1983). Self-care of common illness in Denmark. *Medical Care, 21*, 1012.

DeFriese, G. H., Woomert, A., Guild, P. A., Steckler, A. B., & Konrad, T. R. (1989). From activated patient to pacified activist: A study of the self-care movement in the United States. *Social Science and Medicine, 29*, 195-204.

Dunnell, K., & Cartwright, A. (1972). *Medicine takers, prescribers and hoarders*. London: Routledge and Kegan Paul.

Elliot-Binns, C. (1973). An analysis of lay medicine. *Journal of the Royal College of General Practitioners, 23*, 255.

Fabrega, H. (1973). Toward a model of illness behavior. *Medical Care, 11*, 470.

Farquhar, J., Moccaby, N., & Soloman, D. (1984). Community applications in behavioral medicine. In *Handbook of Behavioral Medicine*. New York: Guilford.

Fraser, G. (1986). *Preventive cardiology*. Oxford: Oxford University Press.

Freer, C. (1980). Self-care: A health diary study. *Medical Care, 18*, 853.

Fryklöf, L. E., & Westerling, R. (Eds.). (1983, November). Self-medication. In *Proceedings from an international symposium, Stockholm*. Stockholm: Swedish Pharmaceutical Press.

Gottlieb, N., & Green, L. (1984). Life-events, social network, life-style, and health: An analysis of the 1979 national survey of personal health practices and consequences. *Health Education Quarterly, 11*, 91.

Graham-Smith, D. (1975). Self-medication with mood-changing drugs. *Journal of Medical Ethics, 1,* 132.

Grandjean, P., Olesen, N., & Hollnagel, H. (1981). Influence of smoking and alcohol consumption on blood lead levels. *International Archives of Occupational and Environmental Health, 48,* 391.

Grimsmo, A. (1984). *Fra å bli syk—til å bli patient* [From being ill to becoming a patient]. Oslo: Statens Institutt for Folkehelse.

Hagerup, L., & Larsen, M. (1971). Tobacco smoking and respiratory symptoms in a Danish population. *Ugeskrift for Læger* [Danish Medical Journal], *133,* 1309.

Hamburg, D., Elliott, G., & Parran, D. (Eds.). (1982). *Health and behaviour: Frontiers of research in the biobehavioral sciences* (Institute of Medicine). Washington, DC: National Academy Press.

Hansen, P. (1977). Epidemiological studies in the Nordic countries: The Glostrup study. *Nordic Council of Arctic Medical Research Reports, 19,* 58.

Harberden, P. van, & Lafaille, R. (1978). Self-help (English mimeo from P. van Harberden & R. Lafaille, Eds., *Selfhup: enn nieuwe vorm van hulpverlening?*). The Hague, the Netherlands: Vurga.

Haro, A. (1975). Health facts and figures. *Scandinavian Review, 63,* 30.

Haug, M. R., Wykle, M. L., & Namazi, K. H. (1989). Self care among older adults. *Social Science and Medicine, 29,* 171-184.

Helman, C. (1978). "Feed a cold, starve a fever": Folk models of infection in an English suburban community and their relation to medical treatment. *Culture, Medicine and Psychiatry, 2,* 107.

Hemminki, E., & Heikkila, J. (1975). Elderly people's compliance with prescriptions, and quality of medication. *Scandinavian Journal of Social Medicine, 3,* 87-92.

Hollnagel, H., Madsen, F., & Larsen, S. (1982). Lungesymptomer, lungefunktionstest, rygevaner og erhvervseksponering blandt 40-årige mænd og kvinder i Glostrup: Indbyrdes relationer [Lung symptoms, lung function tests, smoking habits and occupation among 40-year-old men and women in Glostrup: Reciprocal relationships]. *Ugeskrift for Læger* [Danish Medical Journal], *145,* 118.

Holst, E., & Wagner, M. (1975). Primary health care is the cornerstone. *Scandinavian Review, 63,* 30.

Ibsen, H., Christensen, N., Rasmussen, S., Hollnagel, H., Nielsen, M., & Giese, J. (1981). The influence of chronic high alcohol intake on blood pressure, plasma noradrenaline, concentration and plasma resin concentration. *Clinical Science and Molecular Medicine, 61,* 377.

Kaplan, G. A., & Haan, M. N. (1986). *Socioeconomic position and mortality: Prospective evidence from the Alameda County study.* Paper presented at the American Public Health Association 114th Annual Meeting, Las Vegas.

Kaplan, G. A., & Haan, M. N. (1989). Is there a role for prevention among the elderly? In M. G. Ory & K. Bond (Eds.), *Aging and health care: Social science and policy perspectives.* London: Tavistock.

Kaplan, R. (1984). The connection between clinical health promotion and health status: A critical overview. *American Psychologist, 39,* 1.

Kasl, S., & Cobb, S. (1966). Health behavior, illness behavior and sick role behavior. Behavior I: Health and illness behavior. *Archives of Environmental Health, 12,* 246.

Kleinman, A. (1980). *Patients and healers in the context of culture.* Berkeley: University of California Press.

Kohn, R., & White, K. (Eds.). (1976). *Health care—an international study: Report of the World Health Organization international collaborative study of medical care utilization.* London: Oxford University Press.

Kreiner, S. (1987). Analysis of multidimensional contingency tables by exact conditional tests: Techniques and strategies. *Scandinavian Journal of Statistics, 14,* 19-112.

Langlie, J. (1977). Social networks, health beliefs and preventive health behavior. *Journal of Health and Social Behavior, 18,* 244-260.

Lasates, T., Abrahams, P., et al. (1984). Lay volunteer delivery of a community based risk factor change program. In S. Weiss (Ed.), *Settings for health promotion in behavioral health.* Silver Spring, MD: John Wiley.

Levin, L. (1977). Forces and issues in the revival of interest in self-care: Impetus for redirection in health. *Health Education Monographs, 5,* 115.

Levin, L., Katz, A., & Holst, E. (1976). *Self-care.* New York: Prodist.

Maddox, G. L., & Campbell, R. T. (1985). Scope, concepts, and methods in the study of aging. In R. H. Binstock & E. Shanas (Eds.), *Handbook of aging and the social sciences.* New York: Van Nostrand Reinhold.

Marmot, M. G., Rose, G., Shipley, M., & Hamilton, P. (1978). Employment grade and coronary heart disease in British civil servants. *Journal of Epidemiology and Community Health, 32,* 244.

McEwen, J. (1979). Self-medication in the context of self-care: A review. In J. Anderson (Ed.), *Self-medication.* Lancaster, United Kingdom: MTP Press.

Mechanic, D. (1972). Social psychological factors affecting the presentation of bodily complaints. *The New England Journal of Medicine, 286,* 1132.

Mechanic, D. (1978). *Medical sociology.* New York: Free Press.

Mechanic, D. (1979). Correlates of physician utilization: Why do major multivariate studies of physician utilization find trivial psychosocial and organizational effects? *Journal of Health and Social Behavior, 29,* 387.

Mechanic, D. (Ed.). (1983). *Handbook of health, health care and the professions.* New York: Free Press.

Melgaard, B., Sælan, H., & Hedegaard, L. (1986). Symptoms and signs of polyneuropathy in a normal male population and their relation to alcohol intake. *Acta Neurologica Scandinavica, 73,* 458.

Mossey, J., Havens, B., & Wolinsky, F. (1989). The consistency of formal health care utilization: Physician and hospital utilization. In M. Ory & K. Bond (Eds.), *Aging and health care: Social science and policy perspectives.* New York: Routledge.

Ory, M. (1987-1988). Social and behavioral aspects of drug-taking regimes among older persons. *Journal of Geriatric Drug Therapy, 2*(2-3), 103-114.

Ory, M., & Bond, K. (1989). Health care for an aging society. In M. Ory & K. Bond (Eds.), *Aging and health care: Social science and policy perspectives.* London: Tavistock.

Pearlin, L. T., Lieberman, M. A., Menaghan, E. G., & Mullan, J. T. (1981). Stress process. *Journal of Health and Social Behavior, 22,* 337.

Pedersen, P. (1976). Patienters selvbehandling inden henvendelse til praktiserende læge [Patients' self-treatment prior to consultation with a general practitioner]. *Ugeskrift for Læger, 138,* 1955.

Puska, P., Juomilehti, J., & Salonem, J. (1981). *The North Karelia Project: Evaluation of a comprehensive programme for control of cardiovascular diseases in 1972-77 in North Karelia* (WHO Monograph series). Copenhagen: World Health Organization.

Rakowski, W., Julius, N., Hickey, T., Verbrugge, L., & Holter, J. (1988). Daily symptoms and behavioral responses. *Medical Care, 26,* 278.

Reid, D., Hamilton, P., McCartney, P., Rose, P., Jarett, R., & Keen, H. (1976). Smoking and other risk factors for coronary heart disease in British civil servants. *Lancet, 2,* 979.

Riley, M. (1987). On the significance of age in sociology. *American Sociological Review, 52,* 1.

Riley, M., & Bond, K. (1985). Age strata in social systems. In R. Binstock & E. Shanas (Eds.), *Handbook of aging and the social sciences.* New York: Van Nostrand Reinhold.

Riley, M., Hess, B., & Bond, K. (Eds.). (1983). *Aging in society: Selected reviews of recent research.* Hillsdale, NJ: Lawrence Erlbaum.

Rose, G., & Marmot, M. G. (1981). Social class and coronary heart disease. *British Heart Journal, 45,* 13-19.

Rose, J., Reid, D., Hamilton, P., McCartney, P., Keen, H., & Jarrett, R. (1977). Myocardial ischaemia, risk factors and death from coronary heart disease. *Lancet, 41,* 105.

Rosengren, A., Wilhelmsen, L., & Wedel, H. (1988). Separate and combined effects of smoking and alcohol abuse in middle-aged men. *Acta Medica Scandinavica, 223,* 111.

Rosenstock, I. (1974). The health belief model and preventive health behavior. *Health Education Monographs, 2,* 354.

Rosenstock, I., & Kirscht, J. (1979). Why people seek health care. In G. Stone, F. Cohen, & N. Adler (Eds.), *Health psychology: A handbook.* San Francisco: Jossey-Bass.

Schroll, M. (1982). A ten year prospective study, 1964-1974, of cardiovascular risk factors in men and women from the Glostrup population in 1914. *Danish Medical Bulletin, 29,* 213.

Scott, P. J. W., Stansfield, J., & Williams, B. O. (1982). Prescribing habits and potential adverse drug interactions in geriatric medical service. *Health Bulletin, 40,* 5-9.

Shanas, E., & Maddox, G. (1985). Health, health resources, and the utilization of care. In R. Binstock & E. Shanas (Eds.), *Handbook of aging and the social sciences.* New York: Van Nostrand Reinhold.

Suchman, E. (1967). Preventive health behavior: A model for research on community health campaigns. *Journal of Health and Social Behavior, 8,* 197.

Townsend, P., & Davidson, N. (1982). *Inequalities in health.* London: Penguin.

U.S. Department of Health, Education and Welfare. (1979). *Healthy people: The surgeon general's report on health promotion and disease prevention. Background papers.* Washington, DC: Government Printing Office.

Verbrugge, L. (1985). Gender and health: An update on hypotheses and evidence. *Journal of Health and Social Behavior, 26,* 156-182.

Verbrugge, L., & Ascione, F. (1987). Exploring the iceberg: Common symptoms and how people care for them. *Medical Care, 25,* 539.

Wan, T. (1989). The behavioral model of health care utilization by older people. In M. Ory & K. Bond (Eds.), *Aging and health care.* New York: Routledge.

Wermuth, N., & Lauritzen, S. (1983). Graphical and recursive models for contingency tables. *Biometrika, 70,* 537.

White, K., Andjilkovic, D., Pearson, R., Mabry, J., Ross, A., & Sagan, O. (1967). International comparisons of medical care utilization. *The New England Journal of Medicine, 277,* 516.

Wiley, J., & Camacho, T. (1980). Life-style and future health: Evidence from the Alameda County study. *Preventive Medicine, 9,* 1.

Williamson, J., & Danaher, K. (1980). *Self-care in health.* London: Croom Helm.

Wolinsky, F. (1978). Assessing the effects of predisposing, enabling and illness: Morbidity characteristics on health services utilization. *Journal of Health and Social Behavior, 19,* 384-396.

World Health Organization. (1983, November). *Health education in self-care possibilities and limitations: Report of a scientific consultation.* Geneva: Author.

Zborowski, M. (1958). Cultural components in response to pain. In G. Jaco (Ed.), *Patients, physicians and illness.* New York: Free Press.

Zola, I. (1966). Culture and symptoms: An analysis of patients presenting complaints. *American Sociological Review, 3,* 615.

3

Informal and Formal Health Care Systems Serving Older Persons

GORDON H. DeFRIESE
ALISON WOOMERT

One of the most important considerations in any national policy encompassing the health needs of the older adult population is the matter of the utilization of health services, including attention to levels of need, patterns of voluntary utilization, and the accessibility of appropriate health services. As a backdrop to current policy discussions of the health care needs of the elderly, there are at least two very different points of view, one pessimistic and one optimistic. As first articulated by Fries (1980), older people will spend a smaller and smaller proportion of their lives in ill health as better health care and healthier life-styles combine to postpone incapacitating morbidities and disabilities to the natural end of life. According to Fries, practical approaches to health improvement, especially for our older adult population in the decades ahead, should focus on the reduction of the burden of chronic illness and disability, not on the reduction of mortality. Programs that merit increased emphasis are those that encourage self-care and increased functional capacity, not ones that offer curative services or life-sustaining technologies. Yet others warn that, at least for the current time, the latter years of life—for those who live to be among the "oldest old"—will be characterized by years of disability and dependency with catastrophic health care heroically provided in the last weeks or days of life (Manton, 1982; Schneider & Brody, 1983; Verbrugge, 1989).

These two views can be reconciled by a sociological perspective characterizing the seemingly protracted stage of old age disability as a product of short-range perspectives (Riley & Bond, 1983). This perspective sees life in the more advanced ages characterized by "long years of rolelessness, inactivity, and dependency; by chronic disability; and by lingering death" as a pattern peculiar to the modern world. Riley and Bond (1983) argued that this picture of life for our oldest old "stems from the unprecedented and rapid extension of life expectancy." Now, as never before, we have larger and larger numbers of elderly surviving to the point that they have encountered the disabilities and functional limitations of old age. The recency and enormity of these problems make them seem intractable and inevitable. The current situation, in the view of Riley and Bond, presents a new set of problems, a new and dramatic challenge to find productive and meaningful roles for older adults in families, in communities, or in the work force.

Riley and Bond direct our thinking beyond the "compression of morbidity" thesis. They focus our attention on the positive secular changes that are currently counteracting the tendency for the life of the oldest adults to deteriorate into a protracted life of disability, boredom, and uselessness. Moreover, new scientific evidence suggests that the biological pathway of old age is not monotonic and invariable. We need to avoid the stereotypical images of older people and recognize the heterogeneity of the older adult population (Ory, 1989). Enormous individual differences among older people make generalizations about members of this age group imprecise but also underscore the need for a social policy that is less subject to the charge of "ageism" (Butler, 1975, 1982; Herrick, 1983).

We have generally ignored the importance of personal choice in the determination of the extent to which higher levels of health are realized by individuals in every age group. As we are protected from the likelihood of death from previously common causes, our prospects for a longer life without disability or senescence may also be increased through the practice of prudent patterns of healthful lifestyle and the learning of certain skills necessary for the protection of health and functional independence. We now recognize that the longevity of vital organs is a function of the way they are used and that dysfunction over a lifetime is not the sudden result of disease. We also are beginning to recognize the importance and potential of making genuine structural changes in our society that make it easier and more likely for senior citizens to live a full and rewarding life into their later years.

The implication of these important aging health policy analyses is that the emphasis of health services for an aging population should not be placed predominantly on formal (and certainly not on professional) health care. Rather, a rational and effective approach to the provision of personal health services for the older adult population of the future should include a substantial role for self-care and other informal care arrangements designed to maintain the functional capacities important to independent social life.

THE CONCEPTUAL FRAMEWORK FOR SELF-CARE/INFORMAL CARE

Contemporary Western societies, where formal health care services are in abundant supply, carry the widespread presumption that most illnesses or health limitations will be attended by professional care providers. It is expected that such providers not only will diagnose and define the precise nature of disease symptoms and their presumed causes but will also prescribe appropriate interventions designed to ameliorate these conditions and restore optimal physical and emotional "good health." In the sense that elaborate service industries have developed for most aspects of everyday life (e.g., the maintenance of lawns, the care of automobiles, the care of children, the laundering of clothes, the preparation of food, the cleaning of homes), it is natural to assume a diminished level of expectations with regard to individual initiative in the diagnosis and treatment of illness and the maintenance of health. However, with respect to those long-term "personal care" services that may be required to compensate for chronic limitations in the performance of basic self-care activities, such as meal preparation, housekeeping, bathing, dressing, or shopping, the presumptive role of formal care providers may be less obvious. The care of the vast majority of persons with extreme degrees of functional dependence, such as the frail elderly or the chronically disabled, depends in whole or in part on informal caregivers (Ory & Bond, 1989; Shanas, 1979). It is estimated that nearly three quarters of the noninstitutionalized impaired elderly depend on family and friends, not formal care providers, for all assistance they receive. Less than 10% of the impaired elderly receive services from formal, community-based providers (Doty, 1986).

Definition of Self-Care

Although the terms *informal care* and *self-care* are used interchangeably in the literature pertaining to health and long-term care, these terms have separate and very different conceptual referents. The self-care movement has viewed the actions that laypersons take in their own health interest, or in the health interest of close relatives and friends, as a distinct level of health care that deserves explicit recognition.

The World Health Organization (WHO) convened a scientific working group in 1983 charged to make a set of recommendations for supporting and enhancing effective self-care in the member countries of WHO. This WHO working group advanced the following definition of self-care:

> Self-care in health refers to the activities individuals, families and communities undertake with the intention of enhancing health, preventing disease, limiting illness, and restoring health. These activities are derived from technical knowledge and skills from the pool of both professional and lay experience. They are undertaken by lay people on their own behalf, either separately or in participatory collaboration with professionals. (WHO, 1983)

The conventional triangular depiction of vertically arranged levels of health care services (namely, primary, secondary, and tertiary) is illustrated in Figure 3.1. Self-care appropriately constitutes the broad base of this triangle, representing the level and kind of care most people turn to most of the time. Primary care, in its conventional usage, represents the first level of "formal" health care. Many studies now show that the majority of first responses to illness symptoms are ones defined as "self-care." Additionally, most people who are seen in "formal" primary care practices for common illness symptoms have already attempted to diagnose and treat their illness symptoms through one form or another of self-care (Demers, Altmore, Mustin, Lleinman, & Leonardi, 1980). Less is known, however, about the extent to which age influences one's self-care behaviors (Ory, 1989).

The concepts of self-care and self-help are highly relevant to a discussion of health policy affecting the elderly. The propensity to learn (or acquire) these self-care skills and to practice them in everyday behavior have important implications for the eventual need for other levels and types of both informal and formal care.

Many older people (as well as their caregivers) erroneously interpret a decline in functional health status as a "normal" sign of the aging process, which they associate with a progressive loss of bodily and mental functioning (see Chapter 5 by Leventhal, Leventhal, & Schaefer). For example, a classic study by Townsend and Wedderburn

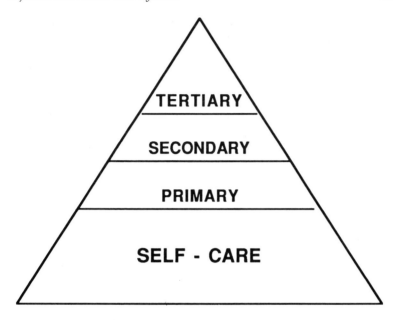

Figure 3.1. Levels of Care

(1965) in the United Kingdom indicated that more than 25% of older persons living at home admitted to difficulties with hearing and nearly one sixth mentioned severe difficulties with sight, although none of them had sought formal medical help for these conditions.

Learning to seek formal medical care appropriately is an important self-care activity that can improve the health status of older persons. This requires learning to redefine changes typically associated with "aging" as abnormal and legitimate reasons for seeking formal health care. Self-care educational programs can play an important role in helping to modify the notion of what constitutes acceptable health for older persons. Most people, whether elderly or not, would prefer to discuss the onset of a symptom with other laypersons before (or in lieu of) raising the issue with their doctors. Slowly developing (i.e., nonacute) illness symptoms and health conditions usually allow plenty of time for information exchange, reflection, and experimentation with one or more methods of symptom relief. When the appearance of symptoms is accompanied by a growing awareness of advancing age, older people may turn to adaptive, instead of help-seeking, behaviors.

The U.S. Self-Care Movement

Organized educational programs have been designed to provide self-care training to individuals who wish to learn how to perform certain health care activities for themselves rather than to completely depend on health professionals for these services. Much of this activity has been seen as an effort to counteract what many have called the "medicalization" of U.S. social life. The U.S. self-care movement can be viewed as having both progressive and conservative elements. On the one hand, this movement reinforces a view of individual responsibility for health. By "empowering" the layperson in his or her encounters with the formal health care system, self-care encourages more self-reliance and self-confidence in making personal health choices and in dealing as an effective partner with the professional provider. On the other hand, the movement has been developed to some extent (by formal care providers and third-party payers) with the idea of minimizing the seemingly "unnecessary" use of formal health care and of reducing the excessive financial pressures on formal systems of health care delivery.

The impetus for the U.S. self-care movement derives from the recognition that, for most people, the initial response to any illness symptom or health limitation is experimentation with one or more learned strategies for symptom relief or seeking lay consultation with respect to alternative ways of dealing with the symptom short of seeking formal care. Self-care curricula offer instruction through which laypersons can acquire the knowledge and experience to diagnose, effectively treat, and/or prevent common illness conditions. Moreover, these curricula stress the importance of health maintenance and the modification of life-style factors that pose serious long-term risks to health. These courses also offer training in how to negotiate with formal health care providers so that communication with professionals is more likely to be clear and genuinely beneficial to health. Panels of health care professionals have concluded that conventional self-care courses in the United States teach self-care skills of low risk that can be performed well by laypersons without professional supervision (DeFriese, Woomert, Guild, Steckler, & Konrad, 1989).

The self-care movement also places considerable emphasis on the management of chronic health conditions after formal health care providers have done all they can do to cure or minimize the pain and discomfort associated with these conditions. Once a condition is no longer in an acute stage, and the focus shifts to maintaining the highest possible level of functioning given the limitation, then self-care can play a critical role. The self-care movement in the United States also includes a substantial emphasis on what is sometimes called "other care" or "cover care," that is, the learning of skills necessary for providing to others the health-related services required by family, neighbors, and other close associates.

While many practitioners of formal health care were at first deeply suspicious of the U.S. self-care movement and its seemingly "countermedical" intentions, in the past several years, there have been literally hundreds of articles in the scholarly and practical periodicals of the health care field written by health professionals advocating the teaching of self-care skills for the management of the long-term consequences of chronic illness and health-limiting conditions. In the process of preparing this chapter, we counted more than 400 references in the clinical literature on one aspect or another of self-care published since 1980. There can be little doubt that the concept of self-care, while once of dubious respect among the health professions in the United States, has now been fully incorporated into the vocabulary and the strategy for formal health care.

The Definition of Informal Care

The concept of "informal care" (in contradistinction to the concept of "formal care") is used primarily as a way of distinguishing the horizontal division of labor between different types of care providers, often offering the same or similar services under slightly different auspices to a client or patient in need (see Figure 3.2). Soldo and Agree (1989), referring to work by Dono et al. (1979), defined informal care as

> personal care provided by a relative, friend, or neighbor (i.e., by members of one's) informal care network, . . . a diffuse primary group characterized by its small size, affectivity, and durable commitment to each other's well-being.

By the same token, a "formal care provider" is a person from outside one's primary group who provides care or help. Hence, the ambiguity and heterogeneity of the category of "formal care provider." It is often not the particular type of care that distinguishes formal from informal care; rather, it is the caregiver (and his or her relationship to the client/patient) that defines one instance as formal and the other as informal. While many would consider a formal care provider to be one who offers services in the name of a structured bureaucracy or organization, others would also include services provided to an individual by a neighbor or volunteer as examples of formal care, so long as that care came from a person or group outside one's primary network.

In sum, the notions of self-care and informal care refer to much the same behaviors, knowledge, and skills. While self-care gives emphasis to the vertical dimension of health care, informal care focuses on the horizontal dimension of health care task and resource allocation. In fact, for purposes of discussion, self-care might be subsumed beneath the rubric *informal care.*

INFORMAL/SELF-CARE: SUPPLEMENT TO OR SUBSTITUTE FOR FORMAL CARE?

One of the more important questions for public policy concerns the extent to which self-care (or informal care) has tended to become "additive to" or a "substitute for" conventional formal health care services. There is substantial controversy within the self-care literature over whether popular curricula for teaching self-care skills to laypersons actually would increase the use of formal health care services. Berg and LoGerfo (1979) examined the actual patterns of health services utilization for specific reasons in a defined panel of families in Seattle, then compared the patterns of use with those recommended by one of the more widely known family self-care textbooks (Vickery & Fries, 1976). These analyses indicated that, had the self-care algorithms been followed, this group of families would have made 45% more physician visits than they actually did.

This finding did not seem reasonable to a number of other researchers and self-care activists. Lorig, Kraines, Brown, and Richardson (1985) employed a "quasi-experimental, staggered intervention, time series design" to study a work-site self-care program offered to more than 15,000 employees at various California businesses and organizations. Educational presentations and self-care instruction manuals (namely, *Take Care of Yourself* by Vickery & Fries, 1976, 1981, and *Taking Care of Your Child* by Vickery, Fries, & Pantell, 1977) were associated with reduced rates of health care visits. The reductions obtained for all ages and educational groups although not for HMO members.

Even greater reductions in the utilization of health care were found by Vickery et al. (1983) in a prospective, randomized trial of a self-care educational intervention in an HMO population. These investigators

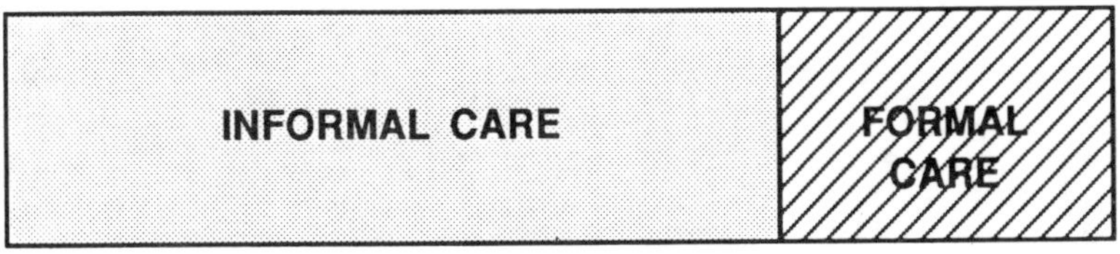

Figure 3.2. Categories of Personal/Health Care: The Horizontal
Dimension

found that subjects in three experimental groups exposed to self-care instruction used ambulatory care services almost 20% less than the control groups. Differences were even greater (i.e., 35% reduction) for visits for minor illness.

In another study, Kemper (1982) demonstrated significant effects on the level of self-care knowledge and per-visit costs among enrollees of another HMO. Participants were randomly allocated to a medical self-care program using *The Healthwise Handbook* (Roberts, Tinker, & Kemper, 1978) or to a control group. However, the Kemper study was unable to show an effect on either the frequency of clinic visits or the total health care costs. Kemper and associates have since developed two self-care educational curricula specifically for seniors, *The Growing Younger Handbook* (Kemper, Deneen, & Giuffre, 1984) and *Growing Wiser* (Kemper, Mettler, Giuffre, & Batzek, 1986). The former deals with such topics as exercise, nutrition, stress management, and health care use. The curriculum features practical approaches to a variety of everyday problems senior citizens encounter with regard to their health and illness concerns. The latter curriculum focuses for the most part on building a positive self-image and creating positive expectations in one's later years as well as on dealing with persons younger than oneself. These courses have been evaluated but the results have yet to be published.

Among the most widely known self-care curricula for older adults is the Self-Care for Senior Citizens (SCSC) program developed by the Dartmouth Institute for Better Health, part of the Dartmouth Medical School in New Hampshire (Nelson et al., 1984). The curriculum was evaluated in two New Hampshire communities, one "test" community of 204 subjects and one "comparison" community with 126 subjects. Volunteer participants were recruited and then surveyed at baseline with regard to demographic characteristics, health status indicators, health knowledge and skills in self-care areas, and personal support needs in the area of activities of daily living (ADL), and health care utilization behavior. Both test and comparison groups were surveyed at 3 months and again at 12 months after the 13-session intervention. During these follow-ups, questions were included to test health skills and knowledge, attempts to change life-style (related to physical fitness, diet and nutrition, stress reduction, and weight loss), health-relevant attitudes, health care utilization, and self-reported indicators of health status and quality of life.

The evaluation indicated that the intervention assisted by this self-care curriculum led to improvements among members of the "test" group (that were sustained for a 12-month period) in health knowledge, in skills performance, and in attitudes of confidence with respect to the performance of these skills. Furthermore, within the first 3 months, there were impressive differences in the proportion of subjects who had made earnest attempts to modify one or more life-style behavior. At 12 months postintervention, these differences seemed to diminish. This study failed to show any influence on the utilization of health or medical care services or on self-reported health status (including measures of functional health). The authors reported that they had few expectations of measurable health status effects from this study due to the short time horizon of the study and the voluntary nature of the study, which would have attracted a "healthier" population as participants. Although disappointed that the intervention did not affect the number of physician visits, the authors reasoned that acute care visits may not respond as well to this type of analysis, because physician-directed visits for chronic health conditions seem to be the more common type of visit among the study population. The intervention did not attempt to enlist physicians to reinforce these utilization objectives of the project.

The Dartmouth curriculum has become the basis for a separate, nationwide educational program for senior citizens, Health Promotion for Older Americans (HPOA), sponsored by the American Red Cross and the American Association of Retired Persons in conjunction with the Dartmouth Institute for Better Health. The central focus of this program is a curriculum titled Staying Healthy After Fifty (SHAF), a course consisting of 11 two-hour sessions. During a two-year period (from 1986 to 1988), 146 separate SHAF courses were offered to more than 2,500 older adult participants in some 70 communities in 24 states and the District of Columbia. The overall rate of completing the course was 85%.

Evaluation data pertinent to the SHAF curriculum were collected in a panel of 13 communities. According to the evaluation report (Simmons et al., 1988):

A typical course participant was a 66-year-old with a high school education. Two-thirds of the course participants were under a physician's care for a chronic problem and over one-third were limited by a health problem.

To assess the benefits derived by program participants, the evaluation identified close friends and associates of the participants who served as a "comparison group" for evaluation purposes. The evaluation did not try to measure the effect of the SHAF curriculum on the health status of participants. However, evaluation data did point to consistent differences between participants and their controls with regard to perceived levels of health skills, health actions, and health behaviors. Apparently, this program's use of personal Self-Change Plans (a form of behavioral contract) had a measurable impact upon life-style-related behaviors and attitudes.

Vickery, Golaszewski, Wright, and Kalmer (1988) reported on the implementation of a "communication-based health education strategy" among the members of an HMO population who were eligible for Medicare. This intervention, using the second edition of Vickery and Fries's well-known self-care reference book (Vickery & Fries, 1981) and other printed materials, including a set of four newsletters on self-care topics, was evaluated using a randomized design. Approximately 1,000 Medicare-enrolled families participated.

This study demonstrated a statistically significant decline of 15% in the total number of medical visits by experimental group members and families at 12 months, along with a corresponding savings of $36.65 per household (Vickery et al., 1988). These results underscore the potential for similar changes in overall health care utilization experience among an elderly population through a self-care intervention. To be sure, selection bias questions may be raised about such a finding in a middle-class, well-educated HMO population, even when experimental and control groups were randomly assigned. Yet these findings lead us to conclude that self-care education can influence overall health care utilization behavior without any demonstrable impact on the level of health of those targeted by these interventions.

Other findings from the self-care literature indicate that medical self-care skills are routinely performed for the less serious conditions and that such care and treatment is both appropriate and effective. The studies conducted in Denmark by Dean (1981), in the United Kingdom by Dunnell and Cartwright (1972), and in the United States by Demers and associates (1980) indicated that, by professional standards, most laypersons both effectively and appropriately practice self-care for specific illness conditions. Moore, LoGerfo, and Inui (1980) reported that, in their randomized study of the self-care behavior of families exposed to a self-care instructional program, many families tended not to use the self-care materials as they were instructed if their own experience or inclination ran counter to professional recommendations. Yet the authors could find no evidence that quality or appropriateness of care were sacrificed through this pattern of use of the self-care materials provided in the course. Moreover, in the study by Vickery and associates (1983) discussed above, the "appropriateness" of minor illness visits was significantly better in the experimental groups, which received self-care material, than in the control groups, which did not. This finding supports the view that laypersons can be trained to perform self-care skills in a manner consistent with professional standards for health care.

The self-care literature reveals the importance of examining the severity of symptoms in drawing conclusions about the efficacy of self-care programs. In another study of the relationship between self-care practices and the use of formal medical care, Fleming, Giachello, Andersen, and Andrade (1984) examined the extent to which persons surveyed in a nationwide study of access to medical care in 1975-1976, and who had experienced a relatively severe episode of illness during the previous 12-month period, practiced either of two forms of self-care (the use of nonprescription drugs or the use of lay consultation). Nearly one third of this national sample had experienced some kind of serious illness during the previous year. There were no significant differences between the proportion of elderly (i.e., those over 65 years of age) who practiced self-care activities versus those less than 65 years of age. Using physician office visits and days in hospital as outcome variables, it appears that those who practice some form of self-care tend to use fewer formal medical care services, a finding that seems to indicate that self-care practice tends to substitute for formal medical care. The domains of formal medical care use and self-care appear to be interdependent: as one increases, the other decreases. These researchers were unable to determine whether self-care practitioners were more or less likely than laypersons who do not practice self-care to use formal health care services "appropriately."

These studies of the impact of self-care educational programs on health services utilization and costs of conventional formal health care have given only mixed support to the notion that a program to educate patients in routine care of common illness conditions can have a cost-reducing effect on the aggregate pattern of formal health care in a defined population. Hence, we cannot clearly determine whether and to what extent self-care practices do in fact substitute for formal health services, for the population in general or for older adults in particular. It does appear that most people tend to use their self-care knowledge and their own resources first, before seeking formal medical care, and, when they resort to self-care, they exercise these skills and judgments appropriately.

FORMAL CARE: SUPPLEMENT TO OR SUBSTITUTE FOR INFORMAL CARE?

While it is important to know whether it is possible through informal/self-care to substitute for the usually more expensive, though not necessarily more appropriate or effective, formal medical care, substitution in the opposite direction is of equal significance. In many instances, formal health and social care programs have been created to meet the needs of a particular population and, in some cases, have substituted for (or replaced) the care and services formerly provided by lay or informal care sources such as families and friends. The best example of this sort of program is the emergence of "home health care" as an administrative label for a type of formal service provided by organizations offering selected types of personal and health care services for those unable to perform these services for themselves (Koren, 1986). It is the intention of such programs not to completely replace currently available informal care arrangements but to add to these in some specific way. While most families and other informal care providers do not withdraw their informal care when these new services become available, it is likely (as in the case of respite care services) that the periodicity or intensity of informal care will change.

Because the number of levels and types of health, social, and personal care needed and available through a variety of public and private agencies have increased dramatically in recent years, the concept of yet another type of administrative control has been introduced. This is the concept of "case management," or the formal role of arranging for the most efficient, appropriate, and effective combination of services and providers for a given client/patient eligible for services under a given insurance or entitlement program. Where individual needs are less than comprehensive, efficiencies and quality of care presumably can be provided only when services are coordinated and access is managed by a third (or fourth) party, the case manager. The role and effectiveness of the case manager is of considerable importance for public policy. The analysis of the effectiveness of case management and home health care services is complicated by the fact that the policy objectives of these programs are not always clear. While some would see their intent and purpose as that of filling gaps in the total spectrum of services available to patients/clients, others would view their purpose as providing substitutable "respite" services intended to relieve overburdened informal caregivers. If one takes the former view, it is important that the process through which access is assured to a multiplicity of community-based and home-based services does not diminish either the availability or the provision of informal care for the frail elderly. If one takes the latter (respite) view, the fact of substitution of formal care for informal care is an indication of the success of the program.

Soldo and Agree (1989) reviewed the literature on the substitutability of formal for informal care among the frail elderly and found "no study indicates that the frail elderly, as a group, receive the bulk of their personal care from formal caregivers." Most care needs of the elderly, particularly the frail elderly, are now and always have been met by informal care providers. Yet the existing studies of these phenomena differ considerably in the way in which both the frailty of the elderly and the formality of care requirements are defined, thus making comparisons among study results difficult. Soldo and Manton (1985) have estimated, using data from the National Long Term Care Survey, that 25% of those persons between the ages of 75 and 84 living in the community are dependent on others with respect to basic activities of daily living. Some studies, such as the work of Branch and Jette (1983), for example, found that two out of every five (or 40%) of the very old frail population are totally dependent on formal health care services. Other studies found a similar need for formal health care services among populations of disabled older adults. Three nationally representative studies (Liu, Manton, Liu, 1985; Soldo, 1985; Stone, 1986) provide evidence that as many as one quarter of all noninstitutionalized elderly who are physically disabled use some type of "formal" personal or health care services (Soldo & Agree, 1989). But most of those who are able to sustain a viable independent living arrangement outside a nursing home have only moderate levels of disability and need for formal health care services. Only about 5% to 10% of the frail elderly are estimated to be completely dependent on formal health and personal care service providers (Liu et al., 1985; Soldo, 1985). For the most part, it appears that formal care services provided in noninstitutional settings are used in conjunction with a variety of types of informal care. It is the "mixture" of the formal and informal care services in what Soldo and Agree (1989) call a "mixed helper network" that defines the model most noninstitutionalized elderly follow when they need personal or health care services that are less than comprehensive.

The issue of the substitutability of formal for informal care is one of several addressed in the National Long Term Care (Channeling) Demonstration (Christianson, 1988). Before the Channeling Demonstration, there had been very little empirical evidence of a substitution effect in public programs for the elderly. Christianson (1988) reviewed only four previous studies known to the Channeling Demonstration research team. One of these studies, by Lewis and associates (1980), found that informal caregivers tend to specialize in the provision of certain types of services and that a diminution of these services depends on which types of services are picked up by more formal programs rather than on a generalized substitution effect. Greene (1983), in a study of 124 persons served by a comprehensive case management program, found some substitution effects: In response to the provision of formal care of a single type, informal caregivers withdrew from 1.35 caregiving areas. In a third study reviewed by Christianson (1988), Talbott, Smith, and Miller (1982) found that informal care decreased by 1.2% when formal services in California's Multipurpose Senior Services Project (MSSP) increased by 10%. With so little previous research in this direction, but using results that did exist, the Channeling Demonstration undertook an examination of the substitution phenomenon.

In 1980, the Channeling project implemented, at 10 sites across the country, a comprehensive case management intervention for frail elderly needing some form of long-term care. In each of the project sites, eligible persons were randomly assigned to either the treatment or a control group. Five of the ten projects provided what was called a "basic case management model" in which clients were assisted in gaining access to needed services already existing in their communities; these projects involved efforts to coordinate access to a range of services available from multiple providers. The remaining five projects also provided case management services but provided an additional, expanded set of services that did not previously exist in these communities. This approach, called the "financial control model," attempted to allocate services and access to resources on the basis of need rather than strictly on the basis of the eligibility requirements of specific programs. The intent of both models was to enable elderly persons to remain in their own homes rather than enter nursing homes or other long-term care facilities. A major concern of this federally funded demonstration was the examination of the extent to which formal, community-based services tended to be used instead of informal care services previously provided by families and friends, thus increasing the outlay of public funds as a substitute for services previously provided at no expense to public agencies.

It is important to note that one of the primary purposes of any community-based formal program of social and health services is to partially relieve those informal caregivers who are currently providing services that enable the elderly client to maintain his or her independent living status. The objective of these services is, to a great extent, to assist the caregivers in being able to continue to provide whatever informal care they now provide for an even longer period of time than might otherwise be the case.

To investigate the impact of the Channeling Demonstration on informal caregiving, elderly persons were interviewed at 6, 12, and 18 months after entry into the demonstration. In addition, their principal caregivers were interviewed at 6 and 12 months after the sample members entered the demonstration.

The data from the Channeling Demonstration did not demonstrate a substitution of formal for informal care in the base case management model, even in areas where increases in formal care services were substantial (e.g., meal preparation, housework, laundry chores, and/or shopping). Only modest substitution effects were observed in the financial control model, and these were very small. For instance, the proportion of clients receiving in-home care increased 21.8%, while the proportion receiving any form of informal care decreased 4.2%. More important, the Channeling project found that these reductions in informal caregiving did not occur for so-called primary caregivers but were mainly associated with the informal care received from friends and neighbors. In fact, the results tended to suggest that the total amount of community caregiving available to these frail elderly actually increased when the services received from both formal and informal caregivers were combined. These findings seem to indicate that the commitment of primary caregivers is relatively high and remains so even when formal care services become available.

The Channeling Demonstration project was of relatively short duration, and case managers seemed to work aggressively to keep informal caregivers highly involved in the overall care planning process. Hence, the extent to which the substitution of formal for informal caregiving might actually have occurred under other circumstances is not entirely clear from this demonstration. It does appear, however, that there is some substitution and that its extent could be manipulated through strategic policy.

These findings are consistent with the review of these issues by Tennstedt and McKinlay (1989), who concluded that

> available data provide no evidence to suggest that families have, or will, withdraw their help in favor of public services. Contrary to assumptions, even when greater needs necessitate more help, informal caregivers provide greater amounts of assistance when compared to utilization of formal services. And in those areas of help where one might expect some shift toward formal services because services are well established and readily available (e.g., personal care, housekeeping, meals), the data reveal larger amounts of informal help associated with larger amounts of formal services, again with the former exceeding the latter. It is *not* the case that informal care complements, or is ancillary to, formal services. Rather, formal services complement, or are ancillary to, a well-established, pervasive and continuing informal system of care.

In a study of 737 elderly patients discharged from Chicago-area hospitals, Jones, Densen, and Brown (1989) found that 60% were assessed as needing help with personal care or housekeeping services upon leaving the hospital, yet fewer than 20% were informed about the existence and mode of access to these services. Although family-provided informal care had always been the mainstay of these elderly persons in meeting their ADL needs, immediately after hospital discharge, there had been an increase in paid (i.e., formal) services use. Likewise, those with ADL dependencies added to the overall family financial burden. In this study, the period of hospitalization tended to rapidly increase the dependence of families on outside formal care for their older adult members. Eight months after discharge, there was a clear trend in the direction of a higher level of formal care dependency, and the trend was even more dramatic for those with ADL dependencies upon discharge from the hospital.

The other major study that has investigated the substitution effect is the National Hospice Study. This project investigated the quality and costs of care for terminally ill cancer patients in three different types of care settings: conventional hospital care, institutional hospice care, and home-based hospice care. One component of this study was an economic investigation of the labor market effects of the caregiving process in each of these three modes of hospice care

(Muurinen, 1986). Caregivers in the home-based care mode were far less likely to have been employed at the outset of the caregiving episode; hence, the choice of that mode of care was probably more feasible from the outset. For caregivers who were employed at the outset of the caregiving episode, the costs of the informal care intensive home-based hospice were too high, making this mode initially infeasible. Given the fact that the daily informal care hours required were 4.8 hours for conventional care, 5.1 hours for institutional hospice, and 10.2 hours for home-based hospice, it is clear that this latter mode is incompatible with full labor market participation by principal caregivers.

Muurinen's (1986) analysis of the labor market effects of hospice care indicates that most informal caregivers in all three modes of hospice experienced some loss of earnings during the episode of caregiving. More than one fourth of those caregivers who were initially employed eventually left the labor force as caregiving obligations increased. Older caregivers and women were more likely to leave the labor force. Muurinen concluded that some of the substantial cost savings of home-centered hospice care must be attributed to the shifting of costs from the formal health care sector to the informal care sector; in this sense, they should not be treated as real cost savings. These findings provide yet another illustration of the importance of including a consideration of the volume and variety of informal care in any assessment of access to personal health care services generally.

The studies reviewed thus far reflect the tendency to view formal and informal care as alternatives (or countervailing forces) to one another. However, the evidence seems to suggest that this view is inadequate for several reasons. First, a complementarity model is more appropriate than one that emphasizes substitutability. Second, informal care is of value in association with formal care throughout the illness experience; informal care is not limited in its relevance to the initial appearance of symptoms (Furstenberg & Davis, 1984). Moreover, it is inadequate to view informal care (or self-care) as a strategy for cost savings with respect to more formal health care services. Where costs have been reduced, they have often simply been shifted to individuals and families who provide services without compensation. Self-care instructional programs have tended to make consumers more sophisticated, but not necessarily less frequent, users of formal health care services. As a strategy for cost savings, self-care instruction may be a hope with little supporting evidence (Coppard, Riley, Macfayden, & Dean, 1984).

It is also clear that within the lay (or informal care) circle are those with more and less expertise and, therefore, greater and lesser capacity for the practice of effective informal health care. There seem to be levels of informal health care specialization, with some laypersons able or willing to practice only certain kinds of self-care skills. Furthermore, certain elements of formal health care depend totally on the interactive reinforcement of informal care processes. For example, it is often the case that long-term, significant modifications in diet, exercise regimen, or other aspects of personal health habits are necessary to manage chronic health conditions effectively. Maintenance of these changes often depends on the support and encouragement of close friends and family. These informal support systems become crucial in getting patients to comply with the recommendations of formal medical care (Furstenberg & Davis, 1984; Ory & Williams, 1989). Among the chronically ill, when "everything medically possible" has been done, the individual is often essentially ignored by formal health care providers. Under such circumstances, a significant decline in functional status is possible unless special effort is made to offset the limitations of the chronic condition. While formal health care tends to focus on abnormality and the deficits associated with physiological or psychological pathology, informal care tends to give emphasis to those processes of human growth and development that act to "normalize" the individual and enable the person to deal with everyday challenges of personal and social life. Then the processes and programs that emphasize informal caregiving can and do have an enhancing effect when combined with formal health care and caregiving services (Coppard et al., 1984).

INFORMAL CARE SYSTEMS AND THE MAINTENANCE OF OPTIMAL FUNCTIONING OF THE ELDERLY

It is both disappointing and surprising that there is so little evidence to substantiate the claim that informal care services and social support have actually aided or improved the functional health status of older Americans. Moreover, there is little evidence to address the value of formal personal care services or case management services on functional health status. What evidence there is with regard to formalized personal care services, such as data from the National Channeling project (Applebaum, Christianson, Harrigan, & Schore, 1988; Kane & Kane, 1987), tend to show that organized case management services do not improve functional health status indicators. In their review of the extant literature on informal care for frail older persons, Tennstedt and McKinlay (1989) pointed out that research on the impact of caregiving has tended to focus almost exclusively on the costs of such care and to almost entirely neglect the benefits. Hence, their own review did not mention a single study as having focused on the health outcomes of informal caregiving. All the studies reviewed focused on the burden of care to the caregiver.

It is true that those older adults with the most severe physical functional limitations tend to be those who receive the largest volume of personal and health care services from both informal and formal caregivers (Branch & Jette, 1983; Tennstedt & McKinlay, 1989). But data do not seem to be available to support the claim that the volume of caregiving available can maintain and/or significantly enhance an individual's functional health status. Despite the lack of data supporting these claims, this remains an important area for further research.

Designing studies to understand the impact of the volume and type of care on patient/client health status is problematic. Manipulation of the supply of care to selected groups of patients, particularly where the effects of the level of disability or functional limitations are controlled, would present considerable ethical problems. There are probably important reasons why studies that would attempt to understand the impact of the volume and type of care on patient/client health status cannot be designed. In addition, there are significant measurement problems associated with the study of self-care behavior and the assessment of the impact of informal care. Given the importance of these issues, the methodological problems associated with this kind of research and policy analysis need further attention.

THE POTENTIAL FOR THE EFFECTIVE INTEGRATION OF FORMAL AND INFORMAL LEVELS OF CARE

There can be little doubt that the phenomena of self-care and informal care represent a fundamentally important segment of the spectrum of health care services available to meet the health care needs of elderly people (Olesen, 1989). Any national health policy that does not give full recognition to this category or level of care will provide only a partial view of the national burden of illness and caregiving responsibilities. But what does "appropriate recognition" really mean? Does it require something more than financial compensation (through direct payments or tax credits) for caregivers?

There are problems, of course, in properly taking into account any consideration of informal care in the allocation of health resources to the care of any population. For one thing, the available volume, let alone the economic value, of these services cannot be easily estimated. Most discussions of caregiver burden tend to focus on the need (and cost) of respite services. It is significant to note that, when asked, most caregivers express a preference for direct relief services instead of monetary compensation for the role they play in caregiving (Horowitz & Shindelman, 1983; Tennstedt & McKinlay, 1989). As we have seen in the review of available research in this chapter, the provision of formal, direct services has a tendency to *reduce* or *substitute for* informal caregiving that might have been taking place before the initiation of formal care arrangements. But the substitution effect seems to be specific to particular types of care, not to caregiving in general. In fact, substitution can have the effect of increasing the overall volume and impact of care. The provision of formal care services can have the effect of allowing informal caregivers to devote their limited energies to the more specialized areas of care that they would prefer or for which they feel most capable (Christianson, 1988; Greene, 1983).

The substitution effect can have two quite different interpretations: On the one hand, it can be seen as a positive indication that formal care services have indeed provided relief to those who are overburdened with caregiver responsibilities; on the other hand, it can be seen as an indication that those with an absolute deficit of care are now better served than before. The interpretation of such findings requires the articulation of a comprehensive social policy related to health and social care for those unable to care for themselves. Evaluation of the impact of such programs must include a consideration of both the costs and the benefits (or outcomes) of care as well as an understanding of the way in which substitution occurs.

Another dimension of the informal-formal care relationship, which we have not explored to any great extent in this chapter, is the potential contribution that informal care or self-care can make to the overall effectiveness of formal medical care. There can be little doubt that the central ideas embodied in the U.S. self-care movement have widespread acceptance within clinical medicine and nursing. Well-organized educational programs for a host of health conditions and diseases are designed to teach patients, as well as their families, to master not only the facts associated with their conditions or limitations but also relevant strategies for prevention, treatment, and management. With the rapid trend toward converting patterns of care from inpatient services to ambulatory care settings, one can expect that self-care strategies will gain increasing acceptance. We are now seeing the emergence of special inpatient units in hospitals called "cooperative care units," where patients are admitted along with an accompanying significant other who agrees to assume partial responsibility for the patient's care during the hospitalization.

Even though these special arrangements for the horizontal linkage of formal and informal care providers in so-called mixed helper networks have received increasing acceptance, there is room for considerably more attention to the role and importance of informal care (and self-care) in the educational preparation of health care professionals. If self-care/other-care skills are to be considered an essential component of the broad spectrum of health care, then surely these essential skills (on the part of laypersons) need to be taught, maintained, and updated periodically. Just as the half-life of all medical science is becoming shorter, so it is with the more technical aspects of lay self-care as well. Curricular development relevant to certain types of informal care/self-care services needs to move beyond simple algorithms pertinent to symptom recognition and triage to other levels of (formal or informal) care. There is a need to disseminate and update information addressing the latest and most practical approaches to the care of persons who are dependent on one or more help/health services to maintain their noninstitutionalized functional status.

Most of these innovations, including experimentation with various forms of case management, are being undertaken with the primary purpose of reducing the cost of providing expensive formal health care services. Few of these experiments have been able to show significant effects of these innovations on the functional health status or well-being of the elderly for whom they were designed. Yet the very fact that such a large (and increasing number) of our elderly will find a need for and benefit from a combination of informal and formal care underscores the need for a better understanding of these services and the conventional patterns of their use. The overall finding that most of these formal programs have not led to measurable improvements in physical and mental health status for elderly or disabled participants should not obscure the potential (and, as yet, largely unexplored) psychosocial benefits derived in the form of life satisfaction, uplifted morale, maintenance of social interaction, and decreased need for some forms of informal caregiving that might otherwise exist. The pervasiveness of informal caregiving for our frail and dependent elderly is an important indication of the basic positive qualities of our society in its modern era.

REFERENCES

Applebaum, R. A., Christianson, J. B., Harrigan, M., & Schore, J. (1988). The evaluation of the national long term care demonstration: 9. The effect of channeling on mortality, functioning, and well-being. *Health Services Research, 23*(1), 143-159.

Berg, A. O., & LoGerfo, J. P. (1979). Potential effects of self-care algorithms on the number of physician visits. *The New England Journal of Medicine, 300*(10), 535-537.

Branch, L. G., & Jette, A. M. (1983). Elders' use of informal long-term care assistance. *The Gerontologist, 23*(1), 51-56.

Butler, R. N. (1975). *Why survive? Being old in America.* New York: Harper & Row.

Butler, R. N. (1982). The triumph of age: Science, gerontology and ageism. *Bulletin of the New York Academy of Medicine, 58*(4), 347-361.

Christianson, J. B. (1988). The evaluation of the National Long Term Care Demonstration: 6. The effect of channeling on informal caregiving. *Health Services Research, 23*(1), 99-117.

Coppard, L. C., Riley, M. W., Macfayden, D. M., & Dean, K. (1984). *Self health care and older people: A manual for public policy and programme development.* Geneva: World Health Organization.

Dean, K. (1981). Self-care responses to illness: A selected review. *Social Science and Medicine, 15A,* 673-687.

DeFriese, G. H., Woomert, A., Guild, P. A., Steckler, A. B., & Konrad, T. R. (1989). From activated patient to pacified activist: A study of the self-care movement in the United States. *Social Science and Medicine, 29*(2), 195-204.

Demers, R. Y., Altmore, R., Mustin, H., Lleinman, A., & Leonardi, D. (1980). An exploration of the dimensions of illness behavior. *Journal of Family Practice, 11*(7), 1085-1092.

Dono, J. E., Falbe, C. M., Kail, B. L., Litwak, E. Sherman, R. H., & Siegel, D. (1979). Primary Groups in Old Age: Structure and Function. *Research on Aging, 1,* 403-433.

Doty, P. (1986). Family care of the elderly: The role of public policy. *Milbank Memorial Fund Quarterly, 64,* 34-75.

Dunnell, K., & Cartwright, A. (1972). *Medicine takers, prescribers and hoarders.* London: Routledge and Kegan Paul.

Fleming, G. V., Giachello, A. L., Andersen, R. M., & Andrade, P. (1984). Self-care: Substitute, supplement, or stimulus for formal medical care services? *Medical Care, 22*(10), 950-966.

Fries, J. F. (1980). Aging, natural death, and the compression of morbidity. *The New England Journal of Medicine, 303*(3), 130-135.

Furstenberg, A. L., & Davis, L. J. (1984). Lay consultation of older people. *Social Science and Medicine, 18*(10), 827-837.

Greene, V. L. (1983). Substitution between formally and informally provided care for the impaired elderly in the community. *Medical Care, 21*(6), 609-619.

Herrick, J. W. (1983). Interbehavioral perspectives on aging. *International Journal of Aging and Human Development, 16*, 95-123.

Horowitz, A., & Shindelman, L. (1983). Social and economic incentives for family caregivers. *Health Care Financing Review, 5*, 25-33.

Jones, E. W., Densen, P. M., & Brown, S. D. (1989, December). Post-hospital needs of elderly people at home: Findings from an eight-month follow-up study. *Health Services Research, 24*(5), 643-664.

Kane, R. A., & Kane, R. L. (1987). *Long-term care: Principles, programs and policies.* New York: Springer.

Kemper, D. W. (1982). Self-care education: Impact on HMO costs. *Medical Care, 20*(7), 710-718.

Kemper, D. W., Deneen, E. J., & Giuffre, J. V. (1984). *The growing younger handbook.* Boise, ID: Healthwise, Inc.

Kemper, D. W., Mettler, M., Giuffre, J., & Batzek, B. (1986). *Growing wiser: The older person's guide to mental wellness.* Boise, ID: Healthwise, Inc.

Koren, M. J. (1986). Home care: Who cares? *The New England Journal of Medicine, 314*(14), 917-920.

Lewis, M. S., et al. (1980, November 24). *The extent to which informal and formal supports interact to maintain the older people in the community.* Paper presented at the 33rd Annual Meeting of the Gerontological Society of America, San Diego, CA.

Liu, K., Manton, K. G., & Liu, B. M. (1985). Home care expenses for the disabled elderly. *Health Care Financing Review, 7*, 51-58.

Lorig, K., Kraines, R. G., Brown, B. W., Jr., & Richardson, N. (1985). A workplace health education program that reduces outpatient visits. *Medical Care, 23*(9), 1044-1054.

Manton, K. G. (1982). Changing concepts of morbidity and mortality in the elderly population. *Milbank Memorial Fund Quarterly, 60*, 183-244.

Moore, S. H., LoGerfo, J. P., & Inui, T. S. (1980). Effect of a self-care book on physician visits. *Journal of the American Medical Association, 243*, 2317.

Muurinen, J. M. (1986). The economics of informal care: Labor market effects in the national hospice study. *Medical Care, 24*(11), 1007-1017.

Nelson, E. C., McHugo, G., Schnurr, P., Devito, C., Roberts, E., Simmons, J., & Zubkoff, W. (1984). Medical self-care education for elders: A controlled trial to evaluate impact. *American Journal of Public Health, 74*(12), 1357-1362.

Olesen, V. L. (1989). Caregiving, ethical and informal: Emerging challenges in the sociology of health and illness. *Journal of Health and Social Behavior, 30*, 1-10.

Ory, M. G. (1989). Considerations in the development of age-sensitive indicators for assessing health promotion. *Health Promotion: An International Journal, 3*(2), 139-150.

Ory, M. G., & Bond, K. (1989). *Health care for an aging society.* In M. G. Ory & K. Bond (Eds.), *Aging and health care: Social science and policy perspectives* (pp. 1-24). London: Routledge.

Ory, M. G., & Williams, T. F. (1989). Rehabilitation: Small goals, sustained interven-tions. *The Annals of the American Academy of Political and Social Science, 503,* 61-76.

Riley, M. W., & Bond, K. (1983). Beyond ageism: Postponing the onset of disability. In M. W. Riley, B. B. Hess, & K. Bond (Eds.), *Aging in society: Selected reviews of recent research* (pp. 243-252). Hillsdale, NJ: Lawrence Erlbaum.

Roberts, T. M., Tinker, K. M., & Kemper, D. W. (1978). *The healthwise handbook.* Boise, ID: Healthwise, Inc.

Schneider, E. I., & Brody, J. A. (1983). Aging, natural death and the compression of morbidity. *The New England Journal of Medicine, 303,* 854-855.

Shanas, E. (1979). The family as a social support system in old age. *The Gerontologist, 19*(2), 169-174.

Simmons, J. J., Nelson, E. C., Benson, L., Roberts, E., Keller, A., Kane-Williams, E., & Salisbury, Z. T. (1988). *Health promotion for older Americans final report.* Hanover, NH: Dartmouth Institute for Better Health.

Soldo, B. J. (1985). In-home services for the dependent elderly: Determinants of current uses and implications for future demand. *Research on Aging, 7,* 281-304.

Soldo, B. J., & Agree, E. M. (1989). The balance between formal and informal care. In M. G. Ory & K. Bond (Eds.), *Aging and health care: Social science and policy perspectives.* New York: Rutledge.

Soldo, B. J., & Manton, K. G. (1985). Health status and service needs of the oldest old: New perspectives and future trends. *Milbank Memorial Fund Quarterly, 63,* 286-319.

Stone, R. (1986). *Aging in the eighties, age 65 and over: Use of community services* (Advance Data No. 124). Hyattsville, MD: National Center for Health Statis-tics.

Talbott, M., Smith, S. A., & Miller, L. (1982, July 30). *Informal instrumental support: Two samples of California's frail, low-income elderly.* Berkeley: University of California, Multipurpose Senior Services Project Evaluation.

Tennstedt, S. L., & McKinlay, J. B. (1989). Informal care for frail older persons. In M. G. Ory & K. Bond (Eds.), *Aging and health care: Social science and policy perspectives.* London: Routledge.

Townsend, P., & Wedderburn, D. (1965). *The aged in the welfare state.* London: Bell and Sons.

Verbrugge, L. M. (1989). Recent, present and future health of American adults. In J. E. Breslow, J. E. Fielding, & L. B. Lave (Eds.), *Annual review of public health* (Vol. 10). Palo Alto, CA: Annual Reviews.

Vickery, D. M., & Fries, J. F. (1976). *Take care of yourself: A consumer's guide to medical care.* Reading, MA: Addison-Wesley.

Vickery, D. M., & Fries, J. F. (1981). *Take care of yourself: A consumer's guide to medical care* (rev. ed.). Reading, MA: Addison-Wesley.

Vickery, D. M., Fries, J. F., & Pantell, R. H. (1977). *Taking care of your child.* Reading, MA: Addison-Wesley.

Vickery, D. M., Golaszewski, T. J., Wright, E. C., & Kalmer, H. (1988). The effect of self-care interventions on the use of medical service within a medicare popu-lation. *Medical Care, 26*(6), 580-588.

Vickery, D. M., Kalmer, H., Lowry, D., et al. (1983). Effect of a self-care education program on medical visits. *Journal of the American Medical Association, 250,* 2952-2956.

Williamson, J. D., & Danaher, K. (1978). *Self-care in health.* London: Croom Helm.

World Health Organization. (1983). *Report of working group on self-care education in health.* Geneva: Author.

4

The Behavior System of Dependency in the Elderly: Interaction with the Social Environment

MARGRET M. BALTES
HANS-WERNER WAHL

The image of long-term care institutions and/or of the elderly person living in an institution is overwhelmingly negative. Goffman's (1961) description of the "total" institution as one in which all of one's physical, social, and psychological needs are provided for under the same roof by the same persons without regard to individual differences has had an overpowering and lasting effect. If one were to describe the negative image of institutions with one concept, "loss of autonomy" would most likely come to mind.

This view has found strong support in research that has documented the negative effects of relocation of the elderly, particularly the move from one's own home to an institution. The increased risks in mortality, health, and well-being have been summarized and discussed extensively (Borup, 1983; Horowitz & Schulz, 1983; Schulz & Brenner, 1977), and ways to alleviate the negative consequences, including preparation and involvement in decision making or in the selection process, have been recommended (i.e., Schulz & Hanusa, 1979, 1980).

AUTHORS' NOTE: The research reported in this chapter was supported by grants from the U.S. Department of Health, Education, and Welfare, the Division of Nursing Research (R02-NU-00578), and from the Volkswagen Foundation awarded to the first author. During the writing of this chapter, Hans-Werner Wahl was research associate on the project "Dependence and Independence in the Elderly: The Role of the Social Environment" funded by the Stiftung Volkswagenwerk. The chapter was completed during the sabbatical of the first author supported by a stipend from the Stiftung Volkswagenwerk.

There is no doubt that long-term care institutions are rarely an avenue back to society. Only a very small minority of old long-term care residents ever return to the community. In fact, an extensive body of literature documents the pervasiveness of social, psychological, and physical impairments among the elderly in institutions (National Center for Health Statistics, 1987; Parmelee, Katz, & Lawton, 1989).

Several explanations have been advanced to account for the origins and consequences of loss of autonomy in the aged person. One of the best known ones, the model of "learned helplessness" espoused by Martin Seligman (1975; Abramson, Seligman, & Teasdale, 1978), has been adopted by a number of psychological gerontologists as a possible mechanism not only describing but also explaining the negative consequences of institutionalization, including loss of control, passivity, dependence, and depression. The tacit assumption that losing control, or a lack of control, means being unhappy and at risk for ill health seems to be supported more and more by research pointing to a strong relationship between control, independence, and health and, conversely, between loss of control, dependence, and illness (Rodin, 1986; Rodin, Timko, & Harris, 1985; see also the chapter in this volume by Rodin & Timko). These authors argued that processes mediating between experience of control and health outcomes can take at least two avenues: a behavioral-cognitive and a biological pathway.

Our own work offers a different explanation, challenging the model of "learned helplessness" (see also Baltes & Wahl, 1987). This chapter will provide an in-depth view of the role of the social environment in institutions in shaping dependent behaviors in the elderly. We draw attention to a highly complementary interaction pattern between the elderly residents and staff called the "dependency-support script." Dependent behavior, while representing a loss in self-care performance, gives the elderly resident a strategy for controlling certain aspects of the social environment. Thus much of the dependence we see in institutions is not to be confused with helplessness or loss of control. We will argue that dependence followed by support in select areas of life might be a product of selection and compensation and thus a necessary prerequisite for successful aging.

Institutions or similar protective or prosthetic settings are needed not only to provide support in the case of failing vitality but also to provide the platform on which successful aging may take place despite ever greater losses in competencies. A prosthetic environment does not need to lead to overcare and learned helplessness; if it is designed so that choice, self-regulation, and self-directedness are not suffocated, successful aging will be possible.

THEORETICAL CONSIDERATIONS

Baltes (1987) argued that, in old age, because of increasing biological vulnerability, the environment may exert a particularly strong influence both in optimizing and in hindering behavioral outcomes. Kahana (1982) has previously linked biological vulnerability to the many disadvantages of the older years, including reduced income, impaired health, and loss of social roles. She argued that all of these losses reduce the options and choices available to the older person in maintaining or finding an environment that is in keeping with his or her preferences. Thus a fitting match between environmental characteristics and individual competence is particularly crucial in old age to maintain the status quo as well as to further development.

The view that behavior is the outcome of person-environment transactions or interactions is no longer an article of debate (Epstein, 1979, 1980; Magnusson & Endler, 1977; Mischel, 1968, 1979). Within gerontology, the awareness of the environment's influence on the aging individual, and thus the beginnings of an ecological aging model, was initiated and fostered by empirical findings (Carp, 1987; Lawton, 1985; Moos & Lemke, 1985; Parmelee & Lawton, 1990). Data on the effects of housing (Howell 1980; Lawton, 1980; Parmelee & Lawton, 1990), of relocation (Borup, 1981; Horowitz & Schulz, 1983; Schulz & Brenner, 1977), of institutionalization (Baltes, Wahl, & Reichert, in press; Langer & Rodin, 1976; Lieberman, 1969; Pincus, 1968; Rodin & Langer, 1977; Schulz, 1976), and of neighborhood (Regnier, 1981) have made the importance of environment in aging only too obvious. These authors have identified issues related to environmental homogeneity, privacy, proximity, totality, gratification of needs, choice, self-directedness, control, and autonomy as having special importance when defining optimal environmental features for the elderly.

Acknowledging the environment's influence on the individual does not in and of itself, however, create a basis for a unifying theory of person-environment relations. The numerous models of person-environment relations span the gamut from cognitively oriented theories (Bronfenbrenner, 1979; Wohlwill, 1973a, 1973b) to more behaviorally oriented models (Moos, 1976; Studer, 1973). Lawton,

Windley, and Byerts (1982) attempted to present the major theories of person-environment relations with special attention to gerontology.

Unresolved issues include the relative power of the two entities, person and environment (Altman & Rogoff, 1987; Parr, 1980), and the directionality of influence as well as reciprocity of the interaction between person and environment (Moos & Lemke, 1985). The debate whether interaction or transaction is the adequate concept to characterize person-environment interactions is ongoing (Parmelee & Lawton, 1990). Furthermore, there is disagreement as to the importance of the objective compared with the subjective environment. At issue is whether behavioral outcomes can be related primarily to objective environmental factors (e.g., Moos, 1976; Wohlwill, 1973a) or to subjective perceptions of such objective environmental factors (e.g., Thomae, 1970). To understand this intersection between person and environment, we cannot, however, analyze the environment by using the person's perception as the sole reference point. Such a subjective indicator for the assessment of environmental properties needs to be supplemented by objective indicators.

Cognitively Oriented Models:
Lawton's Competence-Press Model

Lawton's model of person-environment relations (e.g., Lawton, 1982) is based partly on Murray's "need/press" model (cited in Lawton, 1982) and on Helson's model of adaptation level (cited in Lawton, 1982). Lawton proposed a dynamic interaction between the person and environment, the behavioral outcome of which is determined by the "competence" of the person and the "demand characteristics" of the environment. Recently, Lawton (1989) has introduced the term *proactivity* to support the view that the elderly are not only passive recipients of environmental press and demands but can actively shape their context conditions.

In defining the environment, Lawton paid attention to both the purely external components and the interactional components. Lawton assumed, according to Helson's adaptation-level model, that there is a range of persons fitting one environment or, vice versa, a range of environments fitting one person. Thus a positive fit within a given range exists when person (competence) and environment (demands and opportunities) are in a state of equilibrium.

Most of the time, most people behave in ways that are compatible with or adaptive to the settings they occupy. This is not to say that everyone in the same situation behaves in the same way. It is only suggested that there is a fit between the person and the environment. This fit needs renegotiation when either the environment changes (relocation) or the person changes (illness, losses in motor skills, and so on). Thus loss in competencies (in biological health, sensory/perceptual capacity, motor skills, cognitive capacity, ego strength, and so on) or increase or decrease in environmental demand characteristics will disturb the existing adaptive level. Intervention or coping actions, self- or other-initiated, are necessary to avert negative affect and maladaptive behaviors. Intervention can be based upon therapeutic measures or prosthetic ones depending upon the irreversibility of the loss(es).

The fact that the equilibrium of person-environment relations is frequently disturbed in old age and often highly fragile does not imply that the disturbances are encountered in the same way or at the same time or are caused by the same factors and lead to the same consequences in all old people. Kahana (1982; see also Carp, 1987) elaborated the latter point in her person-environment fit model. She argued that, because of the great interindividual differences and great intraindividual changes in person-environment fit, the question cannot be only: "What is a person's optimum environment?" but "What is the optimum environment for which person at what point in time?"

Behaviorally Oriented Models of Person-Environment Relations

Another cluster of theories, rather than arguing for personality and cognitive processes determining the person-environment relationships, makes the assumptions that (a) each environment—whether physical, personal, or otherwise—may act as a stimulus, facilitating or hindering the occurrence of behaviors, and (b) each environment-person transaction may present a reinforcing or punishing contingency.[1] That is, each environment sets the stage for certain behaviors to occur and for other behaviors to be avoided. Furthermore, each behavior is followed by either supportive or nonsupportive reactions or is ignored. In a responsive environment, consequences are mostly either reinforcing or punishing. This is not to suggest that the person is a passive pawn or that only the person is acted on by the environment. The perspective of person-environment interactions as contingencies provides for a person's acting on the environment in changing environments or choosing those environments in which behaviors and behavioral goals are stimulated and reinforced.

Researchers such as Moos (1976), Patterson (1982), Studer (1973), Willems (1972), and the first author of this chapter (Baltes, 1982, 1988) belong in this theoretical tradition. The work of Barker (1968) and his concept of "behavior setting" plays an important role in the thinking of these scholars. Combining the concept of behavior setting with a social or operant learning framework makes it possible, however, to go beyond a mere classification of behaviors and environments (that is, beyond a behavior mapping strategy) by understanding behaviors and environments as contingencies. This conceptual approach makes it possible to answer questions such as the following: Why do predictable, regular, and different patterns of behavior occur in different settings? Why do people change their behaviors when they go from one setting to another? What mechanisms exist in settings to keep the behaviors of the occupants within the range acceptable to or desirable by "others" and congruent with the setting's physical features?

In our own work (for reviews, see Baltes, 1982, 1988; Baltes & Reisenzein, 1986; Baltes & Wahl, 1987), we have concentrated on the behavioral outcome of "dependence" and its social contingencies in the environment of long-term care institutions by asking the following questions: What aspects of the social environment foster dependence in the elderly resident of a long-term care institution? Do social consequences in institutions for the elderly support dependency or autonomy?

EMPIRICAL FINDINGS ON DEPENDENCE IN INSTITUTIONS USING A BEHAVIORALLY ORIENTED MODEL

Dependence and Its Social Contingencies in Long-Term Care Institutions

Dependence is often mentioned as a product of institutionalization and/or aging. How this effect is achieved, however, has not been identified or described in *behavioral* terms. Accordingly, the basic goal of our research program has been to identify and describe the *behavioral system of dependence* operating in the environment of the elderly. We have focused on the ways social environmental conditions in long-term care institutions may influence the elderly residents' dependent and independent behaviors (for a detailed discussion of the construct dependency, see Baltes & Wahl, 1987). A corollary issue in this context is that of setting specificity; in other words, are the observed behavioral patterns an effect of the institution, or is the chronological age of the inhabitants an essential factor in the dynamics of the interactions?

The main issue—namely, the identification of the extant environmental social contingencies and the determination of their relevance for the development and/or maintenance of dependent and independent behavior—was embedded within two additional target issues of the research program: One addresses the plasticity of behavior in the elderly; specifically, can dependent behaviors of the elderly be modified or reversed by manipulating social contingencies? The second issue relates to the functional validity of the temporal behavior sequences or interactions observed in real life.

These three issues were approached by three distinct research strategies provided by the operant model: the operant-experimental, operant-observational, and operant-ecological strategies (Baer, 1973; Baltes & Lerner, 1980). The operant-experimental research strategy was employed to clarify the issue of modifiability by examining changes in dependent behavior following changes in environmental conditions. To identify existing behavior-consequence relationships, we observed the flow of naturally occurring behavioral sequences (antecedent-consequent relationships) between the actors (elderly) and their social partners. Accordingly, comparative operant-observational studies have been conducted in a number of different settings involving actors of different ages and different social partners. Finally, the issue of functional validity of the temporal behavioral sequences was addressed by using an operant-ecological intervention strategy. Here, interventions into natural settings are designed—based on evidence from operant-experimental and operant-observational work—to change the behavior of either the actor or the social partners observed in the interactions. This latter issue is the main focus of a current research project (Baltes & Neumann, 1987).

Although this chapter focuses on the behavioral system effecting dependency in the elderly, it is essential to note the major findings related to the modifiability issue and the issue of functional validity. As to the modifiability of dependent behavior, operant-experimental work, including our studies as well as those by other operant researchers, has revealed substantial behavioral plasticity in the elderly (for reviews, see Baltes 1982, 1988; Baltes & Barton, 1977, 1979; Hoyer, 1974; Hussian, 1981; Mosher-Ashley, 1986-1987; Patterson &

Jackson, 1980, 1981; Wisocki, 1984). Findings strongly support the possibility that older people's behavior can be modified. The important role of both social and physical environmental factors in influencing the level of functioning of the elderly are underlined. Reversibility of dependent behaviors strengthens the notion that environmental conditions codetermine the acquisition and maintenance of dependency in institutionalized elderly.

The evidence of modifiability of even long-standing dependent behaviors negates the assumption that dependency is primarily the consequence of lack or loss of competence of the elderly, one of the two prerequisites for the model of learned helplessness. On the contrary, the elderly in many cases still display competencies and still possess the basic skills to perform the task at hand when given the opportunity, being prompted, or reinforced.

Additionally, evidence supports the functional validity of the temporal behavior patterns identified in institutions. A doctoral dissertation (Neumann, 1986) using an operant-ecological strategy provided a first indication that independence-supportive behaviors of staff can be effectively increased via a combined cognitive-behavioral training program. Furthermore, as the staff changed their behavior, a change in the behaviors of the elderly was produced; as predicted, more independent behaviors were exhibited. It seems evident, therefore, to interpret the temporal behavior sequences as functional contingencies.

The Ecology in Long-Term Care Institutions

For the identification and analysis of naturally existing social environmental consequences of dependence, we have focused mainly on elderly persons living in institutions. The selection of institutional environments was guided, aside from practical reasons and our interest in institutions per se, by the notion that such environments represent extreme conditions of the social ecology of aging in general. In this vein, we consider them as simulations (P. B. Baltes & Goulet, 1971) or research analogues for socialization into old age.

Technical information about the studies with institutionalized elderly. Six studies to date (Baltes, Burgess, & Stewart, 1980; Baltes, Honn, Barton, Orzech, & Lago, 1983; Baltes, Kindermann, & Reisenzein, 1986; Baltes, Kindermann, Reisenzein, & Schmid, 1987; Barton, Baltes, & Orzech, 1980; Lester & Baltes, 1978) have observed the behavioral and social world of the elderly in institutions. The target populations comprised persons over 65 who were neither completely bedfast nor

Table 4.1
Observation Coding Scheme

Input	Code	Category Name
Source of behavior	1	Target person (with others)
	2	Target Person (alone)
	3	Social partner
Actor identification	10-XX	Target person ID
	01	Staff
	02	Fellow resident
	03	Visitor
	04	Volunteer
	05	Group of social partners
Type of behavior		
Target person	00	Sleeping
	01	Constructively engaged
	04	Independent self-care
	05	Dependent self-care
Social partners	06	Engagement-supportive
	07	Nonengagement-supportive
	08	Independence-supportive
	09	Dependence-supportive
	10	No response
	11	Leaving
Dyadic form of behavior	1	Suggestion, commend, request
	2	Intention
	3	Compliance, cooperation
	4	Refusal, resistance
	5	Conversation
	6	Miscellaneous other

acutely ill but received either intermediate or skilled nursing care. The samples are thus representative of a large portion of the elderly population in long-term care institutions. A total of about 230 institutionalized elderly (summed across all studies) have been observed. The data were collected via an observational coding system using behavior categories based on the findings of a behavior mapping study (Baltes, Barton, et al., 1983). The behavior categories for both the target elderly and their social partners focused exclusively on overt and concrete acts related to everyday independence and dependence in the context of self-care and activities best described as leisure activities (see Table 4.1). Trained observers, using an electronic apparatus (Datamyte or Datapad), coded the flow of naturally occurring behavioral sequences during daily routines repeatedly over a time period of two to three weeks in each setting. Typical behavior sequences or interaction patterns were identified via Sackett's method of sequential lag analysis (Sackett, 1979; Sackett, Holm, Crowley, & Henkins, 1979).

Operant-observational findings with institutionalized elderly. All six studies, including the cross-cultural comparative studies (Baltes, Kindermann, & Reisenzein, 1986; Baltes et al., 1987), replicated the basic patterns of interaction. Comparing the social consequences of dependent versus independent self-care behaviors of elderly persons in long-term care institutions reveals two predominant differences: Dependent self-care behaviors are typically followed by social actions; independent self-care behaviors are not. More specifically, the sole complementary relationship between elderly residents and social partners is dependent self-care behavior followed by dependence-supportive behavior. The social environment responds to dependent self-care behaviors in a task-congruent manner. As to independent self-care, the dominant response of social partners is no response; although this may be adequate according to general social norms, it does not generate a social interaction sequence. Consequently, dependent behaviors in the context of self-care have the highest probability of being followed continuously and immediately by supportive acts from social partners. While the objective of the institutions in which the data were obtained was to "correct" dependency or at least to "maintain" independence as long as possible, in fact, the behavior of the staff tended to reward dependent behavior. There was a definite selection or preference of one pattern—a social script, so to speak— that treated dependent behavior as appropriate. Any weaknesses of the elderly, whether real or expected, were compensated for by the social partner (see Figure 4.1). We have, therefore, labeled this pattern the "dependency-support script."

It should be mentioned that there are other independent behaviors of the elderly resident, such as constructively engaged behaviors (e.g., writing a letter or playing a game with a fellow resident), that are also reinforced by social partners. Yet, compared with dependent self-care behaviors, such reinforcing responses are exhibited in an inconsistent and irregular manner. Such a response pattern can be interpreted as an intermittent reinforcement schedule. Although this schedule is recognized as a "strong" vehicle for the maintenance of behavior, in the environment of the institution, it is a schedule that fails to attract social contact in a reliable and immediate manner. The

Antecedent Behavior of
Elderly

Consequent Behavior

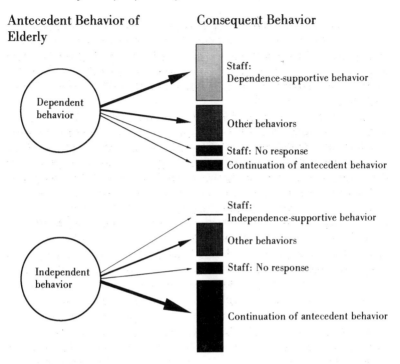

Figure 4.1. The Dependency-Support Script in Long-Term Care
Institutions

NOTE: Dependent behavior of the elderly is firmly associated with staff offering not only physical care but also the primary occasion for social attention and contact. Independent behavior, however, is ignored.

second category of dependent behaviors—namely, nonengaged behaviors, which are the object of frequent complaints by staff—seem to go unnoticed much as independent self-care behaviors do.

So far we have analyzed the question: What behavioral consequences follow behavioral acts of the elderly? A complete analysis of the behavioral system of dependence and independence requires also asking: What behavioral consequences follow behavioral acts of the social partners? The answer is simple: The behaviors of social partners prompt complementary behaviors from the elderly residents. Specifically, dependence-supportive behaviors of social partners are typically followed by dependent self-care behaviors of residents; independence-supportive behaviors, by independent self-care behaviors; engagement-supportive behaviors, by constructively engaged behaviors of residents; and so on. We can deduce that the elderly discriminate very well between the different behaviors of social partners and react "appropriately." Because the behavior sequences from social partners to residents express greater complementarity than the behavior sequences running from residents to social partners, the directionality of the interaction pattern is one-sided and seems to be determined by the social partner and not the resident.

This notion of unidirectionality is underscored when considering both the "control" and the "power" indices of the contingencies (Patterson, 1982). Patterson computed power indices in addition to control (as defined by the presence of contingency) indices to explain the variance of the contingency accounted for by the antecedent event. Thus a behavior A having significant control means it is consistently followed by behavior B; behavior A also having power over behavior B means the occurrence of behavior B is consistently preceded by the behavior A.

Our findings demonstrate that, in the case of the elderly, dependent self-care behaviors have the most control as well as power (Baltes & Reisenzein, 1986). This means that dependent behaviors are typically followed by dependence-supportive behaviors, and dependence-supportive behaviors are typically preceded by dependent behaviors. Constructively engaged behaviors exhibit more power than control; in other words, whereas engagement-supportive behaviors are typically preceded by engaged behaviors of the elderly, the latter often occur without being followed by engagement-supportive behaviors from social partners.

In sum, the least amount of social connectedness is associated with passive or nonengaged and independent self-care behaviors. The highest degree of social connectedness is affiliated with dependent self-care behavior and the second highest with independent constructively-engaged behavior. For the elderly, one behavior—dependent self-care behavior—seems to have the highest probability of securing immediate and reliable support, attention, or actions from social partners. Moreover, the dependent self-care situation represents the only truly reciprocal situation in the world of the institutionalized elderly. The meaning for the elderly appears to be this: If I want to have social contact, there is one sure way to get it, with respect to both the behavioral act (dependent behavior) and the situation (self-care).

These results are underscored by findings about the "dyadic form" of the interaction patterns between residents and social partners (see Table 4.1). Most of the behaviors of the elderly are expressed in the form of compliance or cooperation. In contrast, most of the behaviors of social partners take the form of a request/command/suggestion or cooperation. Rarely did we observe refusal or request on the part of the elderly. This additional information seems to support the notion of dominance and directionality running from the social partner to the elderly resident and not vice versa. The elderly seem to comply with what is requested or selected for by the social environment, whether requested directly by the social partner or indirectly in rules of the institution. There are few interactions in which acts on the part of the resident are aimed at producing a change in the social partner's behavior.

In view of the patterns identified, we contend that the social world in long-term care institutions is highly structured and differentiated. There is evidence for differential contingencies for the behaviors exhibited by the elderly. Specifically, dependent behaviors lead to dependence-supportive behaviors, and independent behaviors lead to no response. In a recent series of discussions (Baltes & Skinner, 1983; Peterson & Raps, 1984; Raps, Peterson, Jonas, & Seligman, 1982), the question of whether institutionalized settings produce learned helplessness was addressed. In line with the current findings, Baltes and Skinner (1983) argued that, for dependent or passive behavior to be labeled "helpless" behavior, one would have to demonstrate "noncontingency" in the institution. In other words, behaviors of the elderly would not be followed by differential consequences. If, however, behavior consistently and differentially produces specific consequences, dependent behavior represents something quite different than learned helplessness.

The institutional environment thus is not one in which helplessness prevails but a world in which specific behaviors generate specific consequences. Dependent rather than independent behaviors, however, are instrumental in securing social consequences, such as social contact. The existence of social contingencies for dependent self-care behaviors raises serious doubts about the link between dependency and the lack of control or the condition of noncontingency. The current findings thus support not only a differentiation between dependent and independent behaviors but also a differentiation between dependency and lack of control, and therewith perhaps a differentiation between dependency and the negative effects predicted by the learned helplessness model.

Comparative data with elderly in the community. The basic notion of distinctly different interaction patterns of elderly residents and their social environment related to independent and dependent

functioning is quite robust. Factors such as length of institutionalization, care status, sex of the resident, or type of institution influence the
frequency of behaviors. However, these factors alter only slightly the
basic patterns of the observed behavior sequences. Thus, within and
across institutions, the patterns seemed pervasive. What about the
generalizability of the findings: Would the same behavior patterns be
apparent in noninstitutionalized elderly? The best way to address
this issue of "setting specificity" would be via a longitudinal study
of old people before and after institutionalization. At this time, we
can offer comparative data with community-dwelling elderly (Wahl
& Baltes, 1990) and with institutionalized (Baltes, Reisenzein, &
Kindermann, 1985) and noninstitutionalized (Kindermann, 1986)
children. Only the first data will be discussed in this context.

Findings with community-dwelling elderly observed during
interactions in self-care contexts (Wahl & Baltes, 1990) indicate
the complementary interaction pattern between dependent and
dependence-supportive behavior to be the dominant pattern here
too. In addition, however, there are two new sequential patterns—
namely, independent behavior being followed by independence-
supportive and, although less frequently, by dependence-supportive
behaviors of partners. In addition, when looking at control and power
of behaviors, we notice more reciprocity (meaning a behavior has
both significant power and control) in interactions between noninstitutionalized elderly and their partners than in interactions between institutionalized elderly and their partners. Despite this and a
display of multiple interaction patterns for the elderly at home too,
dependent behavior is still the most reliable instrument for gaining
social contact.

Conclusions from Empirical Findings

There are three major conclusions: First, when considering the
comparative observational data from elderly at home as well as
the operant-experimental data from the institutionalized elderly, it
seems that an institutional orientation toward expected incompetence rather than real incompetence nourishes the typical interaction
patterns in long-term care institutions. Social partners of the elderly
are likely to react with dependence-supportive behaviors regardless
of the person's competence level. This is true both in institutions (and
thus correspond to Goffman's description of the total institution; see
Goffmann, 1961) and in the private home setting. We talk about an

institutional orientation or a dependency-support script because immediate help is provided by the staff regardless of whether the elderly show dependent behaviors frequently or rarely. Individual sequential analyses performed on randomly selected subjects, who by frequency of behaviors are ranked the most dependent and the most independent, show no differences in the interaction patterns (Baltes, 1979). Thus dependence-supportive behavior is the usual response to dependent self-care behavior of the elderly person, whether he or she is ranked as most independent or most dependent.

Second, an orientation toward dependency has as its basic prerequisite incompetence requiring subsequent compensation by the environment. Institutionalization plays a role in dependency when incompetence and needed compensatory efforts are perceived as essential characteristics of the inhabitants of the institution. Thus we maintain that the social interaction patterns related to independent and dependent functioning identified for the elderly seem to be at least a joint product of old age (more specifically, of perceptions of old age) and of institutionalization. We draw this conclusion from our findings that elderly persons are likely to be treated as dependence-prone even in situations where they might be able to perform the task. The social interaction patterns of the elderly are dominated by the fact of them being "incompetent," which is only reinforced by the fact of institutionalization. This line of argument finds additional support from our data with children, where other clusters of behavior (e.g., constructively engaged behaviors) evoke more complementarity and social connectedness and where dependence-supportive behaviors are tailored to the child's true incompetence.

Finally, reconstructing these findings within the operant learning framework, we have to conclude that, among comparable samples of elderly living in the community and in long-term care settings, dependent behavior exerts the most control and power with regard to social contingencies. When dependency of the elderly is seen as a function of the presence of social contingencies and as rather easily reversible following a change in those contingencies, it raises doubts about the relationship between dependence, helplessness, and lack or loss of control or of self-efficacy as propagated by the learned helplessness model. Furthermore, the fact that the elderly and their social partners participate in a dependency-support script points to the possibility of adaptive selection and compensation processes on the side of the elderly, despite an ensuing loss in self-care performance.

DISCUSSION AND IMPLICATIONS

Our data demonstrate that dependent behaviors of the elderly represent instrumental acts for gaining and securing control over the social environment. Accordingly, the data make a strong argument that dependent behaviors represent an adaptive process to both environmental and biological conditions of aging. The elderly person as well as the social environment restrict the range of interactive behaviors and compensate for real or anticipated weaknesses. This is not to suggest that all dependent behaviors are adaptive or that this kind of adaptation is necessarily healthy or optimal for a person's development at any given point in time. Some dependent behaviors have no doubt been shown to be the result of learned helplessness. On the basis of the operation of diverse behavioral systems, it follows that, theoretically, dependency can have different meanings. In other words, not all dependent behaviors have the same function.

One issue concerning the perspective of dependence as an instrumental act of control needs to be addressed. Our data show that, for the elderly, control through dependent behavior cannot be labeled "active" or "primary control" as defined in the literature by Weisz, Rothbaum, and Blackburn (1984). From our data, we cannot deduce whether the control we observed is to be called "secondary" or "passive control" (Schulz, 1986; Weisz et al., 1984) or is even perceived as control by the elderly. Although Weisz and colleagues differentiated four types of secondary control, all types are passive but differ in the amount or degree of self-involvement versus environment-involvement. In this regard, Schulz used "secondary control" only in the sense that the elderly turn over control from the self to significant others but thereby enhance their own sense of control and also avoid the experience of losing control in the future.

Should all types of secondary control be considered passive control? This is a significant issue, because research has shown that passive control (in the sense of control through no action or inactivity) produces the same ill effects in the long run as no control (Kuhl, 1986). The argument goes as follows: Restriction of and reduction in physical and psychological activity, even in young people (Bortz, 1982), imply disuse of functions, which, in turn, will lead to the loss of such functions. Today, we have a wealth of data showing the negative effects of physical inactivity on a wide variety of health variables in all age groups (for an overview, see Whitbourne, 1985). Of particular importance to old age are data on the effects of physical and mental inactivity on brain function (for a summary, see Bortz, 1982). Thus dependence occurring when the social environment encourages and compensates inactivity in the elderly, as well as when the elderly themselves or others underestimate their existing skills, abilities, and resources, could have ill effects.

Could it be, however, that dependence can have an optimizing function as an instrument for maintaining control in the face of *failing vitality*? One key principle of adaptation to failing vitality in old age has been proposed by one of us under the label *selective optimization with compensation* (M. M. Baltes, 1987; P. B. Baltes, 1987; P. B. Baltes & M. M. Baltes, 1980, 1989, 1990; P. B. Baltes, Dittmann-Kohli, & Dixon, 1984; Dixon & P. B. Baltes, 1986). The model of "selective optimization with compensation" was developed to describe and explain the development of intellectual performance in old age but can be extended to all activities. The basic assumption of the model is that individuals experience increased biological vulnerability as they age. They can maintain or even increase their activity level in some classes of behavior but no longer maintain a general level of high productivity. Which activities to give up (avoid altogether or become "dependent" in) and which to maintain and optimize will vary greatly from person to person, reflecting great interindividual differences or heterogeneity in aging processes. Thus what kind of dependent behaviors an individual would exhibit, to what degree, and in what situations is subject largely to his or her own life history and experiences, current physical and psychological status, and current environmental conditions. All factors together would define the amount and degree of compensatory efforts necessary to remain independent and productive and would determine when and where dependent behaviors are enlisted.

The adaptive task for the aging individual is to select and concentrate on those domains that are high priority and that involve a convergence of environmental demands, individual motivations, skills, and biological capacity. Thus dependent behaviors could present highly adaptive behaviors by which the individual uses his or her environment as a way to bolster other competencies. Skinner (1983) described a whole array of environmental aids that can be used to maintain intellectual performance in old age. Concurrently, other domains would have to be abandoned, resulting possibly in dependent behaviors. In this vein, dependent behaviors play an integral part in successful aging.

Increased vulnerability and age-related reduction in maximal biological functioning strengthen the idea that proactively and reactively selecting less demanding environments and domains becomes increasingly important. Dependent behaviors in an environment with low demands (i.e., a long-term care institution) ideally would allow the elderly to keep autonomy and to selectively optimize in other domains as long as possible. Skinner stated once that the goal of therapy is not to do away with institutions, because some people need prosthetic environments to exist in a more autonomous fashion.

It cannot be emphasized strongly enough, however, that it is an open question whether the current social environment of the elderly, particularly in institutions, provides the stimulation that would enable them to maintain and optimize a few selected activities. The answer more likely will be that, in reality, the social environment of the elderly, especially institutions, tends to provide support and security but often grossly lacks stimulating, development-enhancing qualities.

The major task for existing institutions for the elderly is, therefore, to provide settings and/or occasions that foster not only compensation for weaknesses but also selective optimization of existing strengths. (For further elaboration on this topic, see Baltes, Wahl, & Reichert, in press.) In practice, this would mean replacing a single behavioral system, the dependency-support script, with a number of patterns that address the diverse needs, preferences, competence levels, and so on of the residents. A tailor-made mix combining reinforcement and stimulation of independent behaviors with reinforcement of dependent behaviors would allow the elderly to choose those domains in which to become dependent and those in which to remain independent. The picture of "overcare" (Ransen, 1978, 1981) and of lack of self-directedness and freedom in institutions would be transformed into one of support and stimulation shaped by the needs and preferences of the elderly resident.

NOTE

1. The term *contingency* is a technical term in the literature on operant learning. A contingency refers to the temporal relationship between a behavior and an event that follows the behavior. Note that not all consequences need to be contingent upon the occurrence of a behavior.

REFERENCES

Abramson, L. Y., Seligman, M. E. P., & Teasdale, J. (1978). Learned helplessness in humans: Critique and reformulation. *Journal of Abnormal Psychology, 87*, 49-74.

Altman, I., & Rogoff, B. (1987). World views in psychology: Trait, interactional, organismic, and transactional perspectives. In D. Stokols & I. Altman (Eds.), *Handbook of environmental psychology* (pp. 7-40). New York: John Wiley.

Baer, D. J. (1973). The control of developmental processes: Why wait? In J. R. Nesselroade & H. W. Reese (Eds.), *Life-span developmental psychology: Methodological issues* (pp. 187-193). New York: Academic Press.

Baltes, M. M. (1979). [Comparison of interaction patterns of the most dependent vs. the most independent nursing home residents]. Unpublished raw data.

Baltes, M. M. (1982). Environmental factors in dependency among nursing home residents: A social ecology analysis. In T. A. Wills (Ed.), *Basic processes in helping relationships* (pp. 405-425). New York: Academic Press.

Baltes, M. M. (1987). Erfolgreiches Altern als Ausdruck von Verhaltenskompetenz und Umweltqualität [Successful aging: A consequence of behavioral competence and environmental quality]. In C. Niemitz (Ed.), *Erbe und Umwelt* (pp. 353-376). Frankfurt: Suhrkamp.

Baltes, M. M. (1988). Dependency in the elderly: Three phases of the operant research strategies. *Behavior Therapy, 19,* 301-319.

Baltes, M. M., & Baltes, P. B. (1982). Micro-analytic research on environmental factors and processes in psychological aging. In T. Field, A. Huston, H. C. Quay, L. Troll, & G. E. Finley (Eds.), *Review of human development* (pp. 524-539). New York: John Wiley.

Baltes, M. M., & Barton, E. M. (1977). New approaches toward aging: A case for the operant model. *Educational Gerontology: An International Quarterly, 2,* 383-405.

Baltes, M. M., & Barton, E. M. (1979). Behavioral analysis of aging: A review of the operant model and research. *International Journal of Behavioral Development, 2,* 297-320.

Baltes, M. M., Barton, E. M., Orzech, M. J., & Lago, D. (1983). Die Mikroökologie von Bewohnern und Personal: Eine Behavior-Mapping Studie im Altenheim [The micro-ecology of residents and staff: A behavior mapping study in a nursing home]. *Zeitschrift für Gerontologie, 16,* 18-26.

Baltes, M. M., Burgess, R. L., & Stewart, R. (1980). Independence and dependence in self-care behaviors in nursing home residents: An operant-observational study. *International Journal of Behavioral Development, 3,* 489-500.

Baltes, M. M., Honn, S., Barton, E. M., Orzech, M. J., & Lago, D. (1983). Dependence and independence in elderly nursing home residents: A replication and extension. *Journal of Gerontology, 38,* 556-564.

Baltes, M. M., Kindermann, T., & Reisenzein, R. (1986). Die Beobachtung von unselbständigem und selbständigem Verhalten in einem deutschen Altenheim: Die soziale Umwelt als Einflußgröße [Dependence and independence in a German nursing home: The role of the social environment]. *Zeitschrift für Gerontologie, 19,* 14-21.

Baltes, M. M., Kindermann, T., Reisenzein, R., & Schmid, U. (1987). Further observational data on the behavioral and social world of institutions for the aged. *Psychology and Aging, 2,* 390-403.

Baltes, M. M., & Lerner, R. M. (1980). Roles of the operant model and its methods in the life-span view of human development. *Human Development, 23,* 362-367.

Baltes, M. M., & Neumann, E. (1987). *Erhaltung und Rehabilitation von Selbständigkeit im Alter: Ein Interventionsprogramm für Pflegepersonal. Forschungsprojekt, gefördert von Bundesministerium für Forschung und Technologie* [Maintenance and rehabilitation of independence in old age: An intervention program for staff] (Research Project funded by the Federal Ministry of Research and Technology). Unpublished manuscript, Freie Universität Berlin.

Baltes, M. M., & Reisenzein, R. (1986). The social world in long-term care institutions: Psychosocial control towards dependency? In M. M. Baltes & P. B. Baltes (Eds.), *The psychology of control and aging* (pp. 315-343). Hillsdale, NJ: Lawrence Erlbaum.

Baltes, M. M., Reisenzein, R., & Kindermann, T. (1985, July). *Dependence in institutionalized children: An age-comparative study.* Paper presented at the ISSBD Meetings, Tours, France.

Baltes, M. M., & Skinner, E. A. (1983). Cognitive performance deficits and hospitalization: Learned helplessness, instrumental passivity, or what? *Journal of Personality and Social Psychology, 45,* 1013-1016.

Baltes, M. M., & Wahl, H. (1987). Dependence in aging. In L. L. Carstensen & B. A. Edelstein (Eds.), *Handbook of clinical gerontology* (pp. 204-221). New York: Pergamon.

Baltes, M. M., Wahl, H., & Reichert, M. (in press). Institutions and successful aging for the elderly? *Annual Review of Gerontology and Geriatrics.*

Baltes, P. B. (1987). Theoretical propositions of life-span developmental psychology: On the dynamics between growth and decline. *Developmental Psychology, 23,* 611-626.

Baltes, P. B., & Baltes, M. M. (1980). Plasticity and variability in psychological aging: Methodological and theoretical issues. In G. E. Gurski (Ed.), *Determining the effects of aging on the central nervous system* (pp. 41-60). Berlin: Schering.

Baltes, P. B., & Baltes, M. M. (1989). Optimierung durch Selektion und Kompensation: Ein psychologisches Modell erfolgreichen Alterns [Selective optimization with compensation: A model of successful aging]. *Zeitschrift für Pädagogik, 35,* 85-105.

Baltes, P. B., & Baltes, M. M. (1990). Psychological perspectives on successful aging: A model of selective optimization with compensation. In P. B. Baltes & M. M. Baltes (Eds.), *Successful aging: Perspectives from the behavioral sciences* (pp. 1-34). New York: Cambridge University Press.

Baltes, P. B., Dittmann-Kohli, F., & Dixon, R. (1984). New perspectives on the development of intelligence in adulthood: Toward a dual-process conception and a model of selective optimization with compensation. In P. B. Baltes & O. G. Brim, Jr. (Eds.), *Life-span development and behavior* (Vol. 6, pp. 33-76). New York: Academic Press.

Baltes, P. B., & Goulet, L. R. (1971). Exploration of developmental variables by manipulation and simulation of age differences in behavior. *Human Development, 14,* 149-170.

Bandura, A. (1977). Self-efficacy: Toward a unifying theory of behavioral change. *Psychological Review, 84,* 191-215.

Bandura, A. (1986). *Social foundations of thought and action.* Englewood Cliffs, NJ: Prentice-Hall.

Barker, R. G. (1968). *Ecological psychology.* Stanford, CA: Stanford University Press.

Barton, E. M., Baltes, M. M., & Orzech, M. J. (1980). On the etiology of dependence in nursing home residents during morning care: The role of staff behavior. *Journal of Personality and Social Psychology, 38,* 423-431.

Bortz, W. M. (1982). Disuse and aging. *Journal of the American Medical Association, 248,* 1203-1208.

Borup, J. H. (1981). Relocation: Attitudes, information network, and problems encountered. *The Gerontologist, 21,* 501-511.

Borup, J. H. (1983). Relocation mortality research: Assessment, reply, and the need to refocus on the issues. *The Gerontologist, 23,* 235-242.

Bronfenbrenner, U. (1979). *The ecology of human behavior.* Cambridge, MA: Harvard University Press.

Carp, F. M. (1987). Environment and aging. In D. Stokols & I. Altman (Eds.), *Handbook of environmental psychology* (Vol. I, pp. 329-360). New York: John Wiley.

Dixon, R. A., & Baltes, P. B. (1986). Towards life-span research on the functions and pragmatics of intelligence. In R. J. Sternberg & R. K. Wagner (Eds.), *Practical intelligence: Origins of competence in the everyday world* (pp. 203-235). New York: Cambridge University Press.

Epstein, S. (1979). The stability of behavior: I. On predicting most of the people much of the time. *Journal of Personality and Social Psychology, 37,* 1097-1126.

Epstein, S. (1980). The stability of behavior: II. Implications for psychological research. *American Psychologist, 35,* 790-806.

Goffman, E. (1961). *Asylums: Essays on the social situation of mental patients and other inmates.* Garden City, NY: Doubleday.

Horowitz, M. J., & Schulz, R. (1983). The relocation controversy: Criticism and commentary on five recent studies. *The Gerontologist, 23,* 229-234.

Howell, S. C. (1980). Environments and aging. *Annual Review of Gerontology and Geriatrics, 1,* 237-260.

Hoyer, W. J. (1974). Aging as intra-individual change. *Developmental Psychology, 10,* 821-826.

Hussian, R. A. (1981). *Geriatric psychology: A behavioral perspective.* New York: Van Nostrand Reinhold.

Kahana, E. (1982). A congruence model of person-environment interaction. In M. P. Lawton, P. G. Windley, & T. O. Byerts (Eds.), *Aging and the environment* (pp. 97-121). New York: Springer.

Kindermann, T. (1986). *Entwicklungsbedingungen selbständigen und unselbständigen Verhaltens in der frühen Kindheit: Sozial-ökologische Analyse alltäglicher Mutter-Kind-Interaktionen* [Environmental conditions of dependent and independent behaviors: An ecological analysis of everyday mother-toddler interactions]. Unpublished doctoral dissertation, Freie Universität Berlin.

Kuhl, J. (1986). Aging and models of control: The hidden costs of wisdom. In M. M. Baltes & P. B. Baltes (Eds.), *The psychology of control and aging* (pp. 1-33). Hillsdale, NJ: Lawrence Erlbaum.

Langer, E. J., & Rodin, J. (1976). The effect of choice and enhanced personal responsibility for the aged. *Journal of Personality and Social Psychology, 34,* 191-198.

Lawton, M. P. (1980). *Environment and aging.* Monterey, CA: Brooks/Cole.

Lawton, M. P. (1982). Competence, environmental press, and the adaptation of older people. In M. P. Lawton, P. G. Windley, & T. O. Byerts (Eds.), *Aging and the environment* (pp. 33-59). New York: Springer.

Lawton, M. P. (1985). The elderly in context: Perspectives from environmental psychology and gerontology. *Environment and Aging, 17*, 501-519.

Lawton, M. P. (1989). Behavior-relevant ecological factors. In K. W. Schaie & C. Schooler (Eds.), *Social structure and aging: Psychological processes* (pp. 57-78). Hillsdale, NJ: Lawrence Erlbaum.

Lawton, M. P., Windley, P. G., & Byerts, T. O. (Eds.). (1982). *Aging and the environment*. New York: Springer.

Lester, P. B., & Baltes, M. M. (1978). Functional interdependence of the social environment and the behavior of the institutionalized aged. *Journal of Gerontological Nursing, 4*, 23-27.

Lieberman, M. A. (1969). Institutionalization of the aged: Effects on behavior. *Journal of Gerontology, 24*, 330-340.

Magnusson, D., & Endler, N. S. (Eds.). (1977). *Personality at the crossroads*. Hillsdale, NJ: Lawrence Erlbaum.

Mischel, W. (1968). *Personality and assessment*. New York: John Wiley.

Mischel, W. (1979). On the interface of cognition and personality: Beyond the person-situation debate. *American Psychologist, 34*, 740-745.

Moos, R. (1976). *The human context: Environmental determinants of behavior*. New York: John Wiley.

Moos, R., & Lemke, S. (1985). Specialized living environments for older people. In J. E. Birren & K. W. Schaie (Eds.), *Handbook of the psychology of aging* (pp. 864-889). New York: Van Nostrand.

Mosher-Ashley, P. M. (1986-1987). Procedural and methodological parameters in behavioral-gerontological research: A review. *International Journal of Aging and Human Development, 24*, 189-229.

National Center for Health Statistics. (1987). *Use of nursing homes by the elderly: Preliminary data from the 1985 National Nursing Home Survey* (Advance Data No. 135). Hyattsville, MD: Author.

Neumann, E. (1986). *Modifizierbarkeit von Unselbständigkeit alter Menschen im Altenheim: Eine Interventionsstudie mit Pflegekräften* [Modification of dependence in older nursing home residents: An intervention study with staff]. Unpublished doctoral dissertation, Freie Universität Berlin.

Parmelee, P. A., Katz, I. R., & Lawton, M. P. (1989). Depression among institutionalized aged: Assessment and prevalence estimation. *Journal of Gerontology, 41*, M22-M29.

Parmelee, P. A., & Lawton, M. P. (1990). The design of special environments for the aged. In J. E. Birren & K. W. Schaie (Eds.), *Handbook of the psychology of aging* (3rd ed., pp. 464-488). New York: Academic Press.

Parr, J. (1980). The interaction of persons and living environments. In L. W. Poon (Ed.), *Aging in the 1980s* (pp. 393-406). Washington, DC: American Psychological Association.

Patterson, G. R. (1982). *Coercive family processes*. Eugene, OR: Castalia.

Patterson, R. L., & Jackson, G. M. (1980). Behavior modification with the elderly. In M. Hersen, R. M. Eisler, & P. Miller (Eds.), *Progress in behavior modification* (Vol. 9, pp. 205-239). New York: Academic Press.

Patterson, R. L., & Jackson, G. M. (1981). Behavioral approaches to gerontology. In L. Michelson, M. Hersen, & S. Turner (Eds.), *Future perspectives in behavior therapy* (pp. 293-313). New York: Plenum.

Peterson, L. C., & Raps, C. S. (1984). Helplessness and hospitalization: More remarks. *Journal of Personality and Social Psychology, 46*, 82-83.

Pincus, A. (1968). The definition and measurement of the institutional environment in homes for the aged. *The Gerontologist, 8*, 207-210.

Ransen, D. L. (1978). Some determinants of decline among the institutionalized aged: Overcare. *Cornell Journal of Social Relations, 13*, 61-74.

Ransen, D. L. (1981). Long-term effects of two interventions with the aged: An ecological analysis. *Journal of Applied Developmental Psychology, 2*, 13-27.

Raps, C. S., Peterson, C., Jonas, M., & Seligman, M. E. P. (1982). Patient behavior in hospitals: Helplessness, reactance, or both? *Journal of Personality and Social Psychology, 42*, 1036-1041.

Regnier, V. (1981). *Adaptability and aging: Vol. 2. The neighborhood environment and its impact on the older person.* Paris, France: International Center for Social Gerontology.

Rodin, J. (1986). Health, control, and aging. In M. M. Baltes & P. B. Baltes (Eds.), *The psychology of control and aging* (pp. 139-165). Hillsdale, NJ: Lawrence Erlbaum.

Rodin, J., & Langer, E. (1977). Long-term effects of a control-relevant intervention with the institutionalized aged. *Journal of Personality and Social Psychology, 35*, 897-902.

Rodin, J., Timko, C., & Harris, S. (1985). The construct of control: Biological and psychological correlates. *Annual Review of Gerontology and Geriatrics, 5*, 3-55.

Sackett, G. P. (1979). The lag sequential analysis of contingency and cyclicity in behavioral interaction research. In J. Osofsky (Ed.), *Handbook of infant development* (pp. 623-649). New York: John Wiley.

Sackett, G. P., Holm, R., Crowley, C., & Henkins, A. (1979). Computer technology: A FORTRAN program for lag sequential analysis of contingency and cyclicity in behavioral interaction data. *Behavior Research Methods and Instrumentation, 11*, 366-378.

Schulz, R. (1976). The effects of control and predictability on the psychological and physical well-being of the institutionalized aged. *Journal of Personality and Social Psychology, 33*, 563-573.

Schulz, R. (1986). Successful aging: Balancing primary and secondary control. *Adult Development and Aging News, 13*, 2-4.

Schulz, R., & Brenner, G. (1977). Relocation of the aged: A review and theoretical analysis. *Journal of Gerontology, 32*, 323-333.

Schulz, R., & Hanusa, B. (1979). Environmental influences on the effectiveness of control and competence-enhancing interventions. In L. C. Perlmuter & R. A. Monty (Eds.), *Choice and perceived control* (pp. 315-337). Hillsdale, NJ: Lawrence Erlbaum.

Schulz, R., & Hanusa, B. H. (1980). Experimental social gerontology: A social psychological perspective. *Journal of Social Issues, 36*, 30-46.

Seligman, M. E. P. (1975). *Helplessness: On depression, development, and death.* San Francisco: Freeman.

Skinner, B. F. (1983). Intellectual self-management in old age. *American Psychologist, 38*, 239-244.

Studer, R. G. (1973). Man-environment relations: Discovery or design. In W. E. F. Preiser (Eds.), *Environmental design research* (Vol. 2). Stroudsburg, PA: Dowden, Hutchinson, & Ross.

Thomae, H. (1970). Theory of aging and cognitive theories of personality. *Human Development, 13,* 1-10.

Wahl, H., & Baltes, M. M. (1990). Die soziale Umwelt alter Menschen: Entwicklungsanregende oder-hemmende Pflegeinteraktionen? [The social environment of the elderly: Development-enhancing or inhibiting care interactions?]. *Zeitschrift für Entwicklungspsychologie und Pädagogische Psychologie, 22,* 266-283.

Weisz, J. R., Rothbaum, F. M., & Blackburn, T. C. (1984). Standing out and standing in: The psychology of control in America and Japan. *American Psychologist, 39,* 955-969.

Whitbourne, S. K. (1985). *The aging body.* New York: Springer.

Willems, E. P. (1972). The interface of the hospital environment and patient behavior. *Physical Medicine and Rehabilitation, 53,* 115-122.

Wisocki, P. (1984). Behavioral approaches to gerontology. *Progress in Behavior Modification, 16,* 121-157.

Wohlwill, J. F. (1973a). The environment is not in the head. In W. E. F. Preiser (Ed.), *Environmental design research* (Vol. 2). Stroudsburg, PA: Dowden, Hutchinson, & Ross.

Wohlwill, J. (1973b). *The study of behavioral development.* New York: Academic Press.

PART II

Biopsychosocial Mechanisms Linking Health and Behavior

5

Vigilant Coping and Health Behavior

HOWARD LEVENTHAL

ELAINE A. LEVENTHAL

PAMELA M. SCHAEFER

Over the past decade, we have conducted a series of studies to improve our understanding of the strategies individuals use to protect themselves against health threats. A subsidiary and then an increasingly important goal of our project was to better understand how age—or, more accurately, stage in life—affected this process. In our judgment, we could best advance our understanding if we did not force our participants' mental processes into existent social-psychological models of behavior such as attribution theory (Kelley, 1972), health belief theory (Janz & Becker, 1984), or concepts such as locus of control derived from social learning theory (Rotter, 1966; Wallston & Wallston, 1982). We made this decision because we felt these models obscured both the substance and the process underlying health and illness behavior by recasting people's thoughts and actions into the language of the respective model and assuming that decisions and behavior were directed by the rules of the model rather than rules used by the subject. We adopted, instead, a systems framework (Carver & Scheier, 1982; Kanfer, 1977; Lazarus & Folkman, 1984; Leventhal, 1970), which views individuals as active problem solvers whose instrumental actions are a product of their perception, intellectual understanding, and emotional response to a health threat and the coping procedures used to regulate both the threat and the emotional responses to it. In sum, we have tried to model our subjects'

AUTHORS' NOTE: The aging research reported and preparation of this manuscript were supported by grant AG03501 from the National Institute on Aging.

view of reality because we believe this approach will provide a more complete understanding of both the functions of illness and the mechanisms involved in adapting to it (Leventhal & Nerenz, 1985; Skelton & Croyle, in press; Weinstein, 1988). This type of research has been labeled the study of "illness cognition" or the study of "commonsense models" of illness (Leventhal & Diefenbach, in press; Leventhal, Meyer, & Nerenz, 1980).

Our focus, therefore, is on the cognitive aspects of how people represent or understand illness, their emotional reactions to illness, and their procedures to cope with and appraise its outcome. Because our goal is to understand the processes involved in illness cognition or commonsense modeling of illness threats in real-world settings, we have been forced to attend to three types of contextual factors that set limits upon and shape these cognitive and emotional processes: the disease and its natural history, social context, and stable characteristics or dispositions of the individual (Rosenberg, 1988). The individual's age—that is, his or her place in the life span—is a contextual factor that subsumes a variety of social, psychological, and biological factors that may affect the way an individual represents threats of illness and selects and performs procedures to cope with and evaluate illness episodes. As we will point out later on, this emphasis has important consequences for both theory and methodology and has led to considerable divergence between the line of research reported here and epidemiological studies that compare symptom reports (for example, Verbrugge, 1989) and coping procedures (Brody & Kleban, 1983) among groups varying on the factors of age and gender.

THE COMMONSENSE MODEL AND ITS CONTEXT

Our first task is to provide a picture of the content of commonsense models, that is, to define a substantive framework for the analysis of commonsense thinking. The framework describes the types of social and psychological factors involved in commonsense thinking and provides an overall structure in which to explore their operation. Our second task is to describe the mechanisms and processes that underlie and/or generate the observations that are classified within various components of the framework. This task is essentially one of developing a theoretical model that tells us which operations generate and regulate the factors specified by the framework.

A Framework for Commonsense Models of Illness

The cognitive component. As can be seen in Figure 5.1, our basic framework assumes that situations can be processed in two parallel and partially independent lines, one focused upon the regulation of the perceived world and the other focused upon feelings or emotion (Leventhal, 1970). The basic components of the model (see Figure 5.1) consist first of an underlying processing system whose action transforms stimuli (either internal or external) into representations of a threat and/or emotional reactions. The representation has multiple attributes, including its identity, or the symptoms and the label that indicate the threat; consequences, or perceived physical, psychological, social, and economic impact; time-lines, or time of onset, expected duration, or periodicity (acute, cyclic, or chronic); causes (for example, external disease agent, internal weakness, improper health behavior); and its controllability (Lau & Hartman, 1983; Weinstein, 1988).

The second step in the sequence consists of the procedures used for coping with the threat, or the plans and performances (strategies and tactics) used to control the threat. The plan includes an array of specific response procedures, each of which has (a more or less explicit) expectation regarding its adequacy (response efficacy) for controlling the threat and the individual's beliefs about his or her ability (self-efficacy) to perform the response (Bandura, 1977; Rotter, 1966; Leventhal, 1970). The performance of an action will involve the motor programs for the action, the environmental cues that guide the specifics of the action, and the representation of the threat itself.

The last component in the sequence consists of procedures for the appraisal of response outcomes. These procedures consist of criteria and rules (the type of effect and its time-line) used to evaluate outcomes. While appraisal procedures are generally focused upon the adequacy of specific responses—that is, whether the response has accomplished its intended effect—the comparisons between expected and actual coping outcomes can lead to appraisals of the accuracy of the representation (e.g., whether the disease is controllable, the accuracy of the diagnosis, and so on) and the adequacy of the individual's resources for controlling the threat as well as the appraisal of the adequacy of the coping response.

The emotional component. The emotional response to the threat can be elicited by the very same processes that are involved in constructing the representation of the threat. But emotion can also be elicited by any of the components mentioned earlier; that is, a breakdown in

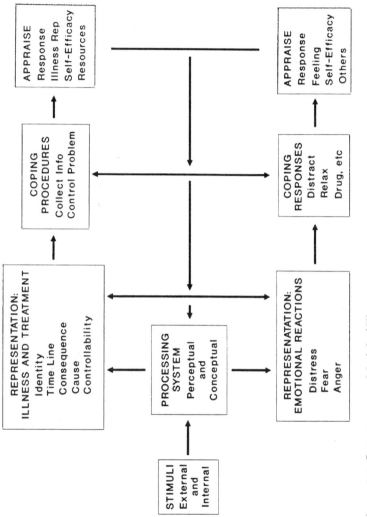

Figure 5.1. Commonsense Model of Illness

coping may provoke fear as may a reappraisal of the threat. There is also a continual interaction or "transaction" between the two parallel lines (Lazarus, 1982; Leventhal & Scherer, 1987). Thus emotional reactions may color or alter the representation of a threat by bringing to mind forgotten examples of consequences and so on (Clark & Teasdale, 1982; Isen, Shalker, Clark, & Karp, 1978), by minimizing the severity of the threat (Croyle & Hunt, in press) or perceived ability to cope with it (Rosen, Terry, & Leventhal, 1982), or by disrupting or in other ways modifying the procedures involved in coping with and appraising coping outcomes.

In sum, representation, coping procedures, and appraisals can elicit different emotions and be affected in turn by these emotions. Although the two parallel lines are in constant interaction, they are represented in parallel, as there may be a substantial degree of separation or independence between the systems developed to cope with the illness threat per se and those used to cope with emotion. Thus, in our prior description of these processes, we termed the representation and control of the threat *danger control* and the experience and control of emotional reactions *fear* (or *emotion*) *control* (Leventhal, 1970; see also Lazarus & Launier, 1978; Rogers, 1983).

Social and Biological Context

Individuals do not react to health threats in a vacuum: Their representations, procedures for coping and appraisal, and emotional responses are a direct reflection of and are constrained by their cultural and biological environments. The implications of this statement are far reaching, affecting the content of behaviors as well as the mechanisms, rules, and/or procedures for processing the information that produces these behaviors.

Social context. The representation of an illness procedure for coping and appraisal is affected by a wide range of special factors ranging from the linguistic environment and mass media, through cultural institutions and roles, to interpersonal exchanges of information. For example, the cultural stereotype of cancer includes pain, disfigurement, and rapid death (Dent & Goulston, 1982a, 1982b; Sutherland, 1967; Weisman, 1976). Indeed, people rarely think about the realities of living with cancer for extended periods of time. Other disease labels may suggest specific symptoms and causes: for example, the term *hypertension* implies that states of behavioral and subjective hyperactivity and emotional and bodily tension are the signs and determinants of hypertension (Blumhagen, 1980). The representation of hypertension as an acute, environmentally induced disorder is reinforced by the information exchanged in the interaction between practitioner and patient that focuses upon symptoms and medications. The interchange parallels in many ways the exchange that would take place for the treatment of acute, non-life-threatening, infectious conditions (Steele & Leventhal, 1982). Thus the practice setting and the practitioner may unwittingly reinforce an acute, symptomatic picture of a disorder that is, in reality, asymptomatic and chronic.

Observation of most TV commercials for over-the-counter remedies also suggests that these messages actively contribute to the formulation of an acute-illness representation: have headache, take product "X," and obtain relief! It is likely that representations and procedures for coping and appraisal are affected by communications, accurate and inaccurate, from family and friends, though far too little is known about the substance and impact of these sources of information (Horwitz, 1978; Leventhal, van Nguyen, & Leventhal, 1985; Robinson, 1971; Suchman, 1965; Wood, Taylor, & Lichtman, 1985).

Biological impact and the disease history. People with different diseases experience different physical symptoms, undergo different diagnostic and treatment procedures, and have different potentials for complete recovery. In addition, individual expectations and knowledge differ for various illnesses. This knowledge base, in interaction with the symptoms and diagnostic and treatment procedures, shapes the individual's emotional and coping behaviors.

While any specific disease, whether hypertension, cancer, or the common cold, may take an idiosyncratic form in a given individual, the temporal pattern for most individuals suffering from the same or a related disease is likely to follow a similar trajectory. This similarity allows us to define phases that are common to individuals and to sets of illnesses. For example, colds and other acute illnesses may begin with minor symptoms, rapidly flare with concrete symptoms, and, with time (and/or treatment), disappear. By contrast, some chronic illnesses have a slow onset with mild, early warning signs coupled with complex procedures for diagnosis and treatments, long-term rehabilitation when appropriate, and a subsequent, lifelong period of vigilance.

The pattern of disease is important in providing a changing landscape of sensations that become translated into moods and feelings of illness or well-being. These feelings are associated with procedures for coping and appraisal that lead to decisions regarding one's health status and need for medical care. Building upon Suchman's work (1965), Safer, Tharps, Jackson, and Leventhal (1979) defined three phases through which this process may travel prior to contact with the medical care system: an appraisal phase, typically initiated by bodily sensations; an illness phase, beginning with the decision that one is definitely ill; and a utilization phase, beginning with the decision to contact a treatment authority and ending in contact with a provider. The phases of illness are important, as they are likely to involve different bodily sensations, different procedures for coping, and different procedures and criteria for appraisal. In sum, the information from this changing biological display and from the cultural environment provides the context and sets the problem upon which the psychological system operates.

STEPS TOWARD A THEORY OF COMMONSENSE MODELS OF ILLNESS

The Constructive Process

Having mapped a framework, we can now ask: How does it work? How are representations of illness threats or a subjective emotional experience constructed and updated or changed, and how are coping procedures brought into play and sustained? What rules or procedures does a person use to appraise how effectively he has altered a perceived threat or his subjective emotion and how does he decide that this representation of the threat and his feelings are reasonable? Finally, how does he determine that he has adequate resources (self and external) for controlling threat and emotional upset?

Our first assumption is that representations and coping are created in an ongoing process. The individual is constantly constructing, updating, or reconstructing representations of settings and feelings, generating and executing procedures for coping, evaluating or appraising outcome.

Second, the system processes information from both the body and the environment. Indeed, during illness, the body often becomes a focus of observation and is experienced as a part of the external environment, separate from the psychological self (Leventhal, 1976; Leventhal, Nerenz, & Leventhal, 1982). The ill person experiences a variety of symptoms or aches and pains that are spatially localized, extended in time, and varying in sensory properties (burning, aching, stabbing, and so on). These sensations are interpreted and become the focus for coping procedures used in planning and acting to deal with health threats.

Information Processing

The processing of information from the external environment and from the body involves matching stimuli to memory structures that determine their meaning and the reactions to them. The function of these maneuvers is to make sense of or define the individual's condition (Cacioppo & Petty, 1983) and to plan, execute, and evaluate ways of eliminating and/or controlling the threat of disease. Performing these control functions verifies or confirms the definition of the threat agent.

Clearly, a close relationship exists between the representation of a threat and the emotional response to it, on the one hand, and the procedures for planning, coping, and appraisal, on the other. The representation and emotional reactions motivate (drive and direct) coping procedures, and the postprocedure appraisal can define the degree of control over an evolving illness episode, lead to the selection of new coping procedures, define new criteria for evaluating outcomes, and change the view one has of a disease. For example, taking aspirin to eliminate a headache can both control the distress of the headache and confirm (within the individual's psychological reality) that the headache is due to minor tension. But, if the headache does not go away after taking aspirin, one might alter one's tentative "self-diagnosis" from a stress headache to a brain tumor, an interpretation that drastically shifts the perceived cause, duration, and consequences of the underlying condition.

Coping and appraisal procedures will also reflect the properties of the information that is to be interpreted, that is, whether it is abstract or propositional (a health warning), sensory or perceptual (a symptom), clear or ambiguous (Anderson, 1983), and familiar to the individual. Seeking medical advice and making various changes in diet and the like may be the more likely reactions to abstract warnings of health threats, while, for example, taking an aspirin or going to sleep early may be the more likely responses to concrete, symptomatic states. We hypothesize that concrete, perceptual information tends to dominate abstract or conceptual information. Thus an intractable symptom can often restimulate attention, thought, and concern, even after being diagnosed as benign.

Procedures also vary in the degree to which they are automatic or conscious and voluntary (Schiffrin & Schneider, 1977). The data available from intensive interview studies are most likely to reveal relatively large or molar procedures that are under voluntary control; because they are extended in time and consciously controlled, they are readily reported. Procedures such as scanning of the body either by eye or by hand to check on criteria such as, for example, symmetry or soreness may occur so automatically and so swiftly that they are virtually unobserved and seldom reported, and it may require direct observation under well-controlled (and ingeniously constructed) conditions to obtain evidence for their existence. These studies show that environmental cues—for example, the presence of a stressor—can shift the interpretation of a symptom from that of illness to an indication of stress (Baumann, Cameron, Zimmerman, & Leventhal, 1989) and that the presence of others with similar screening test results can reduce the perceived severity of a diagnosis (Croyle & Jemmott, in press). The effects of external information are limited, however, by knowledge. When individuals have clear ideas about a disease and its symptoms, their interpretations are less likely to be influenced by external information (Baumann et al., 1989).

We do not assume that illness representations are the only sources of motivation for health and illness behaviors (Kasl & Cobb, 1966). One can engage in protective or curative health actions for nonhealth reasons, for example, to please a parent or spouse (Evans, 1976; Leventhal & Hirschman, 1982; Robberson & Rogers, 1988). But, even when the source of motivation is extrinsic to health, it may affect health behavior by influencing the representation of the threat and the emotional response to it.

Symmetrical Processing

We have suggested that illness representations are constructed by both conceptual (abstract) and schematic (perceptual) processes (Leventhal, 1987). Abstract, semantic information is used to construct the label applied to a threat, while schematic processing generates its concrete representation or "feel," that is, the sensory, locational, and sequential properties of the illness representation (Leventhal, Meyer, & Nerenz, 1980; Leventhal, Nerenz, & Steele, 1984). Indeed, it appears that there is a pressure toward consistency or symmetry between the levels. Thus, when people experience symptoms, they will seek a label; when given a label—told, for example, that they are hypertensives—they will seek symptoms (Meyer, Leventhal, & Gutmann, 1985). The search for symptoms appears to be guided by an underlying concept or schema of the illness, hence each label tends to be associated with a more or less well-defined set of symptoms (Baumann & Leventhal, 1985; Pennebaker, 1982).

External Congruity Checking

Initially, we hypothesized that symmetry was automatic—that is, when someone was diagnosed or labeled *hypertensive*, the search for concrete symptoms such as palpitations, headache, and face flushing occurred instantaneously and with little or no conscious deliberation (Baumann & Leventhal, 1985). Additional observational and experimental data made clear that the procedures used in the "symmetry process" are quite complex and not always automatic. First, we observed that the linkage of symptoms with hypertension increased with time; at their first treatment encounter, 71% of a group of 65 patients believed they could tell their blood pressure was elevated; six months later, 92% of this same group believed they could tell (Meyer et al., 1985). Recordings of the interactions between physicians and patients obtained in a second study (Steele & Gutmann, 1983) suggested that the information exchanged in the visits encouraged this linkage. When patients come for checkups and medication refills, it is typical for the physician and/or nurse to conduct a review of systems, asking about symptoms in each area of the body to locate possible problems and sequelae of hypertension. Unfortunately, the purpose of this review is not always communicated to the patients, and it is quite natural for them to believe these represent potential symptoms of hypertension. In short, hypertensive patients are presented with a "cafeteria" of symptoms that can be checked against their own experience, and they can select from among these symptoms the one(s) that is most frequent or closest in time to a high reading.

The data suggested, therefore, an appraisal process that moves back and forth between the self and the external environment until perceived environmental information confirms, or is congruent with, causal beliefs for the particular illness. At that point, observed symptoms are assumed to be products of the particular disease. The most persuasive evidence that individuals search for concrete symptoms, match them to labels, and check internal symptoms against external, causal cues has been obtained from laboratory experiments (Baumann et al., 1989).

It is clear that a complex interplay exists between symptoms, environmental perceptions, and beliefs about disease causation. It is also apparent that there are both generic prototypes (acute illness, chronic illness) and illness-specific prototypes (for example, mononucleosis, allergies, cardiac disease, cancer, Alzheimer's dementia) stored at both the abstract conceptual and the concrete schematic level (Bishop,

1987; Prohaska, Leventhal, Leventhal, & Keller, 1985). The degree to which an environmental cue can activate and shape judgments depends upon the familiarity with and availability of the underlying schema (Kahnemann & Tversky, 1973). It is worth repeating yet again that these meanings may have no biological validity (Baumann & Leventhal, 1985). Nonetheless, these meanings affect coping procedures, emotional response, and care seeking in important ways; for example, the mass or enlarged lymph node coded as cancer is far more fear provoking than the cough and fatigue attributed to stress and/or a cold, though the former symptoms may be due to a cold and the latter to a cancer.

Temporal Procedures

Because episodes of illness unfold over time, we anticipated and found a number of procedures that assessed time course. These expectations will reflect beliefs about particular classes of illness (for example, acute versus chronic), beliefs relevant to specific anatomic locations (GI, respiratory, and so on), and beliefs specific to particular disorders (for example, food poisoning, flu). And, throughout the illness episode, the individual's processing of information at a concrete, perceptual level for factors such as the intensity or quality of a symptom at a given moment will generate a set of relatively automatic coping and appraisal strategies that are less susceptible to volitional control and, at times, in conflict with the response strategies governed by abstract knowledge.

Data support the existence of two temporal test procedures that operate at the onset of illness episodes. The most obvious of these procedures can be characterized as a rule to "seek help for symptoms of sudden and/or intense onset." Studies by Berkanovic, Telesky, and Reeder (1981) as well as our own data (Cameron, Leventhal, Leventhal, & Schaefer, in submission) show rapid seeking of medical assistance for symptoms that are intense and sudden in onset. Seeking help in this instance appears to be driven both by the cognitive or abstract need for clarity and by the intensity of the concrete sensations and the emotional response they provoke.

The second such temporal procedure can be characterized as a "wait and see" rule. This procedure, which includes information collected by reading and lay consultation, is often the most visible mode of operation during the initial, evaluation phase of an illness episode when the bodily sensations are "vague" and of low intensity (Cameron et al., in submission; Safer et al., 1979). The procedure calls for ongoing observation of symptoms and checking of them against expectations based upon assumptions about the temporal course for the specific disease. Thus the procedure is driven by illness proto-types and schemata, either general (for example, acute to chronic) or specific (for example, flu, cancer) based upon individual experience with illness and exposure to community "folklore."

AGE, HEALTH BEHAVIOR, AND COMMONSENSE MODELS

Having outlined our framework and theoretical model, we can raise two key questions about the relationship of age to both health and illness behaviors. The first, an important descriptive question, asks whether there are differences in the incidence and prevalence of different health behaviors at different ages. Do older and younger people differ in what they think, feel, and do about preventive prac-tices (vitamin ingestion or lower fats and increased fiber in the diet), self-treatment practices, and use of health care? Answers to such questions address main effects and are typical of epidemiological studies. They are important to the formation of social policy, such as the planning for various types of health care facilities given projected changes in the age distribution of the population, but they do not tell us how things happen.

The second key question concerns the determinants of age-related changes in health and illness behavior. If people of different ages act differently, it is reasonable to ask how age affects the mechanisms controlling behavior, as this knowledge will be essential for under-standing and affecting how people utilize health care services. It is clear that age-related developmental changes affect biological, psy-chological, and social contextual variables. This is particularly clear in illness presentations. Diseases present with different symptoms, have different time courses and consequences, and require modified treatment in the elderly (Libow & Sherman, 1981; Reichel, 1978). For example, high blood pressure in the elderly may reflect arterioscle-rotic changes in the media layer of arterial walls rather than the de-velopment of atheromatous plaques of atherosclerosis, the common cause of hypertension in middle age. Second, physical changes ac-companying normal aging can also affect each of the factors discussed in the earlier sections. The representation of illness, coping proce-dures, and appraisal rules may vary over the individual's life his-tory. Thus the older person's expectations about reductions in energy level will affect the selection of procedures for self-management and the prevention and management of illness threats.

Third, the social network also changes over the life span and is likely to be markedly different in old age in comparison with middle and younger adult years. For example, the elderly, particularly elderly women, are typically separated from their children and face a shrinking support system with the demise of spouse, relatives, and friends. The social network may also have different expectations and generate social pressures for the older person that are different than those placed on the young or middle-aged (Schulz & Rau, 1985). An individual's age may also influence treatment decisions; for example, some oncologists may be reluctant to adopt an aggressive chemotherapy regimen for the elderly cancer patient although the evidence suggests treatment is equally effective and little more complicated for the old than for the young patient (DeVita, 1983; E. Leventhal, 1986). In the following section, we describe data from convenience samples of well persons and from samples of patients that are consistent in showing higher levels of preventive behavior and treatment adherence in older than younger persons. We then examine differences in the representation and emotional reactions to illness of older and middle-aged persons to see whether simple main effects (age differences) can account for these behavioral differences. It is only when we hypothesize that older persons may use a common procedure for coping with both emotion and illness that we obtain data providing insight into differences in health and illness behavior for older and younger persons.

ARE THERE AGE DIFFERENCES IN HEALTH AND ILLNESS BEHAVIOR?

Descriptive Data

Does a person's age—that is, his or her place in the life cycle—influence health and illness behavior? Does it affect the frequency and/or type of actions chosen to protect against potential illness threats, and does it affect action taken during illness? If people respond differently, we can ask whether the differences are due to differences in mental representations of illness threats, differences in emotional reactions to these threats, or differences in the procedures used to appraise and to cope with these threats. And, if age does affect these processes, we need to distinguish those components that are due to aging per se from age effects that are due to difference in knowledge, attitudes, and beliefs about disease that are a function of the life history of individuals in a given age cohort (Riley, 1979).

We began our inquiry of age differences and health behaviors with two types of study: (a) surveys of healthy individuals and (b) interview studies of patients in treatment. Because we are concerned with behavioral change over the life span, we collected data from subjects at both younger and older ages and compared both behavior and beliefs of these respondents. If behavior and beliefs were common across age groups, it would imply that we are dealing with culture-wide, stereotypic patterns rather than age-related differences. Finally, we examined age differences across several categories of variables (for example, representations, emotional responses) in the hope that we could relate them to differences in behavior. We also anticipated that the pattern of effects would help us rule out historical or cohort effects and determine how age per se affects health behavior.

Age differences in health behavior. We compared the preventive health behaviors, emotional responses, and illness representations of four samples of "healthy" adults of different ages. These respondents were neither hospitalized nor selected because they were in treatment for a specific disease; they were active and living in the community. The surveys were conducted during a "health fair" held at a large shopping mall during busy, weekend shopping hours. (Fairs of one form or another—for example, antique fairs, craft shows, auto shows—are ongoing events at these centers.) Respondents were approached at random and asked to spend five minutes completing a health questionnaire; the refusal rate was very low, and the sample is very likely representative of the typical shopping center crowd.

A total of 396 respondents answered 15 questions about their preventive health behaviors. These were the lead-off questions for six separate questionnaires, each on a different disease, to which these subjects were randomly assigned. The data showed statistically significant ($p < .01$) differences between the three age groups for 11 items: The 112 older respondents (60 years and older) reported more avoidance of physical exertion and more compliance with healthful dietary practices (for example, eating a balanced diet, avoiding salty food, and eating bran or high fiber foods) when compared with the 173 young (20- to 39-year-old) and 111 middle-aged (40- to 59-year-old) respondents. Older respondents also reported more avoidance of harmful health habits (for example, smoking and excess drinking) and were more attentive to air and water quality. The oldest group also reported a higher frequency of use of medical services (obtaining regular checkups), and both the older and the middle-aged groups reported more frequent use of laxatives, even though these older groups also were less likely to use drugstore remedies. In comparison with both the middle-aged and the oldest group, the youngest expressed much less interest in obtaining information on health problems, either about what others do to prevent illness or medical information on the causes of specific illnesses (Prohaska et al., 1985).

While none of the above differences is of large magnitude, they appear with great consistency across each of the six subsamples in this survey study. But, while they are highly reliable and require explanation, we must caution that the responses to several of these items may be subject to bias as the item wording was very general and contrasted with questions that ask about actual performance of specific behaviors during a defined period of time, for example, today or the past week. The findings are similar, however, to those in data sets where the responses are more specific and objective and less subject to bias (Belloc & Breslow, 1972).

Age differences in treatment behavior. Both subjective and objective data on the illness behaviors of respondents of different ages were collected in two sets of studies of patients under treatment for the same or related diseases. These data allowed us to compare reported behaviors and objective records during well-defined time periods for groups of patients spanning a wide age range, for example, from 40 to 75 years and older. In a hypertension treatment study, we interviewed each of 257 patients, five times, over a nine-month period (Leventhal, Steele, & Gutmann, n.d.). We assessed various aspects of their representations of this disease, asked them about their compliance with medication, and obtained objective data on blood pressure control and dropping from treatment. The one-month follow-up data showed medication misses were reported more often by younger (53% of the patients under 50 years of age) than by middle-aged (44% of those 50 to 59 years old) or old patients (36% of those 60 years and older). The same effects were observable in each of the interviews. An objective indicator, dropping out of treatment during the nine-month period, showed effects similar to the compliance reports: 25% of those under 50 years of age dropped from treatment in comparison with 11% of the 50- to 59-year-olds and only 6% of the over 60-year-olds.

The effect of patients' age was also examined in four of our six studies of chemotherapy treatment for cancer (Nerenz, Love, Leventhal, & Easterling, 1986). We found that older patients were less likely to have considered quitting treatment. For example, when the patients in our longitudinal cancer study of breast and lymphatic cancer were asked, "Have there ever been times when you wanted to quit the treatment?," 52% of those under 50 said yes in comparison with 50% of those 50 to 59 years of age, 41% of those 60 to 69, and 21% of those over 70 years of age. Actual quitting of treatment was virtually a nonevent; across all studies, only 3 of 600 or more participants stopped treatment (Leventhal, Easterling, Coons, Luchterland, & Love, 1986). In summary, the data for both the hypertension and the cancer studies suggest older persons are more compliant with treatment. This finding is congruent with the higher frequencies of preventive health actions reported by older persons in the survey data (Prohaska et al., 1985).

Determinants of Age Differences: The Vigilance Hypothesis

It is important to state that we do not believe that increased use of preventive behaviors and increased compliance with treatment are necessary attributes of aging. Samples drawn from populations in other cultures or in our own culture, at different points in time, might show quite different trends. These differences are descriptive and need not reflect any permanent attribute of aging. But, while these effects are not immutable, the evidence from these samples clearly suggests that, at this point in our cultural history, older persons are more vigilant and responsive to health threats than middle-aged or younger persons.

The challenge is to identify the component(s) of the illness cognition system that mediates the vigilance effect. We first examined whether these behavioral effects reflected differences in the way elderly and middle-aged persons represented illnesses, and we then explored whether they differed in their emotional reactions to illnesses—that is, were the elderly more vigilant because they were more frightened or apprehensive about the onset of illness? As will be seen, there was virtually no evidence for age differences in the representation of illness, and the age differences in emotional reactions to illness threats proved to be the opposite of those suggested above; older persons were less frightened and/or apprehensive about illness (E. Leventhal, 1984). What appears to be critical is that older respondents differ in the procedures they use for coping and appraisal of coping outcomes. Specifically, we hypothesize that, as people grow older, they become increasingly motivated to reduce the level and cost of emotional distress and do so by acting (seeking care) to define and treat health threats, thereby eliminating any emotional distress created by uncertainty. We recognize, of course, that our cross-sectional data can only test hypotheses about age-related differences; testing of "aging" differences requires longitudinal studies.

The cognitive aspect of vigilance. The hypothesis that, in comparison with younger persons, the elderly are more vigilant with respect to health problems has suggested a number of more specific hypotheses. One is that older persons differ in the way they represent diseases. For example, older persons might feel that they are more vulnerable to disease, that disease would have more serious consequences for them, or that diseases are chronic rather than acute and curable. On the other hand, older persons might differ from younger persons in their coping expectations and/or in the appraisals they make of coping outcomes. For example, they might have more confidence in treatment procedures and medical authority and appraise outcomes more favorably. Finally, older persons might be more in tune with preventive health practices and compliance with treatment regimens because they are more anxious or frightened about the dangers of specific diseases. While no single study of ours addressed all of these questions, data from across the entire set provided information respecting most of these possibilities.

Commonalities in abstract beliefs across age cohorts. The data provided its first, consistent set of surprises by showing virtually no differences among our age cohorts on items measuring various attributes of illness representations, appraisals, or coping; this was true for virtually every one of our studies. For example, data from the health behavior survey, which showed more favorable reports for 11 preventive health behavior by the over 60-year subgroup, showed no differences between the age groups for questions regarding the representation or the procedures used for coping and appraisal for each of the six diseases studied: heart attack, hypertension, colon cancer, lung cancer, dementia, and colds. This was true for a series of "abstract" questions asking for judgments of attributes of the representations, such as feelings of personal vulnerability, time perceptions (time to develop, to prevent, or to control), or judgments of the severity of these diseases, including their disruptiveness of daily activities and potential for shortening life. Older respondents saw themselves as more vulnerable to high blood pressure and more susceptible to serious complications from colds. While both responses are concordant with medical reality for elderly patients, these were the only 2 significant effects in 60 statistical comparisons, which clearly need replication. Finally, older and younger respondents were equally confident about their appraisals of self-effectance—that is, their ability to perform protective behaviors—and their appraisal of the diseases as preventable and curable, and they were virtually identical in their appraisal of the efficacy of each of the 15 possible actions for preventing these six diseases (Prohaska et al., 1985).

The above findings were confirmed in a home interview study. It explored the representation of 20 different illnesses for 174 respondents in four age groups from 20 to 75 years and older (E. Leventhal, 1984). To reduce the length of the interview, half the respondents answered questions for each of ten illnesses (Set A: alcoholism, appendicitis, arthritis, lymphatic cancer, cold, colon-rectal cancer, depression, diabetes, emphysema, heart attack; Set B: hypertension, lung cancer, measles, pneumonia, poison ivy, rabies, dementia, stroke, TB, ulcer). Once again, we found no differences among the ratings of the four age groups for the following areas: representation (causes, consequences, identity, time-line, controllable); coping (rehabilitation, treatment); appraisals (hopeful, curable, preventable). For a total of 400 ratings (20 ratings for each of 20 diseases), there were only 7 differences: the two middle-aged groups gave somewhat higher ratings for the more serious illnesses on a "disability scale," and older respondents gave lower ratings of "caused by aging" to high blood pressure, lung cancer, and colds.

Responsiveness to symptoms across age cohorts. Because the data described above reflect responses to relatively abstract questions, we wondered whether our age groups might differ in their reactions to questions focusing on more concrete issues; for example, the interpretation of specific symptoms as signs of disease. Thus, while older persons might be no more likely to report feelings of vulnerability that are highly abstract, they might be more likely to interpret concrete events and everyday symptoms as signs of serious illness. Because people pay attention to concrete symptoms for relatively brief periods of time, they may be stimulated to act when they observe symptoms—hence their reports of higher levels of health behavior— while retaining their beliefs in their invulnerability to serious illnesses. Six groups of respondents in the health behavior survey (the study conducted at a shopping mall) were asked to indicate whether each of 16 symptoms could be considered a warning sign of one of six diseases. The data showed that, in comparison with their younger compatriots, older respondents were less likely to see weakness and aches as signs of illness; these were the two symptoms most readily mistaken for aging. But the older respondents did not differ from the younger in their responses to 14 other symptoms as possible signs of illness, and, once again, the results may be due to chance and should be treated only as suggestive.

A similar effect appeared in the hypertension treatment study: Younger patients (under 50) attributed more symptoms to high blood pressure than did patients in the 50 to 59 age group or patients over 60 years (Leventhal et al., n.d.). Given that older persons are typically more symptomatic than younger persons, it is reasonable to conclude that older people in treatment are less interested in monitoring symptoms as signs of disease. Thus the available data contradict the suggestion that increased vigilance among the elderly is caused by increased attentiveness or monitoring of symptoms or a greater readiness to attribute symptoms to deadly diseases.

The symptom data and reports on feelings of vulnerability suggest that differences in age do not have a dramatic effect on representations of illness, at least not on the more cognitive aspect of common-sense views of illness. Common sense does recognize, however, that chronic diseases are diseases of aging. Thus cancers, heart conditions, strokes, dementia, and so on are correctly seen as more likely among the elderly than the middle-aged or young (Keller, Leventhal, Prohaska, & Leventhal, 1989). This view is shared across age cohorts from 20 to 60 and older. It does not appear, however, that this cultural "stereotype" of illness can account for the higher level of preventive behaviors and treatment adherence in older cohorts as the stereotype includes the assumption that chronic illnesses are relatively uncontrollable, a view that also is shared across age cohorts. In sum, the absence of differences between age cohorts with regard to the representation of diseases, the interpretation of symptoms, or the culture-wide stereotype of chronic illnesses as uncontrollable diseases of aging offers no simple explanation for the increase in preventive behaviors and treatment adherence in older when compared with middle-aged or younger cohorts.

Emotional aspects of the vigilance hypothesis. As cognitive factors (representation, coping, and appraisal) could not readily account for the vigilant health behavior of the elderly, we examined their emotional reactions to potential and current disease threats. As our initial hypothesis, we proposed that, while the elderly are *no* more likely to feel personally vulnerable to illness or to interpret symptoms as signs of illness, they are more vigilant because these cognitive factors provoke more worry and/or emotional upset about the possibility of illness.

The above hypothesis was sharply disconfirmed by the data: In all of our samples, both healthy community-dwelling adults and patient populations and older cohorts as compared with middle-aged and younger cohorts showed fewer signs of emotional distress in response to threats of illness. For example, when the respondents in our shopping center health behavior survey rated their likely emotional reactions to the threats of heart attack, hypertension, colon cancer, lung cancer, senility, and colds, respondents in the oldest cohort felt they would be less angry and frightened should they get sick with any one of these illnesses (Prohaska et al., 1985). The data from the home interview study gave still stronger support for this effect (E. Leventhal, 1984); for example, respondents' ratings of their emotional reactions (anger, shame) to the possibility of contracting each of 20 different illnesses (cancers, diabetes, and so on) showed dramatic, linear declines in emotional response as we moved from younger cohorts to the older cohorts (the mean changes ranged from 1.5 to 2.5 scale points on 7-point scales). Ratings of fear were also lower for older than younger subjects for diseases such as alcoholism dementia and arthritis but *not* for the cancers. These age-related changes in ratings of emotional response were not due to a response set because there were no changes for illnesses such as colds and ulcers that would not be expected to show these age-related declines.

The data on our patient samples were in clear agreement with that for our community samples and in disagreement with the hypothesis that increased compliance in older persons was due to stronger emotional reactions, such as fear or worry, to disease. Data from the hypertension treatment study (Leventhal et al., n.d.) provided only a single clue in this area as we did not query our hypertensives about a wide range of emotional reactions to illness and treatment. An item on anger was included to tap responses to the complex and sometimes annoying routine that is involved in hypertension treatment (hypertension is also presumed to be exacerbated by anger). This item showed significant differences among the age groups: 52%, 33%, and 26% of the patients reported anger, respectively, in the under 50, 51 to 59, and 60 and older age groups.

Data from our longitudinal cancer study revealed still more dramatic and consistent declines in emotional reactions to chemotherapy treatment with age (Coons, Leventhal, Nerenz, Love, & Larson, 1987). Compared with younger patients, older persons reported less anxiety at beginning treatment and less worry, distress, and disruption during treatment; in some instances, the lower ratings occurred only for patients over 70 years of age. A somewhat more surprising aspect of the data was the evidence of fewer drug-induced side effects in the older patients (Nerenz, Leventhal, Easterling, & Love, 1986). In addition, there were dramatic differences among the age groups for three specific side effects: postdrug nausea, postdrug vomiting, and conditioned or "learned" nausea, that is, nausea and vomiting that are elicited by the sight of the hospital, hypodermic needles, and so on (Nerenz et al., 1986), an effect also reported by Morrow (1982, 1984) and Andrykowski, Redd, and Hatfield (1985). The data for conditioned nausea are particularly impressive, declining from a high of 59% for patients under 50 years, through 45% and 28%, respectively, for patients 50 to 59 and 60 to 69, to only 15% in the over 70 group. These differences are striking given that older and younger persons were on the same doses for the same treatment regimens. In summary, older respondents report more frequent health actions and are clearly more compliant when in treatment. But there are no data to suggest that they represent illnesses in a more threatening manner, are more likely to interpret symptoms as signs of illness, have stronger faith in the preventability of diseases or the effectiveness of preventive actions, or believe themselves to be more self-effectant, that is, more able to perform these actions. And there is absolutely no evidence to support the hypothesis that they are more vigilant because they are more fearful, angry, or worried about these health threats. Whatever their imperfections, these studies give little comfort to our original or our revised vigilance hypothesis.

Procedures for minimizing threat and emotional distress. How can we reconcile the apparently contradictory findings showing that, in comparison with younger persons, older persons are cognitively no more concerned with threats to health and are emotionally less responsive to these threats, yet, at the very same time, engage in more preventive actions and are clearly more adherent when in treatment? Do these contrasting effects reflect different mechanisms? Or is it possible that both the decrease in emotional responsiveness and the increase in the frequency of preventive health action reflect a common mechanism?

One frequently mentioned possibility is that older people are simply less involved, hence less emotional, than younger folks and, therefore, more passive and/or prone to ignore events. With the passage of years, they may disengage from the hurly-burly of daily life (Atchley, 1971; Cumming & Henry, 1961) and become more fatalistic and unable to control events and may respond, therefore, with less vigorous emotion. On the other hand, there may be a decline in emotional responsiveness due to a decline in the vigor of the biological system: Diener and Emmons (1985) report a general decline in the intensity of emotional experience with age. A second possibility is that the age-related decline in physical strength and an accumulation of sensory and orthopaedic defects may also encourage older persons to misattribute most physical changes to aging. Thus symptoms of illness may be mistaken for symptoms of age.

While the above hypotheses can account for the reduced emotionality of the elderly and for the less rapid seeking of care for symptoms attributed to age (Prohaska, Keller, Leventhal, & Leventhal, 1987), they are inconsistent with the findings that older persons are more active in taking preventive actions and more adherent when in treatment.

This suggests yet another possibility, which is that older persons may be both more motivated—that is, more risk averse—and more skilled in controlling both illness and emotion. Intense emotional reactions can be exhausting and induce feelings of fatigue, depression, and helplessness. If older persons are more sensitive to the limitations of their energy reserves and the increased time needed to recover from stress and illness, they may be more highly motivated to avoid both the real danger posed by health threats and the emotional distress and exhaustion accompanying these threats. Younger persons, on the other hand, may experience more motivational conflict: Given objective knowledge of health threats, they may be motivated to take protective action but, at the same time, may be fearful and/or anxious about taking such action if the action (and contact with the health care system) might confirm the presence of a life-threatening and untreatable disease. The above analysis suggests that elderly persons may embed both emotion and illness in a common and unified cognitive framework; that is, they view both as debilitating and threatening events that are best dealt with by a common procedure—taking immediate action to control the potential health danger—while middle-aged people have the energy and reserve to maintain a separation between the threat of disease and their fear of it and to prevaricate because of the latter.

Active Coping to Reduce Risk and Stress

Data from the previously mentioned study at the shopping mall provided an important clue respecting the hypothesis that both emotion and illness may be embedded in a unified set of cognitions for older persons. The data showed that older persons reported stronger motivation to control emotional reactions ("I avoid too much emotional distress," "I avoid feelings like anger, anxiety, and depression," "I take things as they come and don't struggle," and "I stay mentally alert and active"; Prohaska et al., 1985). This finding implies that older persons may well be motivated and may have learned how to reduce the intensity of their emotional reactions to avoid both the momentary dysphoria of intense negative affects and the longer-term sense of exhaustion and illness that accompanies extended states of intense arousal. If elderly persons are risk averse and energy conserving, it would account for the high level of preventive behaviors reported by the oldest cohort in the health behavior survey, the relatively low frequencies of thoughts about quitting treatment among older patients receiving chemotherapy in the longitudinal cancer study, and the lower frequency of stopping treatment and noncompliance with medication among older cohorts in the hypertension study. Indeed, for patients under treatment, the strategy appears to include decreased attention to those symptoms that may be stressful reminders of one's current state of illness. Given that older persons may be less emotional for many other reasons, such as the disease being "on time," threatening fewer remaining years of life, and being less disruptive of life goals, new evidence is needed that bears directly on this hypothesis.

Active coping in a clinic sample. The results of one of our recent studies on delay in seeking medical care provided direct support for the active coping hypothesis. It suggested that the reduced levels of emotional responsiveness in older persons may well be a product of more efficient procedures for controlling both emotion and illness that generate a swifter and less conflicted seeking of health care in response to symptoms of questionable seriousness. The participants in this clinic study were interviewed at the time they appeared for an appointment at a general medical clinic. Two samples of patients were interviewed: 80 were 40 to 55 years of age, and 80 were 65 years and older. The first section of the interview determined whether the current visit was spontaneous and self-generated or a physician-determined follow-up. If the most recent visit was in the latter category, the interview reviewed the history of the problem and focused on the initial, spontaneous visit for that problem.

Once a self-generated visit was defined, its history was examined in detail. To ease the recall process, the interview began with the point at which the individual contacted the medical clinic. The questions focused upon the individual's symptoms, his or her interpretation, and his or her feelings and coping procedures at that point in time. The questions then backtracked to the point in time at which the individual had decided he or she had a medical problem and again asked about coping procedures and emotional reactions. The last set of questions focused upon the very first physical sensations and changes at the onset of the episode, the initial coping procedures (talked to someone, self-treated, waited, and so on), and the emotional responses at this early point. The questions allowed us to score three types of delay: total delay, the period from initial notice of change till a call was made to the clinic and its two subdivisions; appraisal delay, the time from first notice of symptoms to the decision that the problem was of a health or medical nature; and illness delay, the time from the decision that one was ill to calling for a clinic appointment (see Safer et al., 1979; Suchman, 1965).

We first examined the relationship between the total delay and the nature of the symptom experience and the patient's age cohort. This analysis showed that all respondents, regardless of age, sought care quickly when symptoms were severe and of sudden onset and less quickly when symptoms were mild. In addition, the older patients delayed less than the middle-aged patients for both the most and the least severe symptoms. When symptoms were of intermediate severity—that is, not so severe as to demand immediate attention but not so mild as to be ignored—the younger cohort delayed more than seven times as long as the older group. It appeared that older patients were less able to tolerate ambiguity and sought care to reduce it.

Our second set of analyses strengthened the above interpretation in two ways. First, the differences in delay in seeking care for symptoms of intermediate and ambiguous severity was most pronounced for the illness delay period, that is, the time from the decision that one has a health problem until calling for an appointment for care. Middle-aged persons delayed more than older persons for intermediate severity symptoms after they decided they had a medical problem; illness delay for the two groups was identical for the most and the least severe symptoms. The middle-aged respondents not only delayed longer in this stage for problems of moderate seriousness than did the elderly respondents but also delayed longer for these moderately serious, uncertain symptoms than they delayed for symptoms they clearly regarded as mild. Moreover, prior research has shown that delay in this period is significantly correlated with anxiety about diagnosis and treatment (Safer et al., 1979), suggesting that anxiety and distress were the source of the delay.

Second, when asked if they had delayed and why, the pattern of responses was consistent with the hypothesis that middle-aged respondents delayed because they were fearful that something serious might be happening. Whereas both the older and the younger cohorts were equally likely to admit to delay for mild problems, the older cohorts did not report delay for severe or ambiguous symptoms, while the middle-aged cohort more frequently reported delay because of fear the problem might be serious. In sum, the over-65 cohort adopted an efficient coping procedure for minimizing both objective threat and uncertainty and emotional distress (Leventhal, Cameron, Leventhal, Schaefer, & Easterling, in preparation).

Misattribution of symptoms to aging—a passive procedure. It would be a mistake to assume that being older is always associated with representations of illness and coping procedures that lead to swift use of health care. Earlier, we mentioned the existence of the "wait and see" procedure, a temporal strategy for interpreting the meaning of symptoms. Kart (1981) hypothesized a specific variant of this passive, wait and see approach to self-diagnosis involving the attribution of symptoms to age instead of to illness. Changes that occur slowly and that are more common with advancing age appear more likely to be attributed to basic alterations in the physical self rather than to temporary, symptomatic changes defined as illness.

There is now evidence for the existence of an attribution strategy that links the interpretation of bodily sensations or symptoms to age. Data in our health behavior survey showed older respondents were less likely to regard weakness and aches as signs of illness, presumably because these symptoms could be seen as signs of aging. Similar patterns appeared in our studies of patients in cancer chemotherapy treatment, where symptoms such as weakness and tiredness appeared to be more distressing to younger than to older patients (Nerenz, Leventhal, et al., 1986; Nerenz, Love, et al., 1986).

Two studies specifically designed to test the misattribution hypothesis (Prohaska et al., 1987) make clear that older persons are indeed somewhat more likely to attribute symptoms to age than to illness, and this attribution delays help seeking regardless of the age of the person who makes it. In one of the studies, respondents ranging in age from 20 to over 60 were randomly assigned to read and evaluate one of four brief "symptom scenarios." One of the scripts described a set of severe symptoms of sudden onset, another described very mild symptoms with sudden onset, and a third described the same mild symptoms and indicated they had come on over a period of several weeks. After reading the descriptions of the symptoms, subjects were asked how they would feel if such an event had happened to them, what they would do about it, and whether they would think the symptoms described would be caused by or related to aging. The results were simple: The symptoms that were mild and of slow onset were somewhat more likely to be seen as signs of aging, and older respondents were somewhat more likely to make this attribution than were younger respondents. When the aging attribution was made, it led subjects to project that they would likely be less upset and less quick to seek medical help. These effects were most clear when a severe symptom was given an aging cause.

As the above findings are from a simulation—that is, the data are taken from reports by well persons guessing how they might act—it was important to look for the same effect in the clinic study reported earlier. Within both the older and the younger cohorts, symptoms that were mild and of slow onset were more likely to be seen as signs of aging than signs of illness. Moreover, the attribution was more frequent among the older than the younger patients, and, when it was made, delay increased, and the increase occurred for both older and younger persons. But, while attributions to aging slow care for both age groups, the older respondents still sought care more swiftly; that is, these are independent, "main" effects. Thus consciously attributing symptoms to aging slows the vigilant coping response typically seen in older persons.

FINAL COMMENTS

We have proposed a complex model for self-regulation in the face of threats to illness. But, complex though it may be, it is also clear we are but at the beginning of the task of specifying the processes involved in the construction of illness representations and identifying the procedures used for coping with illness. Moreover, much work remains to specify more carefully the conditions (personal, biological, and social) responsible for the construction of specific types of representations and the development and use of specific procedures for coping and appraisal. In particular, while the evidence increasingly points to an efficiency procedure for coping with illness among the elderly, it would be a mistake to conclude that this procedure is a consequence of aging per se. This procedure could be more common among older respondents because people who failed to adopt such a strategy suffered an earlier demise. Thus our elderly sample could be a group of survivors who always behaved in an efficient manner.

It is at this point that our approach can be most readily differentiated from that typically practiced in medical/social epidemiology. Where the epidemiologist is concerned with differences in the rates of illness and the rates of health and illness behaviors in different populations—for example, the elderly as compared with the middle-aged and young—our focus is on the psychological mechanisms or algorithms underlying the behavioral differences. Our goal is to define a system by identifying the attributes of representations and procedures for coping and appraisal and to understand how the system works. The epidemiological question is concerned with the prevalence of different representations and procedures in different populations; for example, the efficiency process may be more or less common at different ages and may vary in prevalence across cultures and in the same culture across time. But, once having identified a procedure, our preference is to study its development over time and identify the biological and social factors that generate the experiences needed for its formation rather than studying its distribution over different populations. Prevalence data would be helpful but not essential in this task.

Thus, while epidemiological work is critical to understanding the relationship of behavior to disease in different subpopulations, and, therefore, the formation of policy goals, it is not likely by itself to achieve one of the major objectives of our current work, which is the generation of content and procedures for packaging information to persuade individuals to protect themselves against specific health threats. If we address and answer the questions regarding processes and procedures, we will have the basic raw material needed to develop educational protocols that will convince both older and younger persons of the need to initiate and maintain behaviors that will optimize their potential for remaining alive and vigorous. In short, if we can increase our understanding of how people process information and generate representations, coping responses, and appraisals of health threats, and determine how these constructive processes change with age, we will be provided with a perspective for understanding the dynamic processes involved in changing knowledge, attitudes, and action. We believe that a greater understanding of health and illness behaviors across the life course will contribute to the health and functioning of people at all ages.

REFERENCES

Anderson, J. R. (1983). *Architecture of cognition*. Cambridge, MA: Harvard University Press.

Andrykowski, M. A., Redd, W. H., & Hatfield, A. K. (1985). Development of anticipatory nausea: A prospective analysis. *Journal of Consulting and Clinical Psychology, 53*, 447-454.

Atchley, R. C. (1971). Retirement and leisure participation: Continuity or crisis? *The Gerontologist, 11*, 13-17.

Bandura, A. (1977). Self efficacy: Toward a unifying theory of behavioral change. *Psychological Review, 84*, 191-215.

Baumann, L. J., Cameron, L. D., Zimmerman, R. S., & Leventhal, H. (1989). Illness representations and the symmetry of labels and symptoms. *Health Psychology, 8*, 449-469.

Baumann, L. J., & Leventhal, H. (1985). "I can tell when my blood pressure is up: Can't I?" *Health Psychology, 4*, 203-218.

Belloc, N., & Breslow, L. (1972). Relationship of physical health status and health practices. *Preventive Medicine, 1*, 409-421.

Berkanovic, E., Telesky, C., & Reeder, S. (1981). Structural and social psychological factors in the decision to seek medical care for symptoms. *Medical Care, 19*, 693-709.

Bishop, G. (1987). Lay conceptions of physical symptoms. *Journal of Applied Social Psychology, 17*, 127-146.

Blumhagen, D. (1980). Hyper-tension: A folk illness with a medical name. *Culture, Medicine, and Psychiatry, 4*, 197-227.

Brody, E. M., & Kleban, M. H. (1983). Day-to-day mental and physical health symptoms of older people: A report on health logs. *The Gerontologist, 23*, 75-85.

Cacioppo, J., & Petty, R. (Eds.). (1983). *Social psychophysiology.* New York: Guilford.

Cameron, L., Leventhal, E. A., Leventhal, H., & Schaefer, P. (in submission). *Am I ill? Do I need help?: An analysis of the decision process.*

Carver, C. S., & Scheier, M. F. (1982). Control theory: A useful conceptual framework for personality-social, clinical, and health psychology. *Psychological Bulletin, 92*, 111-135.

Clark, D., & Teasdale, J. (1982). Diurnal variation in clinical depression and accessibility of memories of positive and negative experiences. *Journal of Abnormal Psychology, 91*, 87-95.

Coons, H., Leventhal, H., Nerenz, D., Love, R., & Larson, S. (1987). Anticipatory nausea and emotional distress in patients receiving ciplatin-based chemotherapy. *Oncology Nursing Forum, 14*, 31-35.

Croyle, R. T., & Hunt, J. R. (1990, August). *Coping with health threat: Social influence processes in reaction to medical test results.* Presented in the form of a poster session, "Social Influence Process in the Cognition Appraisal of Health Threat," at the annual convention of the American Psychological Association, Boston.

Croyle, R. T., & Jemmott, J. B., III. (in press). Psychological reactions to risk factor testing. In J. A. Skelton & R. T. Croyle (Eds.), *The mental representation of health and illness.* New York: Springer-Verlag.

Cumming, E., & Henry, E. W. (1961). *Growing old: The process of disengagement.* New York: Basic Books.

Dent, O., & Goulston, K. (1982a). A short scale of cancer knowledge and some sociodemographic correlates. *Social Science and Medicine, 16*, 235-240.

Dent, O., & Goulston, K. (1982b). Community attitudes to cancer. *Journal of Biosocial Science, 14*, 359-372.

DeVita, V. T. (1983). Opening remarks. In R. Yanicih (Ed.), *Perspectives on prevention and treatment of cancer in the elderly* (pp. 1-4). New York: Raven.

Diener, E., & Emmons, R. A. (1985). The independence of positive and negative affect. *Journal of Personality and Social Psychology, 47*, 1105-1117.

Evans, R. I. (1976). Smoking in children: Developing a social psychological strategy of deterrence. *Preventive Medicine, 5*, 122-127.

Horwitz, A. (1978). Family, kin and friend networks in psychiatric help-seeking. *Social Science Medicine, 12*, 297-304.

Isen, A., Shalker, T., Clark, M., & Karp, L. (1978). Affect, accessibility of material in memory and behavior: A cognitive loop? *Journal of Personality and Social Psychology, 36*, 1-12.

Janz, N., & Becker, M. (1984). The health belief model: A decade late. *Health Education Quarterly, 11*, 1-47.

Kahneman, D., & Tversky, A. (1973). On the psychology of prediction. *Psychological Review, 80*, 237-251.

Kanfer, F. H. (1977). The many faces of self-control, or behavior modification changes its focus. In R. B. Stuart (Ed.), *Behavioral self-management: Strategies, Techniques and Outcomes.* New York: Brunner-Mazel.

Kart, C. (1981). Experiencing symptoms: Attribution and misattribution of illness among the aged. In M. R. Haug (Ed.), *Elderly patients and their doctors.* New York: Springer-Verlag.

Kasl, S. V., & Cobb, S. (1966). Health behavior, illness behavior, and sick role behavior: Part 1. Sick role behavior. *Archives of Environmental Health, 12*, 53-541.

Keller, M., Leventhal, H., Prohaska, T., & Leventhal, E. A. (1989). Beliefs about aging and illness in a community sample. *Research in Nursing and Health, 12*, 247-255.

Kelley, H. H. (1972). The process of causal attribution. *American Psychologist, 28*, 107-128.

Lau, R. R., & Hartman, K. A. (1983). Common sense representations of common illnesses. *Health Psychology, 2*, 167-185.

Lazarus, R. S. (1982). Thoughts on the relations between emotion and cognition. *American Psychologist, 37*, 1019-1024.

Lazarus, R. S., & Folkman, S. (1984). *Stress, appraisal, and coping.* New York: Springer-Verlag.

Lazarus, R. S., & Launier, R. (1978). Stress-related transactions between person and environment. In L. A. Pervin & M. Lewis (Eds.), *Perspectives in international psychology.* New York: Plenum.

Leventhal, E. A. (1984). Aging and the perception of illness. *Research on Aging, 6*, 119-135.

Leventhal, E. A. (1986). The dilemma of cancer in the elderly. In J. Varth & J. Meyer (Eds.), *Cancer and the elderly: Frontier on radiotherapy and oncology* (pp. 1-13). Basel: Karger.

Leventhal, H. (1970). Findings and theory in the study of fear communications. *Advances in Experimental Social Psychology, 5*, 119-186.

Leventhal, H. (1976). Comments on the study of smoking and the study of special subcultures and cancer. In J. W. Cullen, B. H. Fox, & R. N. Isom (Eds.), *Cancer: The behavioral dimensions.* New York: Raven.

Leventhal, H. (1982). The integration of emotion and cognition: A view from the perceptual motor theory of emotion. In M. Clark & S. Fiske (Eds.), *Affect and cognition: The 17th Annual Carnegie Symposium on Cognition* (pp. 121-156). Hillsdale, NJ: Lawrence Erlbaum.

Leventhal, H. (1987). Symptom reporting: A focus on process. In S. McHugh & M. T. Vallis (Eds.), *Illness behavior, a multi-disciplinary model: Proceedings of the Second International Conference* (pp. 219-237). New York: Plenum.

Leventhal, H., Cameron, L., Leventhal, E. A., Schaefer, P., & Easterling, D. V. (in preparation). *Cohort differences in coping with health threats: Differential delay in coping with health threats.*

Leventhal, H., & Diefenbach, M. (in press). The active side of illness cognition. In J. A. Skelton & R. T. Croyle (Eds.), *Mental representation in health and illness.* New York: Springer-Verlag.

Leventhal, H., Easterling, D., Coons, H., Luchterhand, C., & Love, R. (1986). Adaptation to chemotherapy treatments. In B. L. Andersen (Ed.), *Women with cancer: Psychological perspectives.* New York: Springer-Verlag.

Leventhal, H., & Hirschman, R. (1982). Social psychology and prevention. In G. Sanders & J. Suls (Eds.), *Social psychology of health and illness* (pp. 183-226). Hillsdale, NJ: Lawrence Erlbaum.

Leventhal, H., Meyer, D., & Nerenz, D. (1980). The common sense representation of illness danger. In S. Rachman (Ed.), *Medical psychology* (Vol. 2, pp. 7-30). New York: Pergamon.

Leventhal, H., & Nerenz, D. (1983). A model for stress research with some implications for the control of stress disorders. In D. Meichenbaum & M. Jaremko (Eds.), *Stress reduction and prevention* (pp. 5-38). New York: Plenum.

Leventhal, H., & Nerenz, D. (1985). The assessment of illness cognition. In P. Karoly (Ed.), *Measurement strategies in health* (pp. 517-554). New York: John Wiley.

Leventhal, H., Nerenz, D., & Leventhal, E. (1982). Feelings of threat and private views of illness: Factors in dehumanization in the medical care system. In J. Singer & A. Baum (Eds.), *Advances in environmental psychology: Vol. 4. Environment and health* (pp. 85-114). Hillsdale, NJ: Lawrence Erlbaum.

Leventhal, H., Nerenz, D., & Steele, D. (1984). Illness representations and coping with health threats. In A. Baum & J. Singer (Eds.), *A handbook of psychology and health* (Vol. 4, pp. 219-252). Hillsdale, NJ: Lawrence Erlbaum.

Leventhal, H., & Scherer, K. (1987). The relationship of emotion to cognition: A functional approach to a semantic controversy. *Cognition and Emotion, 1,* 3-28.

Leventhal, H., Singer, R., & Jones, S. (1965). Effects of fear and specificity of recommendations upon attitudes and behavior. *Journal of Personality and Social Psychology, 2,* 20-29.

Leventhal, H., Steele, D., & Gutmann, M. (n.d.). [Longitudinal trial for compliance to hypertension treatment]. Unpublished data.

Leventhal, H., & Tomarken, A. J. (1986). Emotion: Today's problems. In M. R. Rosenzweig & L. W. Porter (Eds.), *Annual Review of Psychology, 37,* 565-610.

Leventhal, H., van Nguyen, T., & Leventhal, E. A. (1985). Reactions of families to illness: Theoretical models and perspectives. In D. Turk & R. Kerns (Eds.), *Health, illness, and families: A life-span perspective* (pp. 108-145). New York: John Wiley.

Leventhal, H., Watts, J., & Pagano, F. (1967). Effects of fear and instructions on how to cope with danger. *Journal of Personality and Social Psychology, 6,* 313-321.

Libow, L., & Sherman, F. T. (1981). *The core of geriatric medicine*. St. Louis: C. V. Mosby.

Meyer, D., Leventhal, H., & Gutmann, M. (1985). Common sense models of illness: The example of hypertension. *Health Psychology, 4*, 115-135.

Morrow, G. R. (1982). Prevalence and correlates of anticipatory nausea and vomiting in chemotherapy patients. *Journal of National Cancer Institute, 68*, 484-488.

Morrow, G. R. (1984). Clinical characteristics associated with the development of anticipatory nausea and vomiting in cancer patients undergoing chemotherapy treatment. *Journal of Clinical Oncology, 2*, 1170-1176.

Nerenz, D. R., Leventhal, H., Easterling, D. V., & Love, R. R. (1986). Anxiety and drug taste as predictors of anticipatory nausea in cancer chemotherapy. *Journal of Clinical Oncology, 4*, 224-233.

Nerenz, D. R., Love, R. R., Leventhal, H., & Easterling, D. V. (1986). Psychosocial consequences of cancer chemotherapy for elderly patients. *Health Services Research, 20*, 961-976.

Pennebaker, J. (1982). *The psychology of physical symptoms*. New York: Springer-Verlag.

Prohaska, T. R., Keller, M. L., Leventhal, E. A., & Leventhal, H. (1987). Impact of symptoms and aging attribution on emotions and coping. *Health Psychology, 6*, 495-514.

Prohaska, T. R., Leventhal, E. A., Leventhal, H., & Keller, M. L. (1985). Health practices and illness cognition in young, middle-aged, and elderly adults. *Journal of Gerontology, 40*, 569-578.

Reichel, W. (Ed.). (1978). *Clinical aspects of aging*. Baltimore: Williams & Wiltens.

Riley, M. W. (1979). *Aging from birth to death*. Washington, DC: American Association for the Advancement of Science.

Robberson, M. R., & Rogers, R. W. (1988). Beyond fear appeals: Negative and positive persuasion appeals to health and self-esteem. *Journal of Applied Social Psychology, 18*, 277-287.

Robinson, D. (1971). *The process of becoming ill*. London: Routledge & Kegan Paul.

Rogers, R. W. (1983). Cognitive and physiological processes in fear appeals and attitude change: A revised theory of protection motivation. In J. Cacioppo & R. Petty (Eds.), *Social psychophysiology*. New York: Guilford.

Rosen, T. J., Terry, N. S., Leventhal, H. (1982). The role of esteem and coping in response to threat communication. *Journal of Research in Personality, 16*, 90-107.

Rosenberg, S. (1988). Self and others: Studies in social, personality and autobiography. In L. Berkowitz (Ed.), *Advances in experimental social psychology* (Vol. 21, pp. 57-92). New York: Academic Press.

Rotter, J. B. (1966). Generalized expectancies for internal versus external control of reinforcement. *Psychology Monogram, 80*, 609.

Safer, M., Tharps, Q., Jackson, T., & Leventhal, H. (1979). Determinants of three stages of delay in seeking care at a medical clinic. *Medical Care, 17*, 11-29.

Schacter, S., & Singer, J. E. (1962). Cognitive, social and physiological determinants of emotional state. *Psychological Monographs, 69*, 379-399.

Schiffrin, R. N., & Schneider, W. (1977). Controlled and automatic human information processing II: Perceptual learning, automatic attending and a general theory. *Psychological Review, 84*, 127-90.

Schultz, R., & Rau, M. T. (1985). Social support through the life course. In S. Cohen & S. L. Syme (Eds.), *Social support and health*. New York: Academic Press.

Skelton, J. A., & Croyle, R. T. (Eds.). (in press). *Mental representation in health and illness*. New York: Springer-Verlag.

Steele, D. J., & Gutmann, M. C. (1983). *Accomplishing symptomatic representations of hypertension treatment encounters*. Paper presented at the annual meeting of the Society for Applied Anthropology, San Diego, CA.

Steele, D. J., & Leventhal, H. (1982). *Achieving patient mis-education: An ethnography of hypertension treatment encounters*. Paper presented at American Psychological Association Meeting, Washington, DC.

Suchman, E. A. (1965). Stages of illness and medical care. *Journal of Health and Social Behavior, 6*, 114.

Sutherland, A. M. (1967). Psychological observations in cancer patients. *International Psychiatry Clinics, 4*, 75-92.

Verbrugge, L. M. (1989). Gender, aging, and health. In K. S. Markides (Ed.), *Aging and health: Perspectives on gender, race, ethnicity, and class* (pp. 23-78). Newbury Park, CA: Sage.

Wallston, K. A., & Wallston, B. S. (1982). Who is responsible for your health? The construct of health locus of control. In G. S. Sanders & J. Suls (Eds.), *Social psychology of health and illness* (pp. 65-95). Hillsdale, NJ: Lawrence Erlbaum.

Weinstein, N. (1988). The precaution adoption process. *Health Psychology, 8*, 355-386.

Weisman, A. D. (1976). Early diagnosis of vulnerability in cancer patients. *American Journal of the Medical Sciences, 271*, 187-197.

Wood, J. V., Taylor, S. E., & Lichtman, R. R. (1985). Social comparison in adjustment to breast cancer. *Journal of Personality and Social Psychology, 49*, 1169-1183.

6

Coping with Chronic
Illness and Disability

H. ASUMAN KIYAK
SOO BORSON

Over the past 50 years, the profile of illness in the developed world
has shifted from acute disease, with its definitive outcomes of cure or
death, to chronic disease, with waxing and waning symptoms and
more or less lengthy periods of life with impaired function. Cultural
conceptions of the patient's role have been correspondingly rede-
fined. Patients with acute disease must do little more than submit to
the ministrations of time and the professional healer. Patients who are
chronically ill, on the other hand, are faced with a task of considerably
greater complexity. They must develop an ongoing partnership with
health care professionals; they must learn to manage certain symptoms on their own; often, they must make major changes in long-term
goals, in their use of time, and in life-style. Patients with chronic
illnesses must sometimes sacrifice cherished roles, status, income,
and independence to the process of staying alive, which they can no
longer take for granted. During acute exacerbations of disease, these
patients must turn to professional health care providers and cope
with episodic needs for dependence on the health care system. It is in
this context—the long-range adaptation to chronic disease—that the
notion has arisen that behavior may decisively affect the outcomes of
illness. Researchers and clinicians have become increasingly interested in understanding the nature of responses to chronic disease
and in using such understanding to develop interventions that might
alter the course of disease.

AUTHORS' NOTE: This work was supported by a grant from the National Institute
on Aging, Grant No. R01 AG04070, and by the Veterans Administration.

DEFINING COPING

"Coping" may be conceptualized as the sum of adaptive responses that are activated by stressful life events, which mediate their effects on psychological adjustment and well-being. Haan (1974), emphasizing coping as a process, proposed that successful coping encompasses the presence of a compelling stimulus (the stressor), the possibility of behavioral choices, and several psychological competencies. The implication is that coping cannot occur in the absence of a stimulus or stressor. However, the notion of "anticipatory" coping or "coping styles" suggests that people do have a tendency to cope in a particular manner, selecting from a repertoire of coping responses. Competencies include the capacity to change one's mind (flexibility), the capacity to recognize and adhere to the demands of reality (courage and the relative absence of cognitive distortion), and the capacity to express affect (emotional responsiveness). Coping may include preventive actions to avoid a stressful event, and preparation by anticipating an unavoidable event or rehearsing responses to it, to reduce its impact (Cohen & Lazarus, 1979). Cohen and Lazarus described "anticipatory coping" as the characteristic way in which people adapt to and modify their environment. For example, it has been hypothesized that a terminal illness allows caregivers and others in the patient's social network to prepare for the impending death through "anticipatory grief." However, it is not clear whether such preparation ultimately reduces the grief and emotional strain associated with the death (Fulton & Gattesma, 1980; Herriott & Kiyak, 1981).

The ways in which stressors, psychological attributes, and situational conditions combine in a given individual who is faced with a specific stressor at a particular time may be said to define a coping "style." This composite adaptive "fingerprint" has been conceptually related to the outcome of acute medical and surgical events (Cohen & Lazarus, 1979).

FUNCTIONS OF COPING

Coping reactions generally serve two functions: They solve a problem that has produced stress for the individual (e.g., a life event, a role loss or gain, a chronic "hassle"), and they reduce the emotional and physical discomfort that accompanies stressful situations. That is, coping is both a task and a strategy (Hamburg, 1974). Coping responses have been categorized as problem focused and emotion focused (Folkman & Lazarus, 1980; Lazarus & Folkman, 1984). It has been suggested that coping must fulfill both problem-solving and emotion-regulating functions in order to alleviate stress. When the individual focuses only on solving the problem *or* only on dealing with the emotional distress that it creates, the result is often incomplete and costly to his or her well-being.

For example, suppose that an individual responds to the diagnosis of lung cancer by denying it. While this response no doubt reduces emotional distress, the avoidance of emotional reactions may decrease the necessary motivation for treatment and lessen family help mobilized through shared grief. In some situations, people may need to deal first with the anxiety produced by a stressful situation to be able to respond to the problem itself. For example, upon learning that a close friend has a terminal illness, one must first cope with the shock and helplessness that the news creates. Only then can rational decisions be made about what to do to help the dying friend through the last months or weeks of life. In other situations, problem-solving tactics must precede any efforts to deal with feelings. For example, when one happens upon the scene of a serious accident, one first takes action to care for injured people. It may not be until much later that the individual allows his or her emotions to be expressed. In most stressful situations, however, emotion-focused and problem-focused coping take place simultaneously, and the individual must deal with his or her emotions throughout the course of trying to solve the problem.

COGNITIVE ASPECTS OF COPING

Vigilance Versus Avoidance

An early, simple model of coping, proposed by Lazarus and colleagues (Cohen & Lazarus, 1979; Lazarus, 1966; Lazarus & Launier, 1978), dichotomizes coping strategies into vigilance (i.e., heightened attentiveness to details of a stressful situation and seeking information to master it) and avoidance (a tendency to minimize threat by avoiding information that might heighten anxieties). Both may be used in anticipation of an event; they may also be used concurrently and after the problem has abated. Janis (1958/1974) first suggested that vigilant anticipation could enhance coping through repetitive rehearsal of a stressful life event before it happens. Empirical studies of the effect of vigilant coping on the outcome of a discrete stressor (e.g., surgery) have yielded conflicting results. Some investigators have found that efforts to master the situation through information result in less postoperative pain and faster recovery (Egbert, Battit, Welch, & Bartlett, 1964; Janis & Mann, 1977), whereas others have found that vigilance is associated with longer postoperative stays and minor complications (Cohen & Lazarus, 1973). Cohen and Lazarus found no effects of age on coping style in their study of young and middle-aged adults (ages 21 to 60); older individuals were not included in their research.

Lazarus and Folkman (1984) suggested that the effectiveness of vigilance or avoidance as coping styles depends on the situation. For example, avoidance may be more appropriate for patients in a hospital environment, where passivity and dependence are expected. In contrast, avoidance behavior may be maladaptive among outpatients coping with a chronic disease for which useful interventions exist, because avoidance may interfere with necessary collaboration with a health care provider. Others have noted that vigilance and avoidance are both effective strategies but at different stages of a stressful event (Roth & Cohen, 1986). In a review of this literature, personality characteristics such as trait anxiety and need for control have been found to be important intervening variables (Johnston, 1986). Thus patients with high trait anxiety and less self-efficacy or perceived control over their environment tend to cope better by avoiding information about the stressful situation. In a meta-analysis of 43 studies of avoidant or vigilant coping with specific events, Suls and Fletcher (1985) concluded that there was little intrinsic evidence of the superiority of one coping style over the other. Avoidance was associated with better outcomes in the short run, but vigilance resulted in more favorable long-term results.

Cognitive Appraisal

While it is obvious that major losses such as sudden bereavement are generally experienced as significant stressors, the stressfulness of lesser adversities and of day-to-day problems depends on their meaning for the individual. That is, it is important to note that not all humans perceive the same events to be stressful. For example, Lazarus and DeLongis (1983) suggested that cognitive appraisal (i.e., the way in which a person perceives the significance of an encounter) is a major determinant of the event's stressfulness. Cognitive appraisal can minimize or magnify the importance or stressfulness of an event according to the meaning attached to it. If the individual construes the situation as benign or irrelevant, it will not elicit coping responses. If, on the other hand, the individual appraises a situation as challenging, harmful, or threatening, it becomes a stressor and, accordingly, mobilizes adaptive responses. In this model, a stressor is individually determined or defined (McCrae, 1984; Pearlin & Schooler, 1978). Furthermore, one may be able to categorize certain experiences as normative for young and old. Stressors that are normative for an older person may be perceived as less disturbing just because they are expected and do not challenge the individual's self-concept. Chronic illness is more likely to be normative in older persons; therefore, the older person's array of coping responses would be expected to be different than those used by a younger person.

Emotional Valence

Whether a stressor is assessed as positive (i.e., a challenge) or negative (i.e., a threat or loss) is likely to affect how an individual responds to it. For example, an older woman who moves voluntarily to a retirement home may view it as an exciting and much-needed change in her life-style, or she may interpret the change as a major loss that disrupts the quiet continuity of her life and signifies helplessness. In the former case, she may adapt readily and experience no distress; in the latter, she may become clinically depressed. If, however, she views the move as insignificant and expects it to place few demands on her, she may be unpleasantly surprised by the level of stress that she eventually encounters, no matter how minimal.

DIMENSIONS OF COPING

Research into the nature of responses of people with chronic disease has generally relied on self-report measures, using one of several coping scales in the literature. These scales have been developed on the basis of the authors' conceptual models of coping. However, empirical approaches to the systematic study of coping styles and strategies show some commonalities, despite differences in the conceptual models on which they are based. Lazarus and colleagues (Lazarus, Cohen, Folkman, Kanner, & Schaefer, 1980; Lazarus & Folkman, 1984; Lazarus & Launier, 1978) classified coping into four styles: (a) action-oriented behaviors, which include active avoidance, escape, attack, and seeking allies; (b) cognitive or knowledge-seeking behaviors; (c) wish-fulfilling fantasy; and (d) intrapsychic (defensive or accommodative) strategies. The work of Vitaliano, Russo, Carr, Maiuro, and Becker (1985) with the 68-item Ways of Coping Checklist (Folkman & Lazarus, 1980) supports a factor structure similar to that of Folkman and Lazarus, although two of the original factors did not emerge in this study. The dimensions of the revised 39-item scale are (a) problem focused, (b) seeking social support, (c) self-blaming, (d) wishful thinking, and (e) avoidance.

Moos's (1977) classification system, developed with specific reference to coping with physical illness, resembles that of Lazarus and colleagues but elaborates several more behavioral strategies. Coping styles identified in Moos's system include (a) denying or minimizing the seriousness of the problem (as well as projection, suppression, isolation, or dissociation of emotions); (b) seeking relevant information; (c) seeking emotional support and reassurance from others by joining special support groups (e.g., organizations formed by victims of a particular disease and their families); (d) setting goals; (e) rehearsing alternate outcomes of the problem; and (f) searching for a generalized purpose or meaning of the event. Billings and Moos (1981) subsequently revised this classification scheme. A set of 32 coping responses have been analyzed and categorized as appraisal focused (i.e., logical attempts to understand the stressor and its consequences), problem focused (either information seeking or problem solving), and emotion focused (either regulation of stress-related emotions or behavioral expressions of unpleasant emotions).

Kahana and Kahana (1982), studying the impact of institutional relocation, posited four major styles of coping: (a) behavioral or instrumental, (b) intrapsychic, (c) affective, and (d) pathological (including withdrawal, aggression, and hypochondriasis). A subsequent study by Kahana, Kahana, and Young (n.d.) revealed three dimensions in their 22-item coping scale. Labeled (a) instrumental, (b) affective, and (c) escape, these were found to be associated with various outcomes among institutionalized elderly. Instrumental coping was predictive of good health and survival following placement in a nursing home, whereas affective coping had negative consequences. Elderly persons using the latter strategy tended to have lower morale, poorer health, and a higher likelihood of death within three years than did persons using instrumental strategies.

A sociological perspective on coping is provided by the work of Pearlin and Schooler (1978), whose dimensions were derived from a study of the origins of personal stress among 2,300 adults under age 65. Styles were analyzed from responses to open-ended questions about life stress. Factor analyses revealed 17 coping dimensions, 5 of which closely resemble those described above. These dimensions are primarily cognitive and behavioral responses that an individual might use to prevent, avoid, or control stress. They take the form of distinct strategies of coping: (a) working to change the situation, (b) seeking advice, (c) working to control the stress, (d) selectively ignoring the situation, and (e) controlling feelings of stress.

In their studies of coping patterns among middle-aged and elderly adults with chronic illnesses, Felton and colleagues (Felton & Revenson, 1984; Felton, Revenson, & Hinrichsen, 1984) used a questionnaire that included 55 coping responses adapted from the Ways of Coping Checklist (Folkman & Lazarus, 1980) and from Pearlin and Schooler's research (1978). Factor analyses revealed six dimensions, which parallel several categories proposed by the coping theorists described above: (a) cognitive restructuring, (b) emotional expression, (c) wish-fulfilling fantasy, (d) self-blame, (e) information seeking, and (f) minimizing threat. A summary of the dimensions of coping that are common across these studies is presented in Table 6.1.

AGE DIFFERENCES IN COPING

The question of whether coping styles change with age has not been extensively researched. Not only is there a paucity of longitudinal research in this area, but even the few available cross-sectional studies of coping among young and middle-aged persons have generally not reported age differences (Billings & Moos, 1981; Folkman & Lazarus, 1980). Pfeiffer (1977) articulated a widely held view that older persons are more rigid in their thinking than are younger persons and are, therefore, more likely to use a limited range of coping responses, typified by withdrawal, denial, and anxiety. However, the research of Kahana and Kahana (1982), with older people who move to institutions, and Kahana, Kahana, and Young (n.d.), among people with chronic heart disease, does not support this view; their work suggests that older people use a diverse range of coping styles. Similarly, Griffith (1983) found that women aged 55 to 65 in stressful situations use a variety of coping responses. Empirical studies of normal elderly subjects (McCrae & Costa, 1985) show that the capacity for flexible responses to stress is retained into advanced old age.

The work of Felton and colleagues (Felton & Revenson, 1984; Felton et al., 1984; Revenson & Felton, 1985) showed that differences in coping responses among patients stressed by chronic disease are related

Table 6.1
Major Empirical Studies of Coping: Common Dimensions

Authors	Problem focused	Emotion focused	Wish fulfilling	Minimizing threat	Others
Perlin & Schooler (1978)	(1) Change situation (2) Seeking Advice	(1) Control stress (2) Control feelings	—	Selectively ignoring	—
Folkman & Lazarus (1980; Ways of Coping Checklist)					
Jalowiec & Powers (1981)	Problem oriented	Affective[a]	—	—	—
Billings & Moos (1981, 1984; Health and Daily Living Form)	Problem focused	Emotion focused	—	Avoidance	Appraisal focused
Felton, Revenson, & Hinrichsen (1984)	Information seeking	Emotional expression	Wish-Fulfilling	Minimizing threat	(1) Cognitive restructuring (2) Self-blame
Kahana, Kahana, & Young (n.d.; Elderly Care Research Center Coping Scale)	Instrumental	Affective	—	Escape	—
Vitaliano et al. (1985; Revised Ways of Coping Checklist)	Problem focused	—	Wishful thinking	Avoidance	(1) Seek social support (2) Self-blame

a. Some items defined as *affective coping* in this scale have been described as *affective coping* or *avoidance* by other investigators.

148

to specific demands of the illness, illness beliefs, and characteristics of the person but not to age. Most patients, young or old, were found to mobilize coping behaviors that were well suited to the stressor and effective in reducing distress. Research with moderately impaired patients with Alzheimer's disease (Kiyak, Montgomery, Borson, & Teri, 1985), a disorder that directly affects the "organ of coping," demonstrates a restriction in the normal range of coping strategies as well as a tendency to use more primitive coping styles such as denying or ignoring the problem. Age per se does not appear to be a factor. Taken together, data from these studies support the conclusion that the majority of older people appear capable of using a wide repertoire of coping responses and can call upon the most appropriate responses for a given situation. Only in the presence of a significant mental disorder or cognitive impairment should older persons be expected to show diminished effectiveness and breadth of coping responses.

Nevertheless, several studies have suggested that coping styles undergo a natural development across the life span. In a longitudinal study of male Harvard graduates, Vaillant (1977) described a change in coping strategies as the men reached middle age. His findings suggested that people become better copers as they age and are less inclined than in their younger years to distort reality as a means of controlling the stressfulness of events.

McCrae (1982) tested both Pfeiffer's and Vaillant's hypotheses on a sample of 255 healthy men and women aged 24 to 91 in one study, and 150 persons aged 21 to 90 in another study, as part of the Baltimore Longitudinal Studies of Aging, and he found some support for Vaillant's hypothesis. Comparing groups cross-sectionally, McCrae found that older respondents (aged 65 to 91) and middle-aged respondents (aged 50 to 64) reported patterns of coping that differed substantially from those reported by young adults (aged 24 to 40). Older subjects were less likely than younger subjects to endorse coping styles of blaming (either self or others), to resort to escapist fantasy, or to use hostile responses. They were also less likely to use humor and cognitive reappraisal to create an optimistic attitude. Similar results were reported by Irion and Blanchard-Fields (1987) in their cross-sectional study of self-reported coping by adolescents (mean age 15.5), young adults (mean age 20.1), and middle-aged (mean age 43.9) and older adults (mean age 66). Age differences were apparent in all coping strategies in both threat and challenge situations. Middle-aged and older respondents endorsed fewer strategies related to hostile reaction, escape avoidance, and self-blame than did younger respondents. Older persons tended to use more adaptive coping responses than either of the younger groups. These two studies suggest that normal aging is generally accompanied by more mature coping responses and a greater capacity to tolerate negative affective states without losing resilience in the face of stress.

In a study of 75 younger couples (aged 35 to 45) and 141 retired persons (aged 65 to 74), Folkman, Lazarus, Pimley, and Novacek (1987) found that older respondents consistently used more passive, intrapersonal, emotion-focused coping responses, whereas younger respondents were more likely to use active, interpersonal, and problem-focused coping. These differences were consistent across diverse life events and hassles. However, in coping with health problems, the patterns were reversed; in these situations, older persons tended to use confrontive coping more than any other response.

The work of Leventhal and colleagues (reported elsewhere in this book) supports the findings of Folkman and colleagues. In their assessment of 396 persons attending a health fair, these investigators (Prohaska, Leventhal, Leventhal, & Keller, 1985) found more health-promoting practices and avoidance of harmful habits among the oldest respondents. They labeled these people as more vigilant and responsive in preventive coping. In another study of 257 hypertensives aged 40 to 75, Leventhal, Steele, and Gutmann (n.d.) found the best adherence to medication and other physician regimens among patients aged 60 and older, followed by the 50- to 59-year-olds, and the least adherence by people under age 50. It thus appears from this research that people who survive to advanced old age tend to practice more preventive health behaviors and are more likely to adhere to therapeutic regimens than younger persons.

McCrae (1984) found that the meaning of a stressor to the individual (whether the event was defined as a loss, a threat, or a challenge) consistently and significantly affected the choice of coping mechanisms, regardless of the respondent's age. For example, events identified as losses resulted more often in expressions of faith or of feelings for people of all ages, whereas challenges were met with rational action, perseverance, positive thinking, and restraint; these responses were just as likely in older as in young persons coping with similar events. Herein lies a possible explanation for these conflicting findings regarding the influence of age on coping style. The nature of stressful life events changes across the life span; normative stressors in old age differ markedly from normative stressors in youth. For example, the death of a spouse and chronic personal illness are much more likely to occur and to be expected in later life than in young adulthood. It may be these different situations and older persons' appraisals of them, rather than any age-related changes in coping style per se, that account for differences reported in samples of different ages (Folkman & Lazarus, 1980; Siegler & George, 1983). In other words, because the situations are different, the same events evoke different arrays of coping responses at different ages. The recent work of Folkman and associates (1987) provides some support for this interpretation.

It is reasonable to consider whether biological changes associated with the aging process may have a predictable influence on coping. Although research is scarce, one may ask whether normal age-related changes in sensory function, memory, reaction time, stamina, and speed of recovery from physical injuries alter the choice of coping responses selected by an individual in a stressful situation. One might expect a change in the strength or time course of older persons' reactions, both behavioral and emotional. On the other hand, an older person may be expected to have a wider repertoire of coping styles than a young person, because of greater experience with diverse life events and repeated practice in coping with major stressors such as the day-to-day management of serious chronic illness.

But these same losses that could enhance the range of coping for older people may prevent them from employing other coping responses such as the use of social resources. Previously available social supports may no longer exist; one's spouse and confidants may have died; children may have relocated to other communities or become estranged. A survey of 1,841 people over age 60 (Clark, 1982) supported the importance of social resources in the effectiveness of older persons' coping skills. Respondents who reported greater availability of help from family and friends also rated their personal coping effectiveness to be higher than elderly persons lacking such resources.

PERSONALITY AND COPING

Some researchers have suggested that certain personalities are associated with specific coping styles (Geringer & Stein, 1986). The idea of discrete personality types implies differentiable and more or less stable repertoires of preferred coping responses that characterize an individual across the life span. Furthermore, everyday experience suggests that we can predict quite accurately how friends or relatives are likely to respond to a hypothetical stressful event. In other words, we can generally guess *how*, and *how well*, they are likely to cope, because we know their "character," or behavioral characteristics over time.

Despite its intuitive appeal, however, there is little research evidence to support this notion. Shapiro (1965), in his classic monograph on pathological personality types, described characteristic stress responses of patients with obsessive-compulsive, paranoid, hysterical, and impulsive personality types, based on clinical observations. Later work (e.g., Horowitz, 1976) demonstrated how some stress responses may be modified by stable, global personality characteristics.

Neuroticism is one personality trait that may be related to coping style. Costa and McCrae (1980) found that men aged 17 to 97 who scored high on a test of neuroticism were more likely to view all problems as crises and to worry more about their general health and health habits. Age was not associated with health concerns. Recognizing that this group represented a healthy sample of men, one would expect even more difficulty in coping with disease among chronically ill neurotics. This is consistent with previous studies of hypochondriasis and neuroticism (Gianturco & Busse, 1978; Tessler & Mechanic, 1978).

Apart from personality per se, certain attitudes have been successfully correlated with some aspects of coping (see Rodin & Timko, this volume). This has been tested widely with the variable "locus of control," or an individual's beliefs about his or her role in shaping the outcome of stressors. People who believe they have a major role in determining the outcome of stressful life events (i.e., those having an "internal locus of control") appear to adjust more successfully to novel situations than those who see themselves as the passive recipients of environmental stressors (i.e., those with an "external locus of control"; Thomae, 1980). Gutmann (1974, 1977) broadened this concept in describing styles of mastery in response to stressors. The person with a passive mastery style does not feel powerful enough to influence his or her fate directly, whereas one with an active mastery style tends to rely more on personal abilities, to depend less on others for direction, and to feel less helpless.

Felton and Kahana (1974) found that "external locus of control," defined as the belief that institutional staff were in control of what went on in a long-term care facility, was associated with better adjustment among residents of homes for the aged. They suggested that externally oriented elderly were more likely to accept the constraints of institutional living because doing so was consistent with their general beliefs about environmental control.

A subsequent study by Cicirelli (1987) tested this hypothesis in an acute care hospital. Using the Multidimensional Health Locus of Control scale, they measured the locus of control and determined the hospital adjustment of 105 patients aged 60 to 93 with ratings by staff nurses. Consistent with the findings of Felton and Kahana among long-term care residents, those elderly in the acute care settings who believed that powerful others control health outcomes perceived less constraint in the hospital environment. Those who perceived the environment to be constraining were not as well adjusted as the elderly with an external locus. Wolk (1976) suggested that the degree of constraint existing in an institutional setting interacts with locus of control. In this study, adjustment was equally good for externals and internals in a high-constraint retirement home, but internality was a better predictor of adjustment in a low- constraint retirement home.

PSYCHOPATHOLOGY AND COPING

The presence of psychopathology has been found to influence coping responses. Several studies have evaluated statistical samples of patients by selecting subjects with clinical depressive disorders for research on psychopathology and coping style. For example, the research of Moos and Billings (1982), Billings, Cronkite, and Moos (1983), and Foster and Gallagher (1986) consistently found differences in response to a coping inventory between persons diagnosed as depressed and those without a psychiatric disorder. Billings and colleagues (1983) categorized coping into three general styles: appraisal focused, problem focused, and emotion focused. They found that depressed patients (mean age 41) were less likely than nondepressed patients to use problem-solving strategies and more likely to use emotional discharge, which is one subset of emotion-focused strategies. The study by Foster and Gallagher (1986), using similar domains of coping, also found these differences between depressed and nondepressed elderly subjects (with mean ages of 72 and 73, respectively). Depressed older persons were more likely than nondepressed elders to resort to emotional discharge and avoidance behaviors. Depressed elders were also less likely to rate any coping response as helpful in resolving their problems.

SITUATION-SPECIFIC COPING

Many studies have found that certain situations, particularly those having major implications for future functioning, evoke common responses. For example, people with a spinal cord injury (Bulman & Wortman, 1977) or cancer (Weisman & Worden, 1976-1977) display common early emotional responses: shock, denial, and, often, anger at the illness or disability. Such emotional responses occur so predictably after a major negative life event as to be essentially normative. It is not clear whether they should be viewed as a formal part of an individual's coping repertoire or simply as an emotional component of the recognition that a tragic event has occurred. This recognition, a cognitive experience, is essential in laying the groundwork for future coping efforts, but the emotional response may not be. A similar example of consistency of response to a stressful life event is the group of coping processes used in adapting to the news of one's impending death. This model, first conceptualized by Kubler-Ross (1969), consists of five stages that may occur more or less sequentially and that represent different constellations of emotional coping responses. There has been little systematic research with this model. Therefore, although Kubler-Ross presented a rational approach to the process of coping with death, it is unclear how much individual and cultural variations affect this process.

The development of a nonfatal chronic disease represents a stressor less acute than a catastrophic injury or diagnosis. Revenson and Felton (1985) described the characteristic stresses related to four different chronic diseases. It is not surprising that the nature and severity of illness-related stress varied substantially as a function of the specific disease process. In a subsequent publication (Felton et al., 1984), illness characteristics were found to influence the choice of coping strategy, although demographic variables and illness beliefs were more powerful predictors than the nature of the disease itself. This work is reviewed in detail below.

COPING WITH CHRONIC DISEASE

Adaptation to chronic disease is a multifaceted, interactive, and changing task that the patient shares with both personal caregivers (usually members of the family) and professional providers of health services. Each participant brings to the process his or her own set of biases, values, and expectations, many of which are implicit and not clearly articulated. The complexity of the network of individuals involved in managing serious, incurable, and often progressive chronic diseases requires that an analysis of indicators of coping should address each of these several perspectives. For the patient, coping is reflected in maintaining a personal balance between the damaging effects of disease on overall well-being and the destructive effects of its management on life satisfaction. From the viewpoint of the physician, coping is reflected in compliance with a medical regimen that has been tested empirically, and impersonally, in groups of patients more or less similar to this one. For the family caregiver, coping is reflected in the patient's capacity to live with the illness with appropriate degrees of dependence and distress, without jeopardizing the interpersonal relations between the patient, his or her caregiver, and the physician.

Another feature of coping with chronic illnesses among older people is the likelihood of multiple chronic conditions. That is, many people who survive to advanced old age do so with a litany of major diseases, such as arthritis and diabetes and hypertension. Few studies have examined the effects of coping with multiple chronic diseases and/or disabilities simultaneously. Based on our earlier discussion about the effects of practice or experience on subsequent coping, one may conjecture that previous experience in coping with chronic illness can lead to better management of the disabling effects of these diseases and less emotion-focused coping. Instrumental strategies useful in managing a chronic illness (e.g., compliance with medication, exercise, and dietary recommendations) may be more readily undertaken by an older person, who has had time to experience their benefits with other illnesses and has had years of experience with these multiple conditions, than by a younger person newly diagnosed with a chronic illness.

Descriptive Approaches to Evaluating
Coping in Patients with Chronic Disease

As stated earlier, coping may be assessed through self-reports in interviews or paper-and-pencil measures, through physiological measures, or through observations of the individual in specific stressful situations. However, most studies of coping among chronically ill patients have obtained self-reports of coping responses to specific aspects of the illness. For example, Streltzer, Moe, Yanagida, and Siemsen (1983) interviewed 25 patients, ranging in age from 16 to 65, who had end-stage renal disease and who had experienced kidney transplant failure. Based on their open-ended responses to questions about how they were coping with the disease, patients were classified as deniers or grievers. The authors found no differences between the two coping styles in the outcome measures of self-reported depression or adjustment to dialysis. Age differences were not reported.

In another study of hemodialysis patients, Baldree, Murphy, and Powers (1982) interviewed 35 adults aged 21 to 60 (mean age 42) who were undergoing hemodialysis treatment. Patients were asked to describe their coping responses to 29 stressors associated with dialysis, using a scale developed by Jalowiec and Powers (1981). The most frequently used coping styles were hope, maintaining control, prayer, worry, and acceptance. Avoidance or relying on others to solve the problem were least often reported by these patients. Problem-oriented coping was more prevalent than affective coping. No age differences emerged on the total number of stressors or coping measures or on subscales of stressors and coping. However, the length of time on dialysis did influence the types of stressor described.

Similar results were obtained by Jalowiec and Powers (1981) in their study of 25 newly diagnosed hypertensives and 25 emergency room patients aged 20 to 60. Both types of patients reported a predominant use of problem-oriented coping strategies. In particular, attempts to maintain control, to learn more about the situation, and to find alternative means of managing the problem were more often reported than affective or avoidance strategies. Correlations between age and coping style were nonsignificant.

In a study of 89 chronically ill patients aged 18 to 65 who were experiencing a range of disease conditions (e.g., circulatory, metabolic, cardiac, respiratory, or genitourinary disorders), Viney and Westbrook (1982) obtained patients' self-reported strategies of coping. Their measure of coping included six clusters: action, control, escape, fatalism, optimism, and interpersonal coping strategies. The associations between demographic characteristics, life-styles, illness roles, and coping strategies were examined. Education and occupation were associated with the use of fatalism (inversely) and with action (directly). Age interacted with education and occupation to predict the use of fatalism, but age was not significantly associated with any other coping variable. Neither disease nor "objective" degree of disability predicted most coping styles, but patients' perceptions of their handicaps were related to the likelihood of using some strategies. For example, those who perceived their problem as more handicapping in its effects on their function and relationships were more likely to be fatalistic and less likely to be optimistic. Objective disability did relate to the use of control strategies; patients with less disability felt they could control the disease more.

In contrast, other researchers found significant relationships between repressive or defensive coping styles and the nature of the disease with which the patient was coping. For example, Kneier and Temoshok (1984) found that patients aged 40 to 65 with malignant melanoma differed from patients with cardiovascular disease and a healthy comparison group in the same age range. A physiological measure of stress was obtained by assessing electrodermal activity in response to anxiety-provoking statements in an experimental situation; the intensity of the electrodermal response was compared with the amount of anxiety the respondents reported experiencing. A high electrodermal response without a high degree of anxiety defined a pattern labeled *repressive coping*. Melanoma patients showed more repressive coping than the other two groups. It should be noted, however, that, in this study, only repressive coping styles were measured. Furthermore, patients' reactions in an experimental procedure were examined, not their coping strategies with respect to the illness. This study found no age differences. This appears to be a pattern in many studies examining coping with chronic illnesses; age differences are generally not significant or are part of an interaction effect. Thus, within the range examined in these studies (often middle-aged to young-old respondents), age does not influence the range of coping responses to chronic diseases.

COPING WITH ALZHEIMER'S DISEASE: THE EFFECTS OF A PROGRESSIVE BRAIN DISEASE

Alzheimer's disease is an example of a currently incurable disease for which no form of treatment has yet shown reliable benefits. An examination of patients with Alzheimer's disease can illustrate the multifaceted nature of coping and the degree to which coping with a chronic disease involves several elements of a social system. In addition, it provides unique opportunities to assess the effects of cognitive deterioration on coping abilities and on the biology of stress responses. Borson et al. (1989) examined sympathetic nervous system arousal in patients with Alzheimer's disease and normal controls during response to a cognitive challenge. Alzheimer's patients, unlike controls, tended to appraise the cognitive tasks as not very stressful and to evaluate their own performance as better than it was.

During the tasks, which included a simple test of attention (digit span) and more difficult tests of mental effort (serial subtractions), Alzheimer's patients showed blunted autonomic arousal when compared with controls. This study demonstrates the linkage between cognitive appraisal, perceived stress, and physiological response to stress.

In a recently completed study of adaptation to changes associated with Alzheimer's disease (Kiyak, 1988), we examined coping longitudinally in healthy elderly and elderly with cognitive deterioration. Over the course of three years, 59 patients (aged 59 to 82) and their primary caregivers (the majority of which were elderly spouses) were interviewed twice a year. Questions regarding how patients coped with life events, including the changes associated with Alzheimer's disease, were asked of patients and their caregivers. At the initial assessment, 57 of the patients responded to these questions, but, two years later, only 19 patients were alive and intellectually intact enough to respond. Family caregivers were also asked to describe how they coped with the day-to-day problems associated with caring for an Alzheimer's patient. Using a 34-item questionnaire derived from the work of Pearlin and Schooler (1978), Lazarus and Folkman (1984), and Kahana et al. (n.d.), described earlier in this chapter, four dimensions of coping emerged: problem focused, emotion focused, acceptance, and hopefulness.

The primary mode of coping in this sample appeared to be acceptance. This includes items such as "accepted the situation," "made the best of it," and "refused to let it get to you." Patients and caregivers alike consistently endorsed more items on the acceptance dimension of this scale than any other, both initially and two years later. Thus, for example, at the baseline interview, 75% of acceptance items were endorsed by patients and 74% by caregivers. Approximately 50% of emotion-focused items such as "becoming angry," "bitter," or "resentful" were endorsed by both patients and family members. Problem-focused coping and hopefulness were far less frequent styles for these families.

Two years later, we found surprising consistency in the tendency of patients to use acceptance-oriented coping. Even though only one third of the patients interviewed initially could still respond to the questionnaire, they were more likely to report using acceptance than any other style of coping. Thus this group endorsed 74% of the acceptance items but only 15% of the emotion-focused and problem-solving strategies. There was a slight increase in the proportion of hopefulness items endorsed by patients; they agreed with 28% of these items at baseline and with 34% at the two-year follow-up. These changes also highlight a narrowing of the range of coping styles employed by elderly persons as they experience greater cognitive deterioration. There appears to be a loss of active coping responses such as problem solving, information seeking, and expressing emotion. These patients became more passive in their choice of coping responses. This is consistent with the increased passivity of behavior that is often associated with Alzheimer's disease.

An interesting pattern emerged in family members' responses. It should be noted, first, that most respondents were caregivers of moderately impaired patients. There was an increase in the proportion of acceptance items endorsed by caregivers, from 79% initially to 88% at the two-year interview, as one might expect. At the same time, however, there was a notable increase in hopefulness, from 45% initially to 65% two years later. In the follow-up interview, emotion-focused coping remained at about 50% and problem-focused coping was moderately used. The tendency to continue using a variety of coping styles among these caregivers, the majority of whom were over age 65, suggests that aging per se does not necessarily diminish one's coping repertoire, even when the situation with which the older person copes becomes less hopeful.

These findings that show widespread acceptance are not surprising given the chronic and irreversible nature of Alzheimer's disease. Acceptance is probably an effective form of coping with the cognitive deterioration associated with this disease. Our findings regarding emotion-focused coping for both groups are consistent with previous studies, which have shown that emotional reactions often give way to problem solving or acceptance in dealing with major life events. However, the corresponding increase in hopefulness among family members of moderately impaired patients was unexpected. It may be that caregivers become more optimistic about the disease if the patient does not show significant declines in cognitive function and behavior, as appeared to be the case in these patients who remained interviewable two years later.

These results are in some ways consistent with the findings of Segall, Wykle, Namazi, Noelker, and Bryan (1987), who interviewed Black family caregivers of Alzheimer's patients. Using a scale similar to that of Kiyak et al. (1985), Segall and colleagues found that accommodation and religious support (similar to hopefulness) were the most frequently used modes of coping among family members. Active problem-solving modes were least often used. The difference in the importance of religious coping between the two studies may reflect ethnic differences between these samples.

MEASURING OUTCOMES OF COPING WITH CHRONIC DISEASE

The disparate definitions of successful coping in the literature, and the specific behaviors they imply, suggest the multiplicity of measurable outcomes that can be used to assess coping as well as the numerous intervening variables such as situational and personal characteristics. The outcomes of coping responses can include physiological change, psychosocial growth, decline, or no change, although the type of coping response alone rarely determines the outcome. More often, an outcome depends on the interaction between the type of problem and the quality and quantity of internal and external mediators. (The role of social support per se remains controversial; e.g., Simons & West, 1984-1985.)

To illustrate these points: A patient with chronic obstructive pulmonary disease learns that he can slow the progression of tissue damage by giving up cigarettes but that the disease will progress regardless of what he does. He is likely to know from past experience that quitting smoking makes him anxious, irritable, and physically uncomfortable and may even make him cough more. His illness has already deprived him of the physical stamina he long enjoyed, and quitting smoking will now deprive him of the dependable pleasure that he has come to expect from lighting up. What should he do? If he quits, his doctor will view his behavior as adaptive and perceive him as a good patient; if he does not, the physician is likely to see his behavior as indicative of a coping failure and the patient as stubborn or irrational. In contrast, his wife knows that, when he quits, he will be unpleasant toward the grandchildren, withdrawn from her, and hard to get along with; she sees the damage as already done and wonders what is to be gained at this late date. She may see the doctor as naive and insensitive to the hardships of her husband's life, which smoking has done much to soothe. Alternatively, she may have tried for years to get her husband to quit and welcome additional pressure from the physician and the illness; in this case, she is likely to encourage her husband, praise his resolve, and help with his difficult withdrawal period by extra concern and support.

Multidimensional Indicators

Because the concept of coping contains both descriptive and evaluative elements, the use of specific but multidimensional indicators of outcome can help to reduce bias introduced by narrow definitions of coping and by implicit judgments about what kinds of outcomes of coping are desirable. In the following sections, we propose a set of multidimensional indicators of outcome relevant to assessing the quality of coping with chronic disease, and we describe how they may be used to evaluate the current state of knowledge and to target areas for future research emphasis. These outcome variables are listed in Table 6.2.

To date, most formal investigations of the outcomes of coping with chronic illness have used the respondent's self-reported emotional experiences as the dependent variable. Measures have included ratings of mood (particularly depression), self-esteem, and life satisfaction; research has not linked these to measurable illness behaviors or to the course of the disease. Further, these ratings of subjective experience have not been paired with efforts to detect the presence of a clinical psychiatric disorder, such as a major depressive episode, which markedly affects scores on mood and morale scales. As noted in the section on psychopathology and coping, clinically significant depression frequently complicates chronic illnesses (Borson et al., 1986). Although depression may result from maladaptive coping responses, it is not clear that this is always, or even usually, the case; nor is it clear that interventions directed at altering coping will usually relieve a depressive episode. Future research should take into account the fact that mood in chronically ill patients is not a simple reflection of coping style and that a particular coping style may result from depression as often as it causes it.

Measures of the activity of the disease, such as the frequency of acute exacerbations, are sometimes believed by patients and clinicians to be related to stress; to our knowledge, no studies to date have addressed the possibility that coping style can predict these measures. One study of chronically ill older adults attending a clinic (Borson et al., 1986) suggested that inappropriate patterns of health service utilization may be related to clinical depression, but this question requires further investigation to establish the size of this effect and explore the possibility that underutilization of needed services may reflect maladaptive coping. Although some studies have addressed each of the domains listed in Table 6.2, none has incorporated them as outcome variables related explicitly to coping. Such research is a reasonable next step.

Table 6.2
Outcomes of Coping with Chronic Disease

Domain	Variables[a]
Emotional experience	Mood (e.g., anxiety, depression); morale and life satisfaction;
Psychophysiological arousal	Stress hormones (e.g. cortisol, catecholamines)
Disease activity	Physiologic measures of severity (disease-specific); frequency of acute exacerbation; pace of progression
Activities of daily living	Physical self-care; social involvement; leisure activities; use of assistance from others; proportion of time spent in disease-related treatment
Adherence to the prescribed treatment regimen	Proportion of medication actually taken; medical/rehabilitation appointments kept; life-style changes to enhance function (e.g. diet, exercise, drinking, smoking)
Health service utilization	Frequency and type used; "appropriateness" (match between need and supply)
Financial costs of illness	Direct dollar costs; income lost; societal cost of third-party payments
Emergent psychiatric symptoms	Psychiatric diagnoses; symptom scales
Social role and social network function	Family function ratings; role shifts
Perceived value of life	Outlook toward the future; presence/absence, change in purpose/meaning; attitudes about survival

a. This is a partial list of variables.

In reviewing the research on chronic illness and how middle-aged and elderly adults cope with these conditions, we will attempt to examine the outcome variables selected by the researchers within the framework presented above. Table 6.3 summarizes some descriptive studies in this area and the outcome variables utilized by each one.

Relating Coping to Outcome

Several studies (e.g., Billings & Moos, 1981; Felton & Revenson, 1984; Felton et al., 1984; Weisman & Worden, 1976-1977) focused on the outcomes of coping with a chronic illness. Among their findings are that certain types of coping responses may be more effective than others (i.e., result in more positive emotional outcomes). For example, Felton and colleagues (1984) found an association between positive mood and active (cognitive) coping strategies such as cognitive restructuring and information seeking. A negative psychological state was associated with emotional coping responses such as wish-fulfilling fantasy. The duration of the chronic illness was unrelated to coping strategy. Several researchers have suggested that, when a stressor is appraised as "uncontrollable" or has no objective solution, it is more likely to elicit intrapsychic or emotional, rather than behavioral or problem-solving, approaches (Felton et al., 1984; Folkman & Lazarus, 1980; Pearlin & Schooler, 1978). Folkman and Lazarus concluded that health problems regularly evoke emotion-focused responses. However, most chronic diseases and disabilities are partially remediable, or at least manageable, by current medical interventions. We, therefore, propose that emotion-focused coping is a reasonable expectation for patients newly diagnosed with a chronic disease but that its persistence is likely to be maladaptive and to reflect either personal psychopathology or a failure of our current health care system to address behavioral aspects of chronic disease, or both.

The importance of shifting from emotion-focused to behavioral coping for caregivers as well as patients is illustrated in a study of 40 women whose husbands had been hospitalized with a myocardial infarction in the preceding year (Nyamithi, 1987). The investigator found that behavioral, cognitive, and intrapsychic responses were most common during the acute phase of this illness. Respondents indicated a high need for emotional support during their husband's hospitalization, but this need diminished during the convalescence period. Coping responses became more behavioral and were especially focused on monitoring and controlling the effects of the disease.

In a study of caregivers of patients with Alzheimer's disease, Scott, McKenzie, Slack, and Hutton (1987) examined the association between coping styles and caregiver stress. They found that problem-focused coping in the form of seeking information and soliciting of

Table 6.3
Descriptive Studies of Coping with Chronic Illness

Study	Coping definition	Method	Outcome Variables	Results
Baldree, Murphy, & Powers (1982)	Problem oriented versus affective coping	Self-reported coping among dialysis patients: 25 adults aged 21-60	None; descriptive study	Problem oriented (hope, control, prayer, acceptance) more common than affective coping
Streltzer Moe, Yangida, & Siemsen (1983)	Self-reported grief, denial	Open-ended interview of kidney failure patients after transplant rejection	Judgement of psychiatric team as adjusted, accepting	No difference between deniers and grievers
Billings, Cronkite, & Moos (1983)	Appraisal, problem focused, emotion focused	Administered questionnaires to carefully diagnosed depressed versus non-depressed adults	Correlation between mood status and coping behaviors	Nondepressed more likely to use problem solving; depressed patients used information seeking and emotional discharge

| Billings & Moos (1984) | Appraisal, problem focused, emotion focused | Interview and questionnaires to depressive patients entering treatment for depressive disorder, family members, and treatment staff | Severity of depressive symptoms, physical symptoms of stress, self-confidence | Less severe depression, fewer physical symptoms, more self-confidence in patients using logical analysis, information seeking, problem solving and emotional control strategies; emotional discharge associated with dysfunctional health behavior (smoking drinking, overeating) and with more severe depression, more physical symptoms of stress, and less self-confidence |

outside aid were associated with less self-reported stress than were emotion-focused coping styles among these caregivers.

It appears that problem-focused coping can also prevent depression among older people coping with role strains. Essex and Lohr (1986) interviewed 272 women aged 56 to 95 regarding their coping responses to five chronic strains in the areas of health, interpersonal relationships, and daily activities. Women who reported using passive cognitive coping styles (e.g., "accept poor health because it cannot be changed") were significantly more likely to be depressed, while those who coped in a positive cognitive manner (e.g., "reminds self that health is better than others her age") were less likely to be depressed. Thus, if emotion-focused coping can be categorized as a negative coping response, one would predict an association between this pattern and depression.

Using the Coping Strategies Questionnaire developed by Rosenstiel and Keefe (1983) specifically for patients with chronic pain, Rosenstiel-Gross (1986) examined self-reported coping among 48 middle-aged patients (mean age 42) who underwent lumbar laminectomies for lower back pain. She found no relationship between coping strategies and severity or type of back pain as assessed by a medical team. However, the use of two types of coping (self-reliance and loss of control) were associated with fewer self-reports of postsurgical pain and more positive ratings of surgical outcomes in this study.

FROM THEORY TO PRACTICE: TEACHING PATIENTS TO COPE WITH CHRONIC ILLNESS

It has been suggested that coping strategies may be taught to patients as a way of reducing the stressfulness of unpleasant medical procedures for a chronic condition (Hill, 1982; Izzo, 1982; Johnson, Rice, Fuller, & Endriss, 1978). The theoretical basis for such approaches has been articulated by Seligman (1975), who suggested that the acquisition of self-control by behavioral training can reduce an individual's perceptions of helplessness. A sense of mastery has intrinsic stress-reducing functions. According to this theory, patients can rehearse methods to modify distressing events associated with a treatment or with the symptoms of a disease.

These concepts were tested in a study of patients undergoing cataract surgery (Hill, 1982) in which 40 cataract patients aged 50 to

91 were randomly assigned before surgery to one of four types of preparation: (a) behavioral instructions, (b) information about sensory experiences they could expect after surgery, (c) a combination of these two, or (d) information about hospital procedures and the nature of cataracts. Using anxiety, depression, confusion, length of hospital stay, and length of time before going outside after surgery as outcome variables, Hill found no significant differences on most variables across conditions. However, the combination of behavioral and sensory information resulted in a shorter interval before patients ventured out after surgery. Age was correlated with all dependent variables, but the type of preoperative preparation used produced no differential age effects. This result may be interpreted as indicating that a coping intervention can reduce disability after surgery.

Related strategies are beginning to be examined in chronically ill patients. Izzo described an assessment guide for use by health professionals in teaching hypertensive patients to alter their behavior to promote health and prevent complications. It proposes an individualized intervention plan structured around the patient's existing coping skills. Though promising, this tailor-made approach has not yet been tested empirically.

Agle, Baum, Chester, and Wendt (1973) and Fishman and Petty (1981) investigated the effects of a multitargeted rehabilitation intervention on physical functioning, respiratory symptoms, and emotional disturbance in patients with chronic obstructive pulmonary disease. Patients were educated about their disease, taught several cognitive/behavioral strategies for managing shortness of breath, and trained, through systematic physical exercise, to tolerate activity without panic when breathing became difficult. Significant benefits of the intervention on all outcome variables were demonstrated immediately after the completion of the time-limited intervention and one year later. Unfortunately, this systematic approach to modifying patients' ability to cope successfully with their disease has not had the widespread application that its results would appear to justify.

CONCLUSIONS

Systematic research into coping with stressful life events is a relatively new empirical discipline for which a new language has had to be developed. Despite conceptual and methodological variations, coping research has made considerable progress in characterizing and measuring how people adapt to adversity. In addition, it has been possible to demonstrate that certain styles of coping can be related to the quality of adaptation and, in some instances, to the outcome of medical illness.

Research reviewed in this chapter suggests that older persons are capable of using a diverse range of coping responses. These responses are less influenced by the individual's age or personality than by his or her cognitive status and the personal meaning of an event or the person's cognitive appraisal of the situation. Generally, age differences in coping styles are minimal, although older persons appear to use more mature coping styles, to express less optimism in the face of crises, and to place less value on positive events.

It is difficult to measure patients' coping responses to a chronic illness in isolation. Their responses often interact with those of professional health care providers and family members. The types of coping dimension vary also by the nature of the chronic disease. Therefore, it is difficult to describe patterns of coping among all older persons with chronic disease. However, the results of some empirical studies described in this chapter suggest that emotion-focused coping is more common initially, with increasing use of problem-oriented coping styles such as cognitive restructuring and information seeking as the day-to-day problems of the disease emerge. Patients who continue to resort to affective coping experience more problems emotionally and may be more likely to become depressed than those who employ more problem-focused coping styles.

Some attempts to alter coping responses in older persons experiencing surgery or managing chronic pain, with the goal of improving treatment outcomes, have met with encouraging success. However, researchers have primarily examined psychological outcomes of coping rather than outcomes such as physiological indicators of disease progress, health status, or illness behavior. Meaningful coping research is an interdisciplinary endeavor with significant promise of producing testable behavioral interventions for enhancing outcomes in chronic disease and for improving quality of life in the later years.

REFERENCES

Agle, D. P., Baum, G. L., Chester, E. H., & Wendt, M. (1973). Multidiscipline treatment of chronic pulmonary insufficiency. *Psychosomatic Medicine, 35,* 41-49.

Baider, L., & Edelstein, E. L. (1981). Coping mechanisms of postmastectomy women: A group experience. *Israel Journal of Medical Science, 17,* 988-992.

Baldree, K. S., Murphy, S. P., & Powers, M. J. (1982). Stress identification and coping patterns in patients on hemodialysis. *Nursing Research, 31*(2), 107-112.

Billings, A. G., Cronkite, R. C., & Moos, R. H. (1983). Social-environmental factors in unipolar depression: Comparisons of depressed patients and nondepressed controls. *Journal of Abnormal Psychology, 92*, 119-133.

Billings, A. G., & Moos, R. H. (1981). The role of coping responses and social resources in attenuating the stress of life events. *Journal of Behavioral Medicine, 4*, 139.

Borson, S., Barnes, R. F., Kukull, W. A., Okimoto, J. T., Veith, R. C., Inui, T. S., Carter, W., & Raskind, M. A. (1986). Depression in elderly medical outpatients. *Journal of the American Geriatrics Society, 34*, 341-347.

Borson, S., Barnes, R. F., Veith, R. C., Halter, J. B., & Raskind, M. A. (1989). Impaired sympathetic nervous system response to cognitive activity in early Alzheimer's disease. *Journal of Gerontology: Medical Sciences, 41*, M8-M12.

Bulman, R. J., & Wortman, C. B. (1977). Attributions of blame and coping in the "real world": Severe accident victims react to their lot. *Journal of Personality and Social Psychology, 35*, 351-363.

Cicirelli, V. G. (1987). Locus of control and patient role adjustment of the elderly in acute care hospitals. *Psychology and Aging, 2*(2), 138-143.

Clark, A. W. (1982). Personality and social resources as correlates of coping behavior among the aged. *Psychological Reports, 51*, 577-578.

Cohen, F., & Lazarus, R. S. (1973). Active coping processes, coping dispositions, and recovery from surgery. *Psychosomatic Medicine, 35*, 375-389.

Cohen, F., & Lazarus, R. S. (1979). Coping with the stresses of illness. In G. C. Stone, N. E. Adler, & S. Cohen (Eds.), *Health psychology* (pp. 217-254). San Francisco: Jossey-Bass.

Costa, P. T., & McCrae, R. R. (1978). Objective personality assessment. In M. Storandt, I. C. Siegler, & M. F. Elias (Eds.), *The clinical psychology of aging*. New York: Plenum.

Costa, P. T., & McCrae, R. R. (1980). Somatic complaints in males as a function of age and neuroticism: A longitudinal analysis. *Journal of Behavioral Medicine, 3*, 245-257.

Costa, P. T., McCrae, R. R., Andres, R., & Tobin, J. D. (1980). Hypertension, somatic complaints and personality. In M. F. Elias & D. H. P. Streeten (Eds.), *Hypertension and cognitive processes*. Mt. Desert, ME: Beech Hill.

Egbert, L. D., Battit, G. F., Welch, C. E., & Bartlett, M. K. (1964). Reduction of postoperative pain by encouragement and instruction of patients. *The New England Journal of Medicine, 270*, 825-827.

Essex, M. J., & Lohr, M. J. (1986). *Chronic life strains and depression among older women: The differential effectiveness of several coping techniques*. Paper presented at the annual meeting of American Sociological Association, New York.

Felton, B. J., & Kahana, E. (1974). Adjustment and situationally bound locus of control among institutionalized aged. *Journal of Gerontology, 29*, 295-301.

Felton, B. J., & Revenson, T. A. (1984). Coping with chronic illness: A study of illness controllability and the influence of coping strategies on psychological adjustment. *Journal of Consulting and Clinical Psychology, 52*, 343-353.

Felton, B. J., Revenson, T. A., & Hinrichsen, G. A. (1984). Stress and coping in the explanation of psychological adjustment among chronically ill adults. *Social Science Medicine, 18*, 889-898.

Fishman, D. B., & Petty, T. L. (1981). Physical, symptomatic, and psychological improvement in patients receiving comprehensive care for chronic airway obstruction. *Journal of Chronic Disease, 24*, 775-785.

Folkman, S., & Lazarus, R. S. (1980). An analysis of coping in a middle-aged community sample. *Journal of Health and Social Behavior, 21*, 219-239.

Folkman, S., Lazarus, R. S., Pimley, S., & Novacek, J. (1987). Age differences in stress and coping processes. *Psychology and Aging, 2*, 171-184.

Foster, J. M., & Gallagher, D. (1986). An exploratory study comparing depressed and non-depressed elders' coping strategies. *Journal of Gerontology, 41*(1), 91-93.

Fulton, R., & Gattesma, D. G. (1980). Anticipatory grief: A psychosocial concept reconsidered. *British Journal of Psychiatry, 137*, 45-54.

Geringer, J. S., & Stern, T. A. (1986). Coping with medical illness: The impact of personality types. *Psychosomatics, 27*, 251-261.

Gianturco, D. T., & Busse, E. W. (1978). Psychiatric problems encountered during a long-term study of normal aging volunteers. In A. D. Isaacs & F. Post (Eds.), *Studies in geriatric psychiatry*. New York: John Wiley.

Griffith, J. W. (1983). Women's stress responses and coping: Patterns according to age groups. *Issues in Health Care of Women, 4*, 327-340.

Gutmann, D. L. (1974). The country of old men: Cross-cultural studies in the psychology of later life. In R. A. LeVine (Ed.), *Culture and personality: Contemporary readings*. Chicago: Aldine.

Gutmann, D. L. (1977). The cross-cultural perspective: Notes toward a comparative psychology of aging. In J. E. Birren & K. W. Schaie (Eds.), *Handbook of the psychology of aging*. New York: Van Nostrand Reinhold.

Haan, N. (Ed.). (1974). *Coping and defending*. New York: Academic Press.

Hamburg, D. A. (1974). Coping behavior in life-threatening circumstances. *Psychotherapy and Psychosomatics, 23*, 13-25.

Herriott, M., & Kiyak, H. A. (1981). Bereavement in old age: Implications for therapy and research. *Journal of Gerontological Social Work, 3*, 15-43.

Hill, B. J. (1982). Sensory information, behavioral instructions and coping with sensory alteration surgery. *Nursing Research, 31*, 17-21.

Horowitz, M. J. (1976). *Stress response syndrome*. New York: Jason Aronson.

Irion, J. C., & Blanchard-Fields, F. (1987). A cross-sectional comparison of adaptive coping in adulthood. *Journal of Gerontology, 42*(5), 502-504.

Izzo, M. (1982). Assessing the coping abilities of hypertensive patients. *Topics in Clinical Nursing, 4*(2), 33-40.

Jalowiec, A., & Powers, M. J. (1981). Stress and coping in hypertensive and emergency room patients. *Nursing Research, 30*, 10-15.

Janis, I. L. (1974). *Psychological stress*. New York: John Wiley. (Original edition published 1958)

Janis, I. L., & Mann, L. (1977). *Decision making*. New York: Free Press.

Johnson, J. E., Rice, V. H., Fuller, S. S., & Endriss, M. P. (1978). Sensory information, instruction in a coping strategy, and recovery from surgery. *Research in Nursing and Health, 1*, 4-17.

Johnston, M. (1986). Preoperative emotional states and postoperative recovery. *Advances in Psychosomatic Medicine, 15*, 1-22.

Kahana, E. F., & Kahana, B. (1982). Environmental continuity, discontinuity, futurity, and adaptation of the aged. In G. Rowles & R. Ohta (Eds.), *Aging and milieu: Environmental perspectives on growing old.* New York: Academic Press.

Kahana, E., Kahana, B., & Young, R. (n.d.). *Strategies of coping and post-institutional outcomes among the aged: A longitudinal study.* Unpublished manuscript.

Kiyak, H. A. (1988). *Adaptation among elderly persons with Alzheimer's disease* (NIA Grant No. ROI AG04070; Annual progress report). Bethesda, MD: National Institute on Aging.

Kiyak, H. A., Montgomery, R., Borson, S., & Teri, L. (1985). *Coping patterns among patients with Alzheimer's disease and non-demented elderly.* Paper presented at the meetings of the Gerontological Society.

Kneier, A. W., & Temoshok, L. (1984). Repressive coping reactions in patients with malignant melanoma as compared to cardiovascular disease patients. *Journal of Psychosomatic Research, 28*(2), 145-155.

Kubler-Ross, E. (1969). *On death and dying.* New York: Macmillan.

Lazarus, R. S. (Ed.). (1966). *Psychological stress and the coping process.* New York: McGraw-Hill.

Lazarus, R. S., Cohen, J. B., Folkman, S., Kanner, A., & Schaefer, C. (1980). Psychological stress and adaptation: Some unresolved issues. In H. Selye (Ed.), *Selye's guide to stress research* (pp. 90-117). New York: Van Nostrand Reinhold.

Lazarus, R. S., & DeLongis, A. (1983). Psychological stress and coping in aging. *American Psychologist, 38*, 245-254.

Lazarus, R. S., & Folkman, S. (1984). *Stress, appraisal and coping.* New York: Springer.

Lazarus, R. S., & Launier, R. (1978). Stress-related transactions between person and environment. In L. A. Pervin & M. Lewis (Eds.), *Perspectives in interactional psychology* (pp. 287-327). New York: Plenum.

Leventhal, H., Steele, D., & Gutmann, M. (n.d.). *Longitudinal trial for compliance to hypertension treatment.* Unpublished manuscript.

Lieberman, M. A. (1975). Adaptive processes in late life. In N. Datan & L. H. Ginsberg (Eds.), *Lifespan developmental psychology: Normative life crises.* New York: Academic Press.

McCrae, R. R. (1982). Age differences in the use of coping mechanisms. *Journal of Gerontology, 37*, 454.

McCrae, R. R. (1984). Situational determinants of coping responses: Loss, threat and challenge. *Journal of Personality and Social Psychology, 46*(4), 919-928.

McCrae, R. R., & Costa, P. T., Jr. (1985). Personality, stress and coping processes in aging men and women. In R. Anders, E. L. Bierman, & W. R. Hazzard (Eds.), *Principles of geriatric medicine.* New York: McGraw-Hill.

Moos, R. (1977). *Coping with physical illness.* New York: Plenum.

Moos, R. H., & Billings, A. G. (1982). Conceptualizing and measuring coping resources and processes. In L. Goldberger & S. Breznitz (Eds.), *Handbook of stress:Theoretical and clinical aspects.* New York: Macmillan.

Nyamithi, A. M. (1987). The coping responses of female spouses of patients with myocardial infarction. *Heart and Lung, 16*, 86-92.

Pearlin, L., & Schooler, C. (1978). The structure of coping. *Journal of Health and Social Behavior, 19*, 2-21.

Pfeiffer, E. (1977). Psychopathology and social pathology. In J. E. Birren & K. W. Schaie (Eds.), *Handbook of the psychology of aging*. New York: Van Nostrand Reinhold.

Prohaska, T. R., Leventhal, E. A., Leventhal, H., & Keller, M. L. (1985). Health practices and illness cognition in young, middle-aged, and elderly adults. *Journal of Gerontology, 40*, 569-578.

Revenson, T. A., & Felton, B. J. (1985). *Perceived stress in chronic illness: A comparative analysis of four diseases.* Paper presented at the annual meeting of the Gerontological Society of America, New Orleans.

Rosenstiel-Gross, A. (1986). The effect of coping strategies on the relief of pain following surgical intervention for lower back pain. *Psychosomatic Medicine, 48*, 229-241.

Rosenstiel, A. K., & Keefe, F. J. (1983). The use of coping strategies in chronic low back pain patients: Relationship to patient characteristics and current adjustment. *Pain, 17*, 33-44.

Roth, S., & Cohen, L. J. (1986). Approach, avoidance, and coping with stress. *American Psychologist, 41*, 813-819.

Scott, J. P., McKenzie, P. N., Slack, D., & Hutton, J. T. (1987). The role of coping behaviors for primary caregivers of Alzheimer's patients. *Texas Medicine, 83*, 48-50.

Segall, M., Wykle, M., Namazi, K., Noelker, B., & Bryan, J. (1987). *The Black family's experience with dementia.* Paper presented at the meetings of the Gerontological Society of America, Washington, DC.

Seligman, M. E. P. (1975). *Helplessness: On depression, development and death.* San Francisco: Freeman.

Shapiro, D. (1965). *Neurotic styles.* New York: Basic Books.

Siegler, I. C., & George, L. K. (1983). The normal psychology of the aging male: Sex differences in coping and perception of life events. *Journal of Geriatric Psychiatry, 16*, 197-209.

Simons, R. L., & West, G. E. (1984-1985). Life changes, coping resources, and health among the elderly. *International Journal of Aging and Human Development, 20*(3), 173-189.

Streltzer, J., Moe, M., Yanagida, E., & Siemsen, E. (1983). Coping with transplant failure: Grief vs. denial. *International Journal of Psychiatry and Medicine, 13*, 97-106.

Suls, J., & Fletcher, B. (1985). The relative efficacy of avoidant and nonavoidant coping strategies: A meta-analysis. *Health Psychology, 4*, 249-288.

Tessler, R., & Mechanic, D. (1978). Psychological distress and perceived health status. *Journal of Health and Social Behavior, 19*, 254-262.

Thomae, H. (1980). Personality and adjustment to aging. In J. E. Birren & B. Sloane (Eds.), *Handbook on mental health and aging*. Englewood Cliffs, NJ: Prentice-Hall.

Vaillant, G. (1977). *Adaptation to life.* Boston: Little, Brown.

Viney, L. L., & Westbrook, M. T. (1982). Coping with chronic illness: The mediating role of biographic and illness-related factors. *Journal of Psychosomatic Medicine, 26*(6), 595-605.

Vitaliano, P. P., Russo, J., Carr, J. E., Maiuro, R. D., & Becker, J. (1985). The Ways of Coping Checklist: Revision and psychometric properties. *Multivariate Behavioral Research, 20*, 3-26.

Weisman, A., & Worden, J. W. (1976-1977). The existential plight in cancer: Significance of the first 100 days. *International Journal of Psychiatry in Medicine, 7*, 1-15.

Wolk, S. (1976). Situational constraint as a moderator of the locus of control-adjustment relationship. *Journal of Consulting Clinical Psychology, 44*, 420-427.

7

Sense of Control, Aging, and Health

JUDITH RODIN

CHRISTINE TIMKO

It has been suggested that control-relevant processes influence physical health and that the strength of the relationship between control
and health increases with aging. This is based on two hypotheses
regarding changes that accompany old age. First, the elderly are
exposed to a variety of personal and social conditions that challenge
their sense of personal control. Second, older people are undergoing
physiological changes, which make them more vulnerable to the
effects of uncontrollable stressors or to a general loss of control.
Studies have shown that changes in options for control may affect the
emotional and physical health of people of all ages, possibly by
influencing health-related cognitions and behaviors as well as physiological processes. We propose a model in which the control-health
relation grows stronger in old age because aging and age-related
events may have direct effects on both health and perceived control.
It is also true that each of these mechanisms shows much greater
variability in later life; this too increases the potential for stronger
correlations between these variables.

THE CONTROL-AGING RELATIONSHIP

Much has been written on how and why personal control is influenced by growing old. The majority of theorists have hypothesized
that environmental and biological events decrease both perceived

AUTHORS' NOTE: Work on this chapter and the authors' studies described here
were supported by grant AG02455 from the National Institute on Aging to J. Rodin.

and actual control in old age. Rodin (1986a, 1987), for example, suggested that aging frequently lowers perceived control because many environmental events that accompany old age limit the range of outcomes that actually are attainable. These environmental factors include the loss of roles, norms, and appropriate reference groups, losses often created by major life events such as retirement and bereavement (Kuypers & Bengtson, 1973). Weisz (1983) emphasized the association between old age and a loss of actual contingency for a number of important outcomes; for instance, retirement entails a loss of contingency in the world of work, and one's health status depends less on voluntary behaviors and more on biological forces. Indeed, the biological changes that occur in late adulthood, particularly a loss of physical abilities, may induce generalized feelings of lack of control as well as actual helplessness (Rodin, 1980, 1986a, 1987; Schulz, 1980).

Yet another challenge to the older person's sense of control comes from negative stereotypes about the aging process (see Butler, 1970). Labels such as *old* and *institutionalized* connote an inferior status (Avorn & Langer, 1982). Kuypers and Bengtson (1973) argued specifically that elderly persons are quite susceptible to social labeling and that the generally negative stereotypes of aging in Western societies lead to a loss of coping abilities and to a growing sense of incompetence. Similarly, Rodin and Langer (1980) suggested that negative labeling and stigmatization encourage older people to behave in a way that confirms the stereotypes of old age and so leads to lowered self-esteem and diminished feelings of control. In a developmental analysis of self-efficacy, Bandura (1981) described the elderly as a group particularly likely to underestimate their true competence in a number of important life areas. Bandura attributed some of this underestimation to widespread social stereotypes about the aged. He also stated that older people mistakenly come to see themselves as declining intellectually and physically because they use younger groups rather than their peers as a basis for comparison.

Not only do negative stereotypes of aging influence judgments of self-efficacy, but an older person's observations of other, less competent elderly, through the media or personal contact, may lead to modeling of helpless behaviors (Bandura, 1977). Vicarious exposure to dependency and passivity is especially likely to occur in a nursing home setting, where independent activities are rarely reinforced by the staff (Baltes & Reisenzein, 1986). Within and outside of institutions, people in contact with older individuals may be apt to assist them with tasks they formerly performed for themselves. Such assistance, although well intentioned, may undermine the individual's sense of control as well as his or her task performance (Avorn & Langer, 1982; Langer & Imber, 1979).

Unidimensional Versus Multidimensional Concepts of Control

In view of these numerous hypotheses concerning a possible association between growing old and a loss of control, a number of studies have examined the relationship between age per se and people's feelings of control. Many studies in this area have used Rotter's (1966) I-E scale or modifications of it. Rotter's scale treats the locus of control orientation as a unidimensional construct, with beliefs in internal control (i.e., perceiving events as contingent on one's own behavior or personal characteristics) and external control (i.e., perceiving events as resulting from chance, as resulting from the control of powerful others, or as being unpredictable) representing opposite poles of a continuum. Using this scale, investigators found a full range of results—greater internality, greater externality, and no differences between older and younger subjects (Brown & Granick, 1983; Cicirelli, 1980; Duke, Shaheen, & Nowicki, 1974; Fawcett, Stonner, & Zepelin, 1980; Gatz & Siegler, 1981; Hunter, Linn, Harris, & Pratt, 1980; Krantz & Stone, 1978; Kuypers, 1972; Nehrke, Hulicka, & Morganti, 1980; Rotella & Bunker, 1978; Siegler & Gatz, 1985; Wolk, 1976; Wolk & Kurtz, 1975).

Lachman (1986a) and Rodin (1987) suggested that, in studies of control and aging, control may be conceptualized more usefully as a multidimensional construct because age might relate differently to different aspects of control. For example, Lachman (1986a) hypothesized that, because aging sensitizes people to the role of chance and luck in their lives, and because the aged come to see younger people as more powerful than themselves, the elderly should appear more externally oriented on the scales created by Levenson (1974), which measure beliefs that events are controlled by chance or by powerful others. At the same time, because older individuals have accumulated a vast number of mastery experiences in at least a few domains, their belief in internal control may increase. Lachman's own work (1983, 1986b) has not confirmed these hypotheses, however, and other studies using Levenson's multidimensional measure of control (e.g., Ryckman & Malikioski, 1975; Saltz & Magruder-Habib, 1982) have been no more conclusive regarding age-control relationships than studies that used unidimensional measures.

Using other approaches, some investigators have distinguished between self-efficacy and outcome expectations in an effort to elucidate a possible relationship between aging and control (Brim, 1980; Gurin, 1980; Weisz, 1983). Others have focused on studying specific domains in which control may be more or less available and important (Lachman, 1986a; Rodin, 1987).

Actual Versus Perceived Control

The studies just described may have produced inconsistent findings because some measure actual control and others measure perceived control. Taking overt action (behavioral control) without being aware of alternatives may not yield psychologically meaningful consequences. Langer (1983) argued that the person's perception of control, rather than his or her overt responses, is crucial. The distinction between actual and perceived control is an important conceptual issue, especially in the context of aging, and one that demands further empirical investigation.

Studies of the aging-control relationship may also appear contradictory and unclear because age per se does not bear a direct relationship to control expectancies. Rather, age may exert its effects by influencing the relationship between variations in personal control and psychological and physical well-being. If this were the case, we should expect to find correlations between age and the health effects of control-relevant manipulations rather than correlations between age and control per se.

CONTROL-HEALTH RELATIONSHIP IN AGING

Various evidence suggests that a personal sense of control is associated with beneficial health effects among older individuals, whereas a loss of control is related to poor health outcomes. Unfortunately, no studies have as yet directly evaluated the control-health association for subjects of different ages, but we point to the types of studies that need to be done.

Correlational Studies

Most of the studies investigating health correlates of locus of control expectancies among older adults have utilized global self-report measures of health status. Studies by Mancini (1980-1981) and

Brothen and Detzner (1983) found that "internals" reported that they were in better overall health than did "externals." Hunter and colleagues found inconsistent relationships between the locus of control and health measures, including self-report of health, disability, and degree of daily pain (Hunter, Linn, & Harris, 1981-1982; Hunter et al., 1980; Linn & Hunter, 1979). Wolk (1976) found no relationship between perceived control and overall health for subjects living in either high- or low-constraint settings.

Studies conducted by Reid and Ziegler also yielded inconsistent results; they found both positive correlations and no correlations between internality and self-reports of good health (Reid & Ziegler, 1980; Ziegler & Reid, 1979). Ziegler and Reid's (1983) study of elderly persons who relocated to a new residence suggested that locus of control was not correlated with health status 6 months after relocation, but that internals reported better health at the 18-month follow-up.

Brown and Granick (1983) and Hunter and associates (1980) examined the relationship between personal control and specific health-related behaviors and outcomes. Both studies suggested that perceptions of control were not related to the number of previous hospitalizations elderly subjects reported. Brown and Granick found that externals reported a greater number of doctor visits, but, in the Hunter study, the number of times subjects had seen a doctor in the past six months was not related to locus of control. Among Hunter's subjects, externals were more likely to be taking medications and had more problems with their hearing and eyesight, whereas Brown and Granick's external subjects had fewer hearing problems but were more likely to have high blood pressure. Both studies found that subjects' reports concerning a large variety of other health problems and illnesses (e.g., trouble with walking, headaches) were not associated with control perceptions.

Bohm (1983) tested specific health indicators for their relationship to control but added two facets that were not included in other investigations of this issue. First, she specified three different types of perceived control: overall or global control, ability to mobilize support when needed, and perception of how easily needs get met. Second, Bohm statistically controlled for the severity of subjects' actual illness status. Her data showed that people who rated high in global control were less likely to use medications or to visit the doctor. Both global and support-mobilizing control were negatively correlated with number of self-treatments but were positively related to compliance with medication regimens. Finally, perceived ease in getting one's needs met was negatively correlated with number of emergency room visits.

The evidence that internality is associated with better physical health appears relatively weak on the basis of the studies just reviewed. However, the measures of health were not consistent among studies, ranging from broad-based self-reports to experiences with specific health problems to use of the medical care system. Additionally, most studies examining health correlates of control failed to account for severity of illness, which would clearly influence health-related behaviors.

Interventions Using Control

Studies such as those described above, which involve the correlation between health and different measures of control, have suggested interesting, if only modest relationships. However, due to the fact that correlational data cannot be used to test causal hypotheses, other investigators have turned to experimental studies, usually manipulating control via a planned intervention and then assessing effects on health. In contrast to correlational studies, intervention studies with older, and usually infirm, subjects have strongly suggested that increased control benefits subjects' health outcomes.

Relocation studies. In a review and analysis of the literature on relocation of the aged, Schulz and Brenner (1977) presented a conceptual model that emphasized the importance of control and predictability in mediating the damaging effects of relocation on morbidity and mortality. The model posited that one's response to the stress of relocation is determined largely by the perceived controllability and predictability of the move as well as by differences between the pre- and postrelocation environments in terms of the degree of control afforded. Schulz and Brenner found support for their model in numerous relocation studies that commonly used mortality rate as the dependent variable.

Krantz and Schulz (1980) tested one aspect of the model proposed by Schulz and Brenner. They hypothesized that increasing the predictability of the institutional environment for people just entering a long-term care facility would counteract the psychological and physical problems typically associated with relocation. Older people recently admitted to a nursing home were randomly assigned to a control group or to one of two experimental conditions. In one, called the "relevant information condition," new residents received information designed to enhance the predictability of their institution; in the other, the "irrelevant information condition," residents received information that did not help make the environment predictable. After the intervention, subjects in the relevant information group were more likely than control group subjects to say that their physical health had improved in the past two weeks, to be judged by nurses as healthier and as having a greater zest for life, and to participate in activities requiring physical effort. On most measures, the irrelevant information group fell between the other groups and did not differ significantly from either one. Measures taken two months after the intervention found no decline in health or psychological status among subjects provided with predictability-enhancing information.

Bers, Bohm, and Rodin (as described in Rodin, 1986b) also conducted a relocation study that suggested that perceived control over the decision to relocate exerts an important influence on health outcomes. The study sample consisted of hospitalized patients over the age of 65 who were to be discharged to nursing homes within the subsequent week. Half participated in a family interaction task designed to increase feelings of control over the entry decision; the other half received no such treatment. Measures obtained at the time of hospitalization were used to predict which subjects would still be in a nursing home one year later and which subjects would have returned home by that time.

The variable that best discriminated between groups was whether or not subjects believed they had control over deciding to move to the nursing home; having control was a better predictor of ultimate return home than coping style, self-concept, or severity of illness during hospitalization. A multiple regression analysis was performed to predict subjects' health status one year after discharge from the hospital. This analysis also included a group of subjects who had gone directly home from the hospital. The best predictors of poor health status were severity of illness at the time of discharge and entrance to a nursing home following discharge. However, the third best predictor was perceived control over the decision to relocate, with greater control contributing to better health. Thus it appears that the greater the perceived choice an individual has in being relocated, the less negative the effects of the relocation on health outcomes.

Nursing home studies. A different series of field studies, conducted by Rodin and colleagues and by Schulz and colleagues, involving patients already in nursing homes for various periods of time, strongly suggest that decreased control over one's environment is also associated with negative health outcomes, while increased control is associated with positive outcomes.

Langer, Rodin, Beck, Weinman, and Spitzer (1979) randomly assigned elderly nursing home residents to one of three conditions that varied objective control to determine whether enhanced control could slow or reverse declines in memory and health. Residents in one group—the contingent condition—were visited regularly by an experimenter who asked them to seek out and obtain specific information about the nursing home and then to remember it until the next visit so that they could be rewarded with poker chips redeemable for a gift. In a second group—the noncontingent condition—the visits were exactly the same, except that earning the chips was not contingent upon obtaining and remembering the information. In the third, no-treatment condition, subjects were visited once at the beginning and again at the end of the study.

Only the contingent group—the group that was afforded the most control—showed significant improvements on memory tasks and overall health. The memory tasks consisted of tests for immediate memory and for memory of recent and remote events. Health status was assessed from subjects' medical records, vital signs, and use of major tranquilizers and other medications.

In another study, Langer and Rodin (1976) assessed the effects of a different type of manipulation on health and activity. Subjects in one group were called together for a talk by the hospital administrator, who delivered a communication that emphasized the residents' responsibility for themselves, enumerated activities they could take part in, and spelled out when decision making was possible. A second group was given a talk by the administrator that made explicit what was essentially the implicit message in the nursing home, that it was the staff's responsibility to care for them as patients. Residents for whom responsibility had been emphasized became more active and alert, felt less unhappy, and became increasingly involved in a variety of activities in comparison with the group whose feelings of personal control were not explicitly enhanced. These results have been replicated in two other studies (Banziger & Rousch, 1983; Mercer & Kane, 1979). Rodin and Langer (1977) found that most of these group differences remained 18 months later. Additionally, during this 18-month period, the "responsible" patients showed a significantly greater improvement in health; in fact, only 15% of the "responsible" group died within this time, compared with 30% of the "nonresponsible" group.

Using a third type of intervention to increase feelings of control, Schulz (1976) organized visits by college undergraduates to nursing home patients. When the patients were told in advance when the visits would take place, or were given control over the length and timing of the visits, or both, they showed improvements in health, as rated by the staff, and took fewer medications. However, when the visits were both unpredictable and uncontrollable, patients did not show comparable benefits.

MECHANISMS BY WHICH
CONTROL-RELATED INTERVENTIONS MAY WORK

In a follow-up study of the long-term effects of Schulz's (1976) intervention, Schulz and Hanusa (1978) collected data from the same subjects at 24, 30, and 42 months after the end of the intervention. Results showed that health and zest for life, as judged by the staff, declined among subjects who had been told in advance of or given control over the student visits. Schulz and Hanusa's findings stand in sharp contrast to the follow-up results obtained by Rodin and Langer (1977), who found that the positive impact of their intervention persisted over time.

Schulz and Hanusa (1978) offered two possible explanations for the declines exhibited by subjects in Schulz's 1976 study. The first explanation was that subjects' expectation for controlling or predicting events in their lives may have been raised by the interventions and then abruptly violated by the termination of the visits. This explanation suggests that the loss of control may be more damaging than lacking control from the outset (Rodin, 1983, 1986b). Animal studies (e.g., Hanson, Larson, & Snowden, 1976) that experimentally compared a loss of control with a lack of control have indicated that the former exerts more profound effects both physiologically and psychologically. In a later paper, Schulz and Hanusa (1980) suggested further that, for most older individuals, degree of well-being is more likely to reflect relative changes in control opportunities occurring over a short period of time than absolute levels of control. More precisely, it may be only when individuals undergo a sudden change in level of control, as they might with an experimental intervention, that positive or negative outcomes result. Changes in one's level of control are likely to be more salient than one's absolute level, so a loss of control may have a more dramatic effect.

Schulz and Hanusa (1978) also reasoned that different attributional patterns may have been generated among the subjects in Langer and Rodin's (1976) study than among those in Schulz's (1976) study. Langer and Rodin's manipulation may have altered subjects' beliefs about their ability to control outcomes in the institution. That is, the talk given to the experimental group, which emphasized their responsibility for themselves and their outcomes, may have encouraged subjects to believe that their ability to control events would persist over time and across situations. The termination of the experiment need not have affected these beliefs. In contrast, Schulz's intervention may have caused subjects to feel that the opportunity to exercise control was dependent upon an external agent and, therefore, would not remain in other situations or when the agent was removed. This explanation suggests that control may have positive effects only when the locus of control is attributed to internal, stable, and global sources (Abramson, Seligman, & Teasdale, 1978).

A third explanation for the different results of Langer and Rodin (1976) and Schulz (1976) was offered by Ransen (1981), who argued that Langer and Rodin's intervention actually changed the institutional setting, while Schulz's did not. Rodin and Langer (1977) suggested that, because different floors in the nursing home were assigned to different experimental conditions, the probability was enhanced that patterns of interaction among residents and staff members would be affected. In addition, as Ransen noted, Langer and Rodin's agent of change was a full-time member of the institution, and the target behaviors involved many aspects of the setting. By contrast, the agents of change in Schulz's study were outsiders—the student visitors—and the visits were the only target behaviors. Thus, it is likely that in institutional settings, changes in control occur when progressive mutual accommodation made between people and their physical and social environments is altered.

Schulz and Hanusa (1979) attempted an orthogonal manipulation of competence and control as they continued their investigation of the effects of control-relevant interventions. Here, competence corresponds to perceived self-efficacy and control corresponds to the nature of the response-outcome contingencies available. Perceived control and perceived competence were manipulated over a five-week period to test the hypothesis that elderly people who were both made to feel competent and given control over an outcome would exhibit better functioning than subjects exposed to either manipulation alone. Subjects receiving the high-competence manipulation were given positive feedback as they worked on cognitive and social skills tasks; subjects assigned to the low-competence condition received the same amount of feedback as they worked on the tasks, but the feedback was ambiguous. In the high-control condition, subjects were told that their payment for participating in the experiment depended on their performance; in the low-control condition, subjects received payment before beginning the tasks.

According to postintervention self-reports, participants in all treatment conditions felt healthier, more active, and in greater control over daily activities than did subjects in the no-treatment condition. However, subjects who were exposed to either the high-competence or the high-control manipulation demonstrated more improvement in health and greater zest for life, as rated by staff, than subjects who were exposed to both. The unexpected results for the group with both high-competence and high-control, the authors suggested, may have been caused by raising the subjects' expectations for control to too high a level (Lawton, Windley, & Byerts, 1982), with the result that they experienced greater declines in functional ability when their attempts to exercise control were thwarted.

To test their explanation, Schulz and Hanusa (1979) carried out a conceptual replication of the experiment with college freshmen. They chose college students because they assumed that opportunities to exercise competence are virtually limitless in a college environment and that, therefore, the positive effects of control and competence-enhancing interventions should be additive. The results of the college study supported the hypothesis that the combined effects of increased competence and control had a greater positive impact than either intervention alone. These studies suggest that, for enhanced competence to have positive effects, there must be environmental opportunities for exhibiting one's competence. Rodin and Langer (1977) made a similar point in evaluating why their intervention may have had such strong effects. To obtain an appropriate match, the environment may need to be altered to increase opportunities for competent behaviors or to decrease the difficulty of required behaviors so as to prevent expectations for self-efficacy from exceeding actual abilities.

In a different study, Rodin (1983) carried out an intervention consisting of explicit skills training to increase self-regulatory behaviors. Rodin randomly assigned residents of a home for older persons to one of several conditions and examined psychological and physiological outcomes. The experimental group received six training sessions in self-regulatory coping skills from a psychologist. In these sessions, subjects were made aware of their own forms of negative self-statements and were taught and practiced positive self-statements (Meichenbaum, 1974, 1977). Finally, they were given opportunities to apply these new coping techniques while attempting to resolve a number of hypothetical "helplessness-provoking" problems that could be encountered in their daily lives (e.g., an expected visitor suddenly cancels). A second group spent as much time with the psychologist but did not receive explicit skills instruction to enhance control. There was also a no-treatment group. One month after the intervention, subjects in the self-instructional group reported feeling that they had significantly more control and perceived the value of control to be greater than did subjects in the other conditions.

In the same study, Rodin (1983) examined changes in levels of urinary free cortisol as a measure of stress. Subjects in all the groups except the no-treatment controls showed substantial reductions in levels of urinary free cortisol, presumably as a function of reduced stress, from pre- to postintervention measures. However, only the self-regulation skills group was found to have maintained lower cortisol levels at an 18-month follow-up. Declines in cortisol levels were significantly related to subjects' increased participation in active and planned activities, increased energy, perceived freedom to effect change in the environment, and perceived say in determining outcomes.

Whereas, at one month postintervention, none of the groups was judged by a physician to be significantly changed in health, 18 months later, the self-instructional group was judged as showing some improvement. Also, at the 18-month follow-up, in comparison with preintervention, the self-instructional group was taking fewer analgesics, major and minor tranquilizers, and sleeping pills, while the other groups were taking more. The self-instruction group subjects also reported significant decreases in dizziness, headaches, weakness, urinary infections, and gastrointestinal problems.

Taken together, the control-related interventions described above support three broad conclusions. First, increased control over the environment and greater perceived self-efficacy have a positive impact on the physical and psychological status of the institutionalized aged. Second, this effect may be obtained with different approaches to control. Third, predictable positive events also have a positive impact on health and psychological variables. Thus, various types of intervention aimed at increasing control often appear to mitigate environmental challenges to the older person's adaptive resources.

Benefits of Interventions in Community Populations

The extent to which the same findings pertain to elderly people living outside of nursing homes has yet to be adequately studied. Slivinske and Fitch (1987) examined the effects of a control-related intervention among elderly residents of independent and assisted retirement communities. Over a 10-week period, the experimental group attended a series of classes designed to assist participants in mastering their environment; the control group attended group activities unrelated to mastery. During the course of the study, when compared with the control subjects, the experimental group gained significantly more on measures of perceived control and physical well-being. Control group members tended to remain stable or even decline slightly on the perceived control and health assessments. Although subjects in this study were not under skilled nursing care, they had to observe many administrative rules and regulations (e.g., hours and locations of group meals, hours during which noise was prohibited) that potentially limited perceived personal control. It is still uncertain, therefore, whether the positive effects of increased control found in intervention studies are due simply to the highly restricted environments of residences for the elderly (Rodin, 1986a).

MECHANISMS MEDIATING THE EFFECTS OF CONTROL ON HEALTH

Although intervention studies suggest that increased control often benefits the psychological and physical functioning of older people, they do not necessarily specify the mechanisms by which control brings about positive outcomes. Some studies have attempted to test possible mediating mechanisms. In general, this work suggests that control contributes to better physical and psychological functioning, through the mechanisms of behavioral and cognitive change, and through physiological adaptations.

Behavioral and Cognitive Mechanisms

Perceptions of control may influence whether actions are taken to prevent and to remedy health problems. These actions include gathering health-related information, engaging in self-care behaviors, being active in interactions with medical providers, and showing better compliance with medical regimens. The intervention studies reviewed above indicate that subjects afforded relatively high control tended to improve their health status more than those with lower levels of control. We are suggesting here that, given equally serious illnesses, people high in perceived control are more likely than people low in perceived control to take action to enhance their health status.

Some health-related measures do not adequately separate the effects of severity of illness from the effects of taking an active role in one's health enhancement; for example, an increased number of physician visits may indicate the presence of an illness or may be a sign that the individual has decided to participate more actively in his or her own health care. Research investigating the control-health relationship in aging must address this measurement issue more clearly.

Research on the construct of health locus of control (Wallston & Wallston, 1982) supports the hypothesis that individuals with higher levels of perceived control take greater responsibility for meeting their health needs. For example, one study of information-seeking found that people classified as internals who highly valued health indicated a greater willingness to read information on hypertension than did externals who also highly valued health (Wallston, Maides, & Wallston, 1976). In a similar study, willingness to read hypertension information did not differ between young adult internals and externals, but older adult internals were more willing to read the information than were externals of the same age (Toner & Manuck, 1979). A study of information seeking by renal dialysis patients suggested that internals, as compared to externals, knew more about their condition, desired to know even more, and were more willing to attend patient education classes (Sproles, 1977). Among participants in an exercise program, internals were less likely than externals to drop out (Dishman, Ickes, & Morgan, 1980); among people trying to quit smoking, internals were more successful than externals in reducing cigarette consumption and in maintaining the reduction (Kaplan & Cowles, 1978; Shipley, 1980; Wildman, Rosenbaum, Framer, Keane, & Johnson, 1979). Studies of compliance and health beliefs showed that hypertensive internals reported better dietary compliance (Wallston & McLeod, 1979) and better medication compliance (Lewis, Morisky, & Flynn, 1978) than did externals. Similarly, dialysis patients with an internal locus of control adhered more closely to their prescribed diet and were more likely to restrict weight gain (Levin & Schulz, 1980). These studies indicate that feelings of control may directly affect health-related behavior, which in turn can improve health or modify disease.

Research based on Bandura's theory of self-efficacy provides further support for behavioral change as a mediator of the relationship between feelings of control and health outcomes. The suggestion that self-judgments of efficacy determine a person's choice of behaviors implies that attempts to reduce the consumption of drugs, alcohol, or cigarettes, for example, could be affected by such judgments. Because self-efficacy also affects the amount of effort devoted to a task, and the length of persistence, adherence to medical regimens might be more consistent and longer lasting among people with high expectations of self-efficacy. These types of hypotheses have been confirmed in research on the construct of self-efficacy. Studies on smoking cessation have shown that perceived self-efficacy is a reliable predictor of whether relapses occur and of the circumstances surrounding relapses (e.g., Condiotte & Lichtenstein, 1981). Studies using overweight subjects have similarly shown that perceptions of self-efficacy regarding eating and weight management predict success at weight reduction attempts (e.g., Chambliss & Murray, 1979). Beliefs in one's ability to manage pain have been found to increase both laboratory and clinical tolerance of pain (e.g., Manning & Wright, 1983; Neufeld & Thomas, 1977), while recovery from myocardial infarction is facilitated by enhancing patients' and their spouses' judgments of their cardiac and physical capabilities (e.g., Ewart, Taylor, Reese, & Debusk, 1983; Taylor, Bandura, Ewart, Miller, & Debusk, 1984). These results strongly uphold the notion that one's perceived competence to engage in preventive and curative health behaviors increases the likelihood of both undertaking and continuing health-enhancing actions.

We propose that the tendency for individuals with lower perceived control to engage in fewer health-protective behaviors may become stronger in old age. Weaker beliefs in personal control might be especially likely to decrease health-promoting activity among older people because, as Rodin (1978) suggested, physical decline is frequently viewed as an unalterable part of the aging process. When physical symptoms are attributed to aging, the person may see them as inevitable and nonmodifiable and thus not undertake remedial steps that could be beneficial. In two studies, large proportions of the elderly subjects chose not to report physical symptoms, including severe conditions such as congestive heart failure and correctable functional impairments such as hearing deficiencies, because they ascribed their conditions to advancing age (Brody & Kleban, 1981; Williamson et al., 1964). In another study, older respondents were more likely than younger subjects to attribute physical symptoms produced by an illness to their age and then to cope by monitoring, accepting, or denying and minimizing the symptoms or by postponing or avoiding medical attention for them (Leventhal & Prohaska, 1986; see also Chapter 5, Leventhal, Leventhal, & Schaefer). In old age, health problems may be underattributed to situational factors such as the occurrence of environmental or stress-inducing events.

Rodin and Langer (1980) found that encouraging plausible environmental attributions for physical problems (e.g., slippery floors create difficulty in walking) was associated with better health in a nursing home sample.

Contact with the medical care system itself may lower perceived control. The treatment of illness and disease, especially if hospitalization is required, restricts opportunities for control for patients of all ages (Lorber, 1975; Taylor, 1979). However, more frequent participation in the health care system, likely to be necessitated by declining health and older age, may heighten the effects of this restriction (Rodin, 1986a). Health professionals, until recently, have preferred the most manageable and treatable (i.e., compliant and deferential) patients (Wills, 1978). In some nursing homes, staff members foster manageability and treatability by encouraging residents to become dependent and to relinquish personal control over daily tasks and social interactions (Timko & Rodin, 1985). Among medical outpatients, physicians are less responsive (i.e., information giving, questioning, supportive) to topics raised by elderly patients rather than by younger patients (Greene, Hoffman, Charon, & Adelman, 1987), and elderly individuals are more accepting and less challenging of physicians' authority than are younger persons (Haug, 1979; Haug & Ory, 1987).

A cognitive mechanism by which control may be linked to health involves the labeling of symptoms. Extensive work has been done on how people come to experience and label bodily sensations as symptoms relevant to health or illness (e.g., Leventhal & Everhart, 1979; Mechanic, 1972; Pennebaker, 1982; Schachter & Singer, 1962), and control appears to be one variable that influences the labeling process. When the level of perceived control over environmental events is manipulated experimentally, subjects who are given low or no control report more physical symptoms than those who feel more in control (Matthews, Scheier, Brunson, & Carducci, 1980; Pennebaker, Burnam, Schaeffer, & Harper, 1977; Weidner & Matthews, 1978). It is possible that the loss of control caused by situational changes of aging (e.g., retirement) elicits bodily preoccupation, symptom monitoring, and entrance into the sick role (Levkoff, Cleary, & Wetle, 1987).

There are at least three possible explanations for the results concerning symptom perception and labeling. First, experiences of uncontrollability may influence people's cognitive strategies so that they try harder and pay more attention (Matthews et al., 1980), with the "psychic cost" of the increased attention being experienced physiologically (Pennebaker, 1982). Second, experiences of loss of control may cause individuals to adopt symptom-relevant schemas and then selectively search their bodies in greater detail for symptoms (Pennebaker, 1982). This second hypothesis is based on the assumption that people adopt schemas that direct their search and the processing of information. Those who are aroused and upset, as they would be in an uncontrollable situation, often attribute their distress to being ill (Mechanic, 1972). The third explanation for the relationship between a loss of control and increased symptomatology is that a failure to control the environment affects physiological activity in both the neuroendocrine and immune systems. Thus, the individual may actually experience more symptoms as a function of physiological activation.

Physiological Mechanisms

Efforts to link loss of control to physiological processes were pioneered by the work of Engel and Schmale (Engel & Schmale, 1967; Schmale & Engel, 1967). They suggested that giving up in response to situations of loss may precede the development of illness of all types. According to their view, if feelings of helplessness or hopelessness develop in patients who have experienced an actual, threatened, or symbolic loss, these feelings would facilitate the development of existing somatic predispositions or increased vulnerability to external pathogens, either of which would result in disease. Although Engel and Schmale emphasized the occurrence of loss, it seems that what is fundamental to the sense of loss they described is a feeling of lack of control—the inability to cope in the face of negative environmental events (Rodin, 1986b).

The hypothesis that increased control may directly affect a large variety of physiological states has been supported by the results of numerous laboratory studies in both humans and animals. In studies with humans, for example, Glass, Reim, and Singer (1971) found that subjects given perceived control over the termination of aversive noise exhibited significantly less autonomic reactivity (vasoconstriction) than subjects who did not have perceived control over the noise. An experiment by Geer and Maisel (1972) showed that subjects given control over aversive stimuli displayed lower galvanic skin response reactivity than did subjects who did not have control.

Neuroendocrine responses. Other studies indicate that the experience of uncontrollability results in activation of the sympathetic adrenal-medullary system and the pituitary-adrenal-cortical axis (see Chapter 8). Both catecholamines, secreted by the sympathetic system, and corticosteroids, secreted by the pituitary system, have been shown to increase in response to uncontrollability. Fluctuations in these hormones influence bodily systems of relevance to the development of coronary disease and to the suppression of the immune system.

The association between catecholamine levels and control has been demonstrated in both human and animal studies. Focusing on studies of people, Frankenhaeuser and colleagues strongly showed that uncontrollable stress elevates peripheral levels of catecholamines (Frankenhaeuser, 1975; Frankenhaeuser, Lundberg & Forsman, 1978; Lundberg & Frankenhaeuser, 1978). Peripheral catecholamine secretions are associated with a rise in blood pressure and heart rate, elevation of blood lipids, induction of myocardial lesions, and provocation of ventricular arrhythmias (Krantz, Glass, Contrado, & Miller, 1981). Thus, the catecholamine increase that occurs in response to uncontrollability may be one mechanism accounting for the reported relationship between coronary disease and control-related variables.

The response to uncontrollability is one of the most significant contributors to stress and to the Type A pattern of behavior (i.e., competitive striving for achievement, sense of time urgency, and hostility), which in turn are the most promising psychosocial risk factors for cardiovascular disease (Engel, 1978; Friedman, Byers, Diamant, & Rosenman, 1975; Glass, Krakoff, Contrada, et al., 1980; Glass, Krakoff, Finkelman, et al., 1980; Greene, Moss, & Goldstein, 1974). It is interesting, however, that, while aspects of Type A behavior may increase the risk of heart disease, Type As are apparently at less risk for mortality after a heart attack (Ragland & Brand, 1988). Presumably, this is because Type As take greater control and change their behavior patterns, or they follow the prescribed regimen more carefully.

In a typical study showing the effect of loss of control on corticosteroids in humans, subjects were able to choose among noise intensities while their yoked partners were exposed to the same noise levels (Lundberg & Frankenhaeuser, 1978). The yoked group that was unable to choose its own intensity secreted significantly more cortisol. Like catecholamines, pituitary-adrenal secretions have been implicated in the development of cardiovascular disease. Corticosteroids regulate the metabolism of cholesterol and other lipids involved in the atherosclerotic process and play a role in regulating electrolyte balance and blood pressure. Because corticosteroids are elevated in response to a lack of control and are a factor in heart disease, they may mediate the control-disease relationship.

Frankenhaeuser (1975) argued that the controllability of a task is a major determinant of the degree of effort expended and/or the distress experienced and hence of the balance between sympathetic adrenal and pituitary-adrenal arousal, as measured by catecholamine and cortisol excretion. In laboratory experiments using demanding tasks, Frankenhaeuser and colleagues showed that effort is related to catecholamine secretion, whereas distress is related to cortisol secretion. Personal control appears to be the important modulating factor in these tasks because it tends to reduce the negative and enhance the positive aspects of arousal, thereby changing the balance between sympathetic adrenal and pituitary-adrenal activity.

Immunological responses. While the psychoendocrine effects of control variations have been replicated and extended by numerous laboratories, the relationship between control and responses of the immune system is currently less well understood. There are several possibilities for the mechanism whereby a lack of control could cause changes in the functioning of a person's immune system. As discussed above, uncontrollable stressors produce higher levels of circulating corticosteroids than controllable stressors (Davis et al., 1977; Weiss, Stone, & Harrell, 1970). Another possibility involves endogenous opioids, the body's natural pain-reducing substances. Shavit, Lewis, Terman, Gale, and Liebeskind (1983) found that conditions that produced opioid analgesia were immunosuppressive, whereas conditions that produced nonopioid analgesia were not. Cells in the immune system, especially lymphocytes and neutrophils, possess opiate receptors (Hazum, Chang, & Cuatrecacas, 1979).

A relationship between control and immune function may play a dramatic role in the health of aged people in particular. Environmental and psychosocial stressors that have been shown to affect immunity may be more common among the elderly; bereavement and overcrowding are examples (Palmblad, 1981). As we review below, the immune system itself also clearly changes with aging (Siskind, 1981). Because immunological function is affected by aging and processes relevant to control, it is possible that, with age, which brings a general loss of immunological competence, the relation between lack of control and suppression of the immune system may become stronger. This would suggest that, all other things being equal, the incidence of disease related to immune function would be expected to increase when individuals perceive a lack of control and that this would happen to a greater extent in older rather than younger people. Given other differences among age groups in health status, however, it is often difficult to make a just comparison (Rodin, 1986a).

In general, loss of immunological competence in the aged reflects both intrinsic deficiencies in the competence of specific cell populations and extrinsic deficiencies in the environment of the cells. For example, it has been suggested that suppressor T cells—thymus-dependent cells with immunosuppressive properties—increase in number and/or activity with age and also that this increase plays a major role in the age-related decline of immune potential. Whereas the response to exogenous antigens decreases with age, the reverse occurs with respect to endogenous antigens, thus leading to an increase in the incidence and severity of the so-called autoimmune diseases (Timiras, 1972).

Numerous studies have shown that the rates of secretion and metabolism of adrenocortical hormones decline with age, possibly in relation to decreases in weight and alteration in tissue components of the cortex (Grad, Kral, Payne, & Berenson, 1967; Romanoff, Morris, Welch, Grace, & Pincus, 1963; Serio et al., 1969). It has also been reported that cortisol may disappear from the circulation of older subjects at a slower rate than in younger persons (West et al., 1961). Some data have suggested that elevated levels of cortisol can reduce immune functioning, because corticosteroids display immunosuppressive properties (Munck, Guyre, & Holbrook, 1984). There have also been reports of an adverse relationship between corticosterone level and the capacity of the spleen to synthesize antibodies (Gabrielson & Good, 1967; Gisler, 1974). In healthy people, homeostatic regulatory mechanisms usually counteract the suppressive properties of corticosteroids; but, in chronically ill or aged individuals, homeostatic regulatory mechanisms may be less effective (Timiras, 1972).

Age changes that occur in immune and neuroendocrine functioning suggest that loss of control may have an especially debilitating effect on the health of elderly persons through its effects on the pituitary-adrenal system (Rodin, 1980, 1983, 1986b). One segment of Rodin's longitudinal study (unpublished data) was designed to test this hypothesis. A subsample of subjects, free of endocrine disease (e.g., diabetes) and the most obvious immunological diseases (e.g., cancer, rheumatoid arthritis), was tested at the baseline period for immunocompetence (see Rodin, 1986b, for details). A first type of analysis related the baseline immunological parameters to the psychosocial data, also collected at baseline. Results revealed that the strongest correlates of immunosuppression were the effects of major stressful life events on subjects' sense of control. The major impact of feeling a lack of control over stressors was to suppress the number of helper cells and to lower the ability of T cells to mobilize an effective response to an antigen challenge.

Rodin also examined subjects who experienced a significant stressor during the course of the study to date. Prestressor to poststressor changes in scores of biological measures show that the number of helper cells fell in response to stress and that this reduction was related to both health and nutritional status, as well as to the psychological variables of expectancy and control. The ability to mobilize a response to an antigen was strongly reduced by these psychological parameters. From these preliminary data, it may be tentatively concluded that perceived losses in predictability and control of a highly stressful event are related to reductions in the number of helper T cells and to the body's reduced efficiency in counteracting a foreign antigen. It is important to recognize that the actual occurrence of a stressor may not determine effects on the immune system, but that its predictability and its effects on perceived control, in combination and/or interaction with health and nutritional status, may.

VARIABILITY IN PREFERENCE FOR CONTROL WITH AGING

Although we have emphasized the benefits to be derived from increased personal control for older people, in particular, we must also emphasize that we are not suggesting that it is universally beneficial to feel increased control. People differ in their desires for personal control, and there are some conditions in which perceived control is more likely to induce stress than to have a beneficial impact (Averill, 1973). Consistent with our proposal that variations in control may be most important for the aged, we further propose that their individual preferences for control may show greater variability than is seen in younger groups. Moreover, we speculate that, in situations in which having control is stress inducing, the negative effects may be more disruptive for older than younger people. It is important, therefore, that future research determine the interactions among age, individual preferences for control, situational factors, and variations in opportunities for control that produce positive psychological and physical outcomes.

There is evidence that individuals' preferences for control vary widely. In laboratory studies, a minority of subjects always opt for uncontrollable rather than controllable aversive events when they are given a choice (e.g., Averill & Rosenn, 1972). Field experiments in health care settings have shown that some individuals benefit more than others from being highly informed about and/or involved in their own medical treatment. In studies that either made patients more active participants in treatment (e.g., Cromwell, Butterfield, Brayfield, & Curry, 1977) or heightened their sense of choice (e.g., Mills & Krantz, 1979), or provided for self-monitoring or self-care (Berg & Logerfo, 1979), individual reactions to treatment interventions differed substantially. We suspect that variability in optimal or preferred levels of control increases with age in line with increasing variability in perceptions of control (Lachman, 1986b).

Research has indicated that medical patients whose treatments offer options congruent with their control beliefs show the best psychological and physical adjustment (Cromwell et al., 1977; Lewis, Morisky, & Flynn, 1978; Wallston et al., 1976). If it is true that people's preferences for control increase in variability with aging, then it becomes more difficult to match an elderly individual's expectancies of control and the levels of actual control afforded by the environment. It is also important to note that, among both institutionalized and noninstitutionalized elderly, options for exerting control that are offered by the environment are likely to be reduced, as may be the array of responses a particular individual is able to make. For some individuals, both of these factors may widen the gap between preferred level of control and actual level of control.

THE COSTS OF EXCESSIVE CONTROL

Engaging in futile attempts to control events that are actually uncontrollable is likely to have psychological and physiological costs (Janoff-Bulman & Brickman, 1980; Schulz & Hanusa, 1980; Wortman & Brehm, 1975). Excessive feelings of responsibility may be aversive (Averill, 1973; Rodin, Rennert, & Solomon, 1980; Thompson, 1981); and personal control often places heavy demands on people in the form of a major investment of time, effort, and resources, as well as the risk of the consequences of failure. A lack of sufficient information to support effective control over an outcome has also been proposed to decrease the desirability of control (Rodin et al., 1980). Finally, it has been suggested that the psychological cost of control may be greater for older people because they may experience more extreme reactions to stress than other age groups and because stress may accelerate the aging process (Eisdorfer & Wilkie, 1977).

The possible physiological costs of control also merit attention. Specifically, there is evidence that, in some individuals, excessive efforts to assert control can have negative effects on many of the same physiological systems that show benefits with increased control. The work of Glass (1977), for example, considers Type A individuals who are so hard driving that they continue to try to exercise control even in the face of maladaptive outcomes or uncontrollable situations. Glass postulates that this repeated and frustrated desire for control may be related to increased catecholamine output, which in turn contributes to atherosclerosis. The effects of control-relevant self-regulation on biological processes are not simple and straightforward. Research has yet to fully explore the conditions under which exercising control is beneficial and those under which it is not.

CONCLUSIONS

Environmental and personal factors associated with growing old appear to diminish opportunities for control in later life. Although these factors tend to become more numerous as one grows old, they do not necessarily lead to strong associations between perceived control and chronological age per se, because older people vary in the extent to which they desire control and in the nature of the environmental and personal factors to which they are exposed.

Aging-related events, we hypothesized, can influence perceptions of both personal competence and response-outcome contingencies. Indeed, the degree of biologically mandated decline with aging has been overestimated largely because events occurring in old age so commonly produce a loss of one's sense of control. Currently, little is known about how people combine judgments of self-competence and contingency to form an overall judgment of the level of perceived control (Weisz, 1983), and this is clearly an area in which research is needed. It is possible that the weight a person assigns to each component of control changes developmentally or that the combinatorial process itself undergoes changes over the life span.

Evidence suggests that manipulations of control have a strong impact on health outcomes, including symptoms, morbidity, and mortality. Health-related cognitions and behaviors, symptom labels, and physiological processes appear to mediate the control-health relationship, and the elderly may be most vulnerable to the negative health effects of loss of control because old age strongly influences each of these mediators. Older people may diminish health-promoting activity because physical decline is frequently attributed to the irreversible aging process. The perception of oneself as undergoing the inevitable decline of aging might also lead older people to have a greater tendency to label their bodily sensations as symptoms of disability or illness. The aged may be more likely to focus on bodily sensations not only because they may intentionally search for physical signs of aging but also because they may have less environmental stimulation, particularly if they are institutionalized. In addition, many elderly people actually experience symptoms due to biological changes, regardless of their attentional focus. Neuroendocrine and immune system changes head the list of the numerous physiological changes that occur with aging, but it also includes DNA damage and changes in protein synthesis, cells, and tissues (Schimke, 1981).

Future research is needed to explore the hypothesis that the negative effects of loss of control on health are most profound for the aged by comparing different age groups in the same study and to clarify the mechanisms by which increased control benefits the health of persons of all ages. Studies are also needed to specify how different aspects of control relate to different health-relevant outcomes. In all the work we reviewed, the assumption has been that control influences health outcomes. It is interesting that little work has been done to test the alternative view that changes in health affect beliefs about control (and/or actual control). Longitudinal work, which follows naturally occurring changes in health and control, would be ideal to address this type of question. Based on our current understanding, however, we may conclude that both perceived competence and environmental contingency figure importantly in the health and well-being of older people. The clinical and social significance of these observations is considerable. They point to a need to exact substantial changes in the health care system as it affects older people while remaining mindful of the specific conditions under which control may be expected to exert positive or negative effects on health.

REFERENCES

Abramson, L. Y., Seligman, M. E. P., & Teasdale, J. D. (1978). Learned helplessness in humans: Critique and reformulation. *Journal of Abnormal Psychology, 87,* 49-74.

Averill, J. R. (1973). Personal control over aversive stimuli and its relationship to stress. *Psychological Bulletin, 80,* 286-303.

Averill, J. R., & Rosenn, M. (1972). Vigilant and non-vigilant coping strategies and pathophysiological stress reactions during the anticipation of electric shock. *Journal of Personality and Social Psychology, 23*, 128-141.

Avorn, J., & Langer, E. J. (1982). Induced disability in nursing home patients: A controlled trial. *Journal of the American Geriatric Society, 30*, 397-400.

Baltes, M. M., & Reisenzein, R. (1986). The social world in long-term care institutions: Psychosocial control toward dependency? In M. M. Baltes & P. B. Baltes (Eds.), *Aging and the psychology of control*. Hillsdale, NJ: Lawrence Erlbaum.

Bandura, A. (1977). Self-efficacy: Toward a unifying theory of behavioral change. *Psychological Review, 84*, 191-215.

Bandura, A. (1981). Self-referent thought: A developmental analysis of self-efficacy. In J. H. Flavell & L. Ross (Eds.), *Social cognitive development: Frontiers and possible futures* (pp. 200-239). New York: Cambridge University Press.

Banziger, G., & Rousch, S. (1983). Nursing homes for the birds: A control-relevant intervention with bird feeders. *The Gerontologist, 23*, 527-531.

Berg, A. O., & Logerfo, J. P. (1979). Potential effect of self-care algorithms on the number of physician visits. *The New England Journal of Medicine, 300*, 535-537.

Bohm, L. C. (1983). *Social support and well-being in older adults: The impact of perceived control*. Unpublished doctoral dissertation, Yale University.

Bradley, R. H., & Webb, R. (1976). Age-related differences in three behavior domains. *Human Development, 19*, 49-55.

Brim, O. G. (1980). *How a person controls the sense of efficacy through the life span*. Paper presented at the Social Science Research Council Conference on the Self and Perceived Control Through the Life Span, New York.

Brody, E. M., & Kleban, M. H. (1981). Physical and mental health symptoms of older people: Who do they tell? *Journal of the American Geriatrics Society, 29*, 442-449.

Brothen, T., & Detzner, D. (1983). Perceived health and locus of control in the aged. *Perceptual and Motor Skills, 56*, 946.

Brown, B. R., & Granick, S. (1983). Cognitive and psychosocial differences between I and E locus of control aged persons. *Experimental Aging Research, 9*, 107-110.

Butler, R. (1970). Myths and realities of clinical geriatrics. *Image and Commentary, 12*, 26-29.

Chambliss, C. A., & Murray, E. J. (1979). Efficacy attribution, locus of control, and weight loss. *Cognitive Therapy and Research, 3*, 349-353.

Cicirelli, V. G. (1980). Relationship of family background variables to locus of control in the elderly. *Journal of Gerontology, 35*, 108-114.

Condiotte, M. M., & Lichtenstein, E. (1981). Self-efficacy and relapse in smoking cessation programs. *Journal of Consulting and Clinical Psychology, 49*, 648-658.

Cromwell R. L., Butterfield, D. C., Brayfield, F. M., & Curry, J. J. (1977). *Acute myocardial infarction: Reaction and recovery*. St. Louis: C. V. Mosby.

Davis, H., Porter, J. W., Livingstone, J., Herrman, J., MacFadden, L., & Levine, S. (1977). Pituitary-adrenal activity and lever press shock escape behavior. *Physiological Psychology, 5*, 280.

Dishman, R. K., Ickes, W., & Morgan, W. P. (1980). Self-motivation and adherence to habitual physical activity. *Journal of Applied Social Psychology, 10*, 115-132.

Duke, M. P., Shaheen, J., & Nowicki, S. (1974). The determination of control in a geriatric population and a subsequent test of the social learning model for interpersonal distances. *Journal of Psychology, 86*, 277-285.

Eisdorfer, C., & Wilkie, F. (1977). Stress, disease, aging and behavior. In J. E. Birren & K. W. Schaie (Eds.), *Handbook of the psychology of aging* (pp. 251-275). New York: Van Nostrand Reinhold.

Engel, G. E. (1978). Psychological stress, vasodepressor (vasobasal) syncope, and sudden death. *Annals of Internal Medicine, 89*, 403-412.

Engel, G. E., & Schmale, A. H. (1967). Psychoanalytic theory of somatic disorder: Conversion, specificity, and the disease onset situation. *Journal of the American Psychoanalytic Association, 15*, 344-365.

Ewart, C. K., Taylor, C. B., Reese, L. B., & Debusk, F. F. (1984). Effects of early postmyocardial infarction exercise testing on self-perception and subsequent physical activity. *American Journal of Cardiology, 51*, 1076-1080.

Fawcett, G., Stonner, D., & Zepelin, H. (1980). Locus of control, perceived constraint, and morale among institutionalized aged. *International Journal of Aging and Human Development, 11*, 13-23.

Frankenhaeuser, M. (1975). Experimental approaches to the study of catecholamines and emotion. In L. Levi (Ed.), *Emotions: Their parameters and measurement.* New York: Raven Press.

Frankenhaeuser, M., Lundberg, U., & Forsman, L. (1978). *Dissociation between sympathetic adrenal and pituitary-adrenal responses to an achievement situation characterized by high controllability: Comparison between Type A and Type B males and females* (Tech. Rep. No. 540). Stockholm, Sweden: University of Stockholm.

Friedman, M., Byers, S. O., Diamant, J., & Rosenman, R. H. (1975). Plasma catecholamine response of coronary-prone subjects (Type A) to a specific challenge. *Metabolism, 24*, 205-210.

Gabrielson, A. E., & Good, R. A. (1967). Chemical suppression of adapted immunity. *Advances in Immunology, 6*, 90-229.

Gatz, M., & Siegler, I. C. (1981, August). *Locus of control: A retrospective.* Paper presented at the meeting of the American Psychological Association, Los Angeles.

Geer, J., & Maisel, E. (1972). Evaluating the effects of the prediction-control confound. *Journal of Personality and Social Psychology, 23*, 314-319.

Gisler, R. H. (1974). Stress and the hormonal regulation of the immune response in mice. *Psychotherapy and Psychosomatics, 23*, 197-208.

Glass, D. C. (1977). *Behavior patterns, stress and coronary disease.* Hillsdale, NJ: Lawrence Erlbaum.

Glass, D. C., Krakoff, L. R., Contrada, R., Hilton, W. C., Kehoe, K., Mannucci, E. G., Collins, C., Snow, B., & Elting, E. (1980). Effects of harassment and competition upon cardiovascular and plasma catecholamine response in Type A and Type B individuals. *Psychophysiology, 17*, 453-463.

Glass, D. C., Krakoff, L. R., Finkelman, J., Snow, B., Contrada, R., Kehoe, J., Mannucci, E. G., Isecke, W., Collins, C., Hilton, W. F., & Elting, E. (1980). Effect of task overload upon cardiovascular and plasma catecholamine responses in Type A and Type B individuals. *Basic and Applied Social Psychology, 1*, 199-218.

Glass, D. C., Reim B., & Singer, J. (1971). Behavioral consequences of adaptation to controllable and uncontrollable noise. *Journal of Experimental Social Psychology, 7*, 244-257.

Grad, B., Kral, V. A., Payne, R. C., & Berenson, J. (1967). Plasma and urinary corticoids in young and old persons. *Journal of Gerontology, 22*, 66.

Greene, M. G., Hoffman, S., Charon, R., & Adelman, R. (1987). Psychosocial concerns in the medical encounter: A comparison of the interactions of doctors with their old and young patients. *The Gerontologist, 27,* 164-168.

Greene, W. H., Moss, A. J., & Goldstein, S. (1974). Delay, denial, and death in coronary heart disease. In R. S. Eliot (Ed.), *Stress and the heart.* Mont Kisco, NY: Futura.

Gurin, P. (1980). *The situation and other neglected issues in personal causation.* Paper presented in the Thematic Minutes V of the Social Science Research Council Conference on the Self and Perceived Personal Control Through the Life Span, New York.

Hanson, J. D., Larson, M. E., & Snowden, C. T. (1976). The effects of control over high intensity noise of plasma cortisol levels in rhesus monkeys. *Behavioral Biology, 16,* 333.

Haug, M. (1979). Doctor patient relationships and the older patient. *Journal of Gerontology, 34,* 852-860.

Haug, M., & Ory, M. G. (1987). Issues in elderly patient-provider interactions. *Research on Aging, 9,* 3-44.

Hazum, E., Chang, K. J., & Cuatrecascas, P. (1979). Specific non opiate receptors for beta-endorphin. *Science, 205,* 1033-1035.

Herberman, R. B., Nunn, M. E., Holden, H. T., Staal, S., & Djeu, J. Y. (1977). Augmentation of natural cytotoxic reactivity of mouse lymphoid cells against syngeneic and allogeneic target cells. *International Journal of Cancer, 19,* 555-564.

Hunter, K. I., Linn, M. W., & Harris, R. (1981-1982). Characteristics of high and low self-esteem in the elderly. *International Journal of Aging and Human Development, 14,* 117-126.

Hunter, K. I., Linn, M. W., Harris, R., & Pratt, T. (1980). Discriminators of internal and external locus of control orientation in the elderly. *Research on Aging, 2,* 49-60.

Janoff-Bulman, R., & Brickman, P. (1980). Expectations and what people learn from failure. In N. T. Feather (Ed.), *Expectancy, incentive and action.* Hillsdale, NJ: Lawrence Erlbaum.

Kaplan, G. D., & Cowles, A. (1978). Health locus of control and health value in prediction of smoking reduction. *Health Education Monographs, 6,* 129-137.

Krantz, D. S., Glass, D. C., Contrado, R., & Miller, N. E. (1981). Behavior and health. In *The five-year outlook on science and technology* (Vol. 2). Washington, DC: National Science Foundation, Government Printing Office.

Krantz, D. S., & Schulz, R. (1980). Personal control and health: Some applications to crises of middle and old age. In A. Baum & J. E. Singer (Eds.), *Advances in environmental psychology* (Vol. 2, pp. 23-57). New York: Academic Press.

Krantz, D. S., & Stone, V. (1978). Locus of control and the effects of success and failure in young and community-residing aged women. *Journal of Personality, 46,* 536-551.

Kuypers, J. A. (1972). Internal-external locus of control, ego functioning, and personality characteristics in old age. *The Gerontologist, 12,* 168-173.

Kuypers, J. A., & Bengtson, V. L. (1973). Social breakdown and competence. *Human Development, 16,* 181-201.

Lachman, M. E. (1983). Perceptions of intellectual aging: Antecedent or consequence of intellectual functioning? *Developmental Psychology, 19*, 482-498.

Lachman, M. E. (1985). Personal efficacy in middle and old age: Differential and normative patterns of change. In G. H. Elder (Ed.), *Life-course dynamics: Trajectories and transitions, 1968-1980*. Ithaca, NY: Cornell University Press.

Lachman, M. E. (1986a). Personal control in later life: Stability, change, and cognitive correlates. In M. M. Baltes & P. B. Baltes (Eds.), *Aging and the psychology of control*. Hillsdale, NJ: Lawrence Erlbaum.

Lachman, M. E. (1986b). Locus of control in aging research: A case for multidimensional and domain-specific assessment. *Psychology and Aging, 1*, 34-40.

Langer, E. J. (1983). *The psychology of control*. Beverly Hills, CA: Sage.

Langer, E. J., & Imber, L. (1979). When practice makes perfect: The debilitating effects of overlearning. *Journal of Personality and Social Psychology, 37*, 2014.

Langer, E. J., & Rodin, J. (1976). The effects of choice and enhanced personal responsibility for the aged: A field experiment in an institutional setting. *Journal of Personality and Social Psychology, 34*, 191-198.

Langer, E., Rodin, J., Beck, P., Weinman, C., & Spitzer, L. (1979). Environmental determinants of memory improvement in late adulthood. *Journal of Personality and Social Psychology, 27*, 2000-2013.

Laudenslager, M. L., Ryan, S. M., Drugan, R. C., Hyson, R. L., & Maier, S. F. (1983). Coping and immunosuppression: Inescapable but not escapable shock suppresses lymphocyte proliferation. *Science, 221*, 568-570.

Lawton, M. P., Windley, P. G., & Byerts, T. O. (1982). *Environment and aging: Theoretical approaches*. New York: Springer.

Levenson, H. (1974). Activism and powerful others: Distinctions within the concept of internal-external control. *Journal of Personality Assessment, 38*, 377-383.

Leventhal, E. A., & Prohaska, T. R. (1986). Age, symptom interpretation, and health behavior. *Journal of the American Geriatrics Society, 34*, 185-191.

Leventhal, H., & Everhart, D. (1979). Emotion, pain, and physical illness. In C. F. Izard (Ed.), *Emotions and psychopathology*. New York: Plenum.

Levin, A., & Schulz, M. A. (1980). *Multidimensional health locus of control and compliance in low and high participation hemodialysis*. Unpublished manuscript, University of Wisconsin, Madison.

Levine, S., & Coover, G. D. (1976). Environmental control of suppression of the pituitary-adrenal system. *Physiology and Behavior, 17*, 35-37.

Levkoff, S. E., Cleary, P. D., & Wetle, T. (1987). Differences in the appraisal of health between aged and middle-aged adults. *Journal of Gerontology, 42*, 114-120.

Lewis, F. M., Morisky, D. E., & Flynn, B. S. (1978). A test of the construct validity of health locus of control: Effects of a self-reported compliance for hypertensive patients. *Health Education Monographs, 6*, 138-148.

Linn, M. W., & Hunter, K. (1979). Perception of age in the elderly. *Journal of Gerontology, 34*, 46-52.

Lorber, J. (1975). Good patients and problem patients: Conformity and deviance in a general hospital. *Journal of Health and Social Behavior, 16*, 213-225.

Lundberg, U., & Frankenhaeuser, M. (1978). Psychophysiological reactions to noise as modified by personal control over stimulus intensity. *Biological Psychology, 6*, 51.

Mancini, J. A. (1980-1981). Effects of health and income on control orientation and life satisfaction among aged public housing residents. *International Journal of Aging and Human Development, 12*, 215-220.

Manning, M. M., & Wright, T. L. (1983). Self-efficacy expectancies, outcome expectancies, and the persistence of pain control in childbirth. *Journal of Personality and Social Psychology, 45*, 421-431.

Matthews, K., Scheier, M. F., Brunson, B. I., & Carducci, B. (1980). Attention, unpredictability and reports of physical symptoms. *Journal of Personality and Social Psychology, 38*, 525-537.

Mechanic, D. (1972). Social psychologic factors affecting the presentation of bodily complaints. *The New England Journal of Medicine, 268*, 1132-1139.

Meichenbaum, D. (1974). Self-instructional strategy training: A cognitive prosthesis for the aged. *Human Development, 17*, 273.

Meichenbaum, D. (1977). *Cognitive-behavior modification: An integrative approach.* New York: Plenum.

Mercer, S., & Kane, R. A. (1979). Helplessness and hopelessness among the institutionalized aged: An experiment. *Health and Social Work, 4*, 90-116.

Mills, R. T., & Krantz, D. S. (1979). Information, choice and reactions to stress: A field experiment in a blood bank with laboratory analogue. *Journal of Personality and Social Psychology, 37*, 608-620.

Monjan, A., & Collector, M. (1977). Stress induced modulation of the immune response. *Science, 196*, 307-308.

Munck, A., Guyre, P. M., & Holbrook, N. J. (1984). Physiological functions of gluco-corticoids in stress and their relation to pharmacological actions. *Endocrine Reviews, 5*, 25-43.

Nehrke, M. F., Hulicka, I. M., & Morganti, J. B. (1980). Age differences in life satisfaction, locus of control, and self-concept. *International Journal of Aging and Human Development, 11*, 25-33.

Neufeld, R. W. J., & Thomas, P. (1977). Effects of perceived self-efficacy of a prophylactic controlling mechanism on self-control under painful stimulation. *Canadian Journal of Behavioral Science, 9*, 224-232.

Oehler, J. R., & Herberman, R. B. (1978). Natural cell-mediated cytotoxicity in rats. Effects of immunopharmacologic treatments on natural reactivity and on reactivity augmented by polyinosinic-polycytidylic acid. *International Journal of Cancer, 21*, 221-229.

Palmblad, J. (1981). Stress and immunologic competence: Studies in man. In R. Ader (Ed.), *Psychoneuroimmunology* (pp. 229-257). New York: Academic Press.

Pennebaker, J. W. (1982). *The psychology of physical symptoms.* New York: Springer-Verlag.

Pennebaker, J. W., Burnam, M. A., Schaeffer, M. A., & Harper, D. (1977). Lack of control as a determinant of perceived physical symptoms. *Journal of Personality and Social Psychology, 35*, 167-174.

Pross, H. F., & Barnes, M. G. (1977). Spontaneous human lymphocyte-mediated cytotoxicity against tumour target cells. I. The effect of malignant disease. *International Journal of Cancer, 18*, 593-604.

Ragland, D. R., & Brand, R. J. (1988). Type A behavior and mortality from coronary heart disease. *The New England Journal of Medicine, 318*, 65-69.

Ransen, D. L. (1981). Long-term effects of two interventions with the aged: An ecological analysis. *Journal of Applied Developmental Psychology, 2,* 13-27.

Reid, D. W., & Ziegler, M. (1980). Validity and stability of a new desired control measure pertaining to psychological adjustment of the elderly. *Journal of Gerontology, 35,* 395-402.

Rodin, J. (1978). Somatopsychics and attribution. *Personality and Social Psychology Bulletin, 4,* 531-540.

Rodin, J. (1980). Managing the stress of aging: The role of control and coping. In S. Levine & H. Ursin (Eds.), *NATO conference on coping and health.* New York: Academic Press.

Rodin, J. (1983). Behavioral medicine: Beneficial effects of self-control training in aging. *International Review of Applied Psychology, 32,* 153-181.

Rodin, J. (1986a). Aging and health: Effects of the sense of control. *Science, 233,* 1271-1276.

Rodin, J. (1986b). Health, control and aging. In M. M. Baltes & P. B. Baltes (Eds.), *Aging and the psychology of control.* Hillsdale, NJ: Lawrence Erlbaum.

Rodin, J. (1987). Personal control through the life course. In R. Abeles (Ed.), *Implications of the life span perspective for social psychology.* Hillsdale, NJ: Lawrence Erlbaum.

Rodin, J., & Langer, E. J. (1977). Long-term effects of a control-relevant intervention with the institutionalized aged. *Journal of Personality and Social Psychology, 35,* 897-902.

Rodin, J., & Langer, E. J. (1980). Aging labels: The decline of control and the fall of self-esteem. *Journal of Social Issues, 36,* 12-29.

Rodin, J., Rennert, K., & Solomon, S. K. (1980). Intrinsic motivation for control: Fact or fiction. In A. Baum & J. E. Singer (Eds.), *Advances in environmental psychology* (Vol. 2, pp. 131-148). Hillsdale, NJ: Lawrence Erlbaum.

Romanoff, L. P., Morris, C. W., Welch, P., Grace, M. P., & Pincus, G. (1963). Metabolism of progesterone: 4-c in young and elderly men. *Journal of Clinical and Endocrine Metabolism, 23,* 286.

Rotella, R. J., & Bunker, L. K. (1978). Locus of control and achievement motivation in the active aged (65 years and over). *Perceptual and Motor Skills, 46,* 1043-1046.

Rotter, J. B. (1966). Generalized expectancies for internal versus external control of reinforcement. *Psychological Monographs: General and Applied, 80,* (Whole No. 609), 1-28.

Ryckman, R. M., & Malikioski, M. X. (1975). Relationship between locus of control and chronological age. *Psychological Reports, 36,* 655-658.

Saltz, C., & Magruder-Habib, K. (1982, November). *Age as an indicator of depression and locus of control among non-psychiatric inpatients.* Paper presented at the meeting of the Gerontological Society of America, Boston.

Schachter, S., & Singer, J. (1962). Cognitive, social and physiological determinants of emotional state. *Psychological Review, 69,* 379-399.

Schimke, R. T. (1981). *Biological mechanisms in aging* (NIH Publication No. 81-2194). Bethesda, MD: National Institutes of Health.

Schmale, A. H., & Engel, G. H. (1967). The giving up-given up complex illustrated on film. *Archives of Behavioral Psychiatry, 17,* 135-145.

Schulz, R. (1976). Effects of control and predictability on the physical and psychological well-being of the institutionalized aged. *Journal of Personality and Social Psychology, 33,* 563-573.

Schulz, R. (1980). Aging and control. In J. Garber & M. E. P. Seligman (Eds.), *Human helplessness: Theory and applications* (pp. 261-277). New York: Academic Press.

Schulz, R., & Brenner, G. (1977). Relocation of the aged: A review and theoretical analysis. *Journal of Gerontology, 32,* 323-333.

Schulz, R., & Hanusa, B. H. (1978). Long-term effects of control and predictability-enhancing interventions: Findings and ethical issues. *Journal of Personality and Social Psychology, 36,* 1194-1201.

Schulz, R., & Hanusa, B. H. (1979). Environmental influences on the effectiveness of control- and competence-enhancing interventions. In L. C. Perlmutter & R. A. Monty (Eds.), *Choice and perceived control* (pp. 315-337). Hillsdale, NJ: Lawrence Erlbaum.

Schulz, R., & Hanusa, B. H. (1980). Experimental social gerontology: A social psychological perspective. *Journal of Social Issues, 36,* 30-46.

Serio, M., Piolanti, P., Capelli, G., Magistris, L., Ricci, F., Anzalone, M., & Giusti, G. (1969). The miscible pool and turnover rate of cortisol in the aged, and variations in relation to time of day. *Experimental Gerontology, 4,* 95.

Shavit, Y., Lewis, J. W., Terman, G. W., Gale, R. P., & Liebeskind, J. C. (1983). Endogenous opioids may mediate the effects of stress on tumor growth and immune function. *Proceedings of the Western Pharmacology Society, 8,* 53-56.

Shipley, R. H. (1980). *Effect of follow-up letters on maintenance of smoking abstinence.* Paper presented at the meeting of the Midwestern Psychological Association, St. Louis.

Siegler, I. C., & Gatz, M. (1985). Age patterns in locus of control. In E. Palmore, J. Nowlin, E. Busse, I. Siegler, & G. Maddox (Eds.), *Normal aging* (Vol. 3). Durham, NC: Duke University Press.

Siskind, G. (1981). Immunological aspects of aging: An overview. In R. T. Schimke (Ed.), *Biological mechanisms in aging* (NIH Publication No. 81-2194, pp. 455-466). Bethesda, MD: National Institutes of Health.

Sklar, L. S., & Anisman, H. (1979). Stress and coping factors influence tumor growth. *Science, 205,* 513-515.

Slivinske, L. R., & Fitch, V. L. (1987). The effect of control enhancing interventions on the well-being of elderly individuals living in retirement communities. *The Gerontologist, 27,* 176-181.

Sproles, K. J. (1977). *Health locus of control and knowledge of hemodialysis and health maintenance of patients with chronic renal failure.* Unpublished manuscript, Virginia Commonwealth University.

Taylor, C. B., Bandura, A., Ewart, C. K., Miller, N. H., & Debusk, R. F. (1984). *Raising spouse's and patient's perception of his cardiac capabilities following a myocardial infarction.* Unpublished manuscript, Stanford University.

Taylor, S. E. (1979). Hospital patient behavior: Reactance, helplessness, or control? *Journal of Social Issues, 35,* 156-184.

Thompson, S. (1981). Will it hurt less if I can control it? A complex answer to a simple question. *Psychological Bulletin, 90,* 89-101.

Timiras, P. A. (1972). *Developmental physiology and aging.* New York: Macmillan.

Timko, C., & Rodin, J. (1985). Staff-patient relationships in nursing homes: Sources of conflict and rehabilitation potential. *Rehabilitation Psychology, 30,* 93-108.

Toner, J. B., & Manuck, S. B. (1979). Health locus of control and health-related information seeking at a hypertension screening. *Social Science and Medicine, 13A,* 823.

Visintainer, M. A., Volpicelli, J. R., & Seligman, M. E. P. (1982). Tumor rejection in rats after inescapable or escapable shock. *Science, 216,* 437-439.

Wallston, B. S., Wallston, K. A., Kaplan, G. D., & Maides, S. A. (1976). Development and validation of the health locus of control (HLC) scale. *Journal of Consulting and Clinical Psychology, 44,* 580-585.

Wallston, K. A., Maides, S., & Wallston, B. S. (1976). Health-related information seeking as a function of health-related locus of control and health value. *Journal of Research in Personality, 10,* 215-222.

Wallston, K. A., & McLeod, E. (1979). *Predictive factors in the adherence to an anti-hypertensive regimen among adult male outpatients.* Unpublished manuscript, Vanderbilt University.

Wallston, K. A., & Wallston, B. S. (1981). Health locus of control scales. In H. Lefcourt (Ed.), *Research with the locus of control construct* (Vol. 1). New York: Academic Press.

Wallston, K. A., & Wallston, B. S. (1982). Who is responsible for your health? The construct of health locus of control. In G. S. Sanders & J. Suls (Eds.), *Social psychology of health and illness.* Hillsdale, NJ: Lawrence Erlbaum.

Weidner, G., & Matthews, K. (1978). Reported physical symptoms elicited by unpredictable events and the Type A coronary-prone behavior pattern. *Journal of Personality and Social Psychology, 36,* 1213-1220.

Weiss, J. M. (1970). Somatic effects of predictable and unpredictable shock. *Psychosomatic Medicine, 32,* 397-409.

Weiss, J. M. (1971). Effects of coping behavior with and without a feedback signal in stress pathology in rats. *Journal of Comparative and Physiological Psychology, 77,* 22-30.

Weiss, J. M. (1972). Psychological factors in stress and disease. *Scientific American, 226,* 104-113.

Weiss, J. M., Stone, E. A., & Harrell, N. (1970). Coping behavior and brain norepinephrine level in rats. *Journal of Comparative and Physiological Psychology, 72,* 153-160.

Weisz, J. R. (1983). Can I control it? The pursuit of veridical answers across the life span. *Life-Span Development and Behavior, 5,* 233-300.

West, C. D., Brown, H., Simons, E. L., Carter, D. B., Kumagi, L. F., & Englert, E. (1961). Adrenocortisol function and cortisol metabolism in old age. *Journal of Clinical and Endocrine Metabolism, 21,* 1197.

Wildman, H. E., Rosenbaum, M. S., Framer, E. M., Keane, T. M., & Johnson, N. G. (1979). *Smoking cessation: Predicting success with the health locus of control scale.* Paper presented at the meeting of the Association for the Advancement of Behavior Therapy, San Francisco.

Williamson, J., Stokoe, I. H., Gray, S. Fisher, M., Smith, A., McGhee, A., & Stephenson, E. (1964). Old people and their unreported needs. *The Lancet, 1,* 1117-1120.

Wills, T. H. (1978). Perceptions of clients by professional helpers. *Psychological Bulletin, 85,* 968-1000.

Wolk, S. (1976). Situational constraint as a moderator of the locus of control-adjustment relationship. *Journal of Consulting and Clinical Psychology, 44,* 420-427.

Wolk, S., & Kurtz, J. (1975). Positive adjustment and involvement during aging and expectancy for internal control. *Journal of Consulting and Clinical Psychology, 43,* 173-178.

Wortman, C. B., & Brehm, J. W. (1975). Responses to uncontrollable outcomes: An integration of reactance theory and the learned helplessness model. In L. Berkowitz (Ed.), *Advances in experimental social psychology* (Vol 8). New York: Academic Press.

Ziegler, M., & Reid, D. W. (1979). Correlates of locus of desired control in two samples of elderly persons: Community residents and hospitalized patients. *Journal of Consulting and Clinical Psychology, 47,* 977-979.

Ziegler, M., & Reid, D. W. (1983). Correlates of changes in desired control scores and in life satisfaction scores among elderly persons. *International Journal of Aging and Human Development, 16,* 135-146.

8

Aging, Stress, and Illness:
Psychobiological Linkages

THOMAS M. VOGT

Health is, ultimately, a product of complex interactions among social, psychological, and biological phenomena. Few people deny that the mind has something to do with physical health. Most people accept the notion that there is a vague something labeled "stress" that can adversely affect health and that other factors in the physical and social environment can interact to alleviate or intensify the effects of that stress. Yet, in daily practice, we have not made that conceptual leap. We treat diseases as a mechanical malfunction. Clinicians rarely consider treatments aimed at modifying the effects of stress or other social or psychological phenomena. We lack adequate measurements and a synthesizing conceptual model of how stress-inducing and stress-relieving factors interrelate with one another, with perceptions of health, and with objective measures of health. Finally, the interaction between age and responses to social and psychological stimuli is rarely adequately addressed in relating such phenomena to health outcomes (Kasl & Berkman, 1981).

LIMITATIONS IN PREVIOUS RESEARCH

The literature relating social and psychological characteristics to health has contributed to the development of concepts of disease causation that interrelate social, biological, environmental, and genetic factors (Bahnson, 1974; Cassel, 1974, 1976; Henry, 1982). But the

AUTHOR'S NOTE: Work on this chapter and the author's studies described herein were supported by Grant No. 5 R01 AG05682 from the National Institute on Aging.

precise mechanisms by which social and psychological conditions affect health are not well defined, although increasingly elaborate physiological response pathways have been identified. The interaction of health-related behaviors and health state at the time of measurement with both social factors and health outcomes is well documented (Kaprio & Koskenvuo, 1988; Unden & Orth-Gomer, 1989; Wiley & Camacho, 1980). McQueen and Siegrist (1982, p. 365) examined a broad range of social factors as etiologic agents and concluded that what is needed is "approaches which are multidisciplinary and which focus on the interplay" of the various factors that might be etiologically important.

Most studies in this area have been cross-sectional or case control in design and have focused on conceptually unclear predictor variables and disease-specific outcomes (e.g., the relation of life events to heart disease or of hopelessness to cancer). Cassel (1974a, 1974b) has challenged the disease-specific outcome approach, arguing that specific manifestations of disease are a function of the genetic predisposition of the individuals and the nature of the physiochemical or microbiological insults they encounter; that is, the effects of social and psychological factors are not disease specific—at least not as disease is classically defined.

Conversely, Krause (1986) argued that our tendency to empirically group predictor events such as life events may obscure relationships. He found, for example, that social supports did not buffer the impact of a global measure of stressful life events among elderly residents in a community. However, when the events were separated into categories, he found strikingly different results. Social supports moderated the negative effects of crisis events (e.g., divorce, unemployment) and of crime and legal problems. Social support, however, had a negative impact on bereavement, which appeared to be worse where supports were higher, and had no impact whatsoever on financial stress.

LaRocco, House, and French (1980) reanalyzed data previously reported by Pinneau (1975) to show no evidence that social support networks buffer job stress. The reanalysis found pervasive evidence of highly selective effects that were not examined in the first study. It determined that mental and physical health effects of job stress were buffered, primarily by coworker support, and that job strain (worker perception of job load and strain) was reduced by social supports whether or not stress was present. Weinberger, Tierney, Booher, and Hiner (1980) found that specific social support dimensions, notably self-esteem, were associated with functional status among elderly arthritics. O'Reilly and Thomas (1989) examined the role of social support in maintaining improved cardiovascular health status after the end of a national trial. They found that specific components of social support were related to maintenance of reduced risk states, and they suggested that various social support components were specific to different disease outcomes. This specificity of predictor and outcome relationships is a dividing point among many researchers and may explain why literature reviews can be so confusing. Zuckerman, Kasl, and Ostfeld (1984), for example, reported that a variety of social characteristics are significant predictors of mortality, while Reed, McGee, Katsuhiko, and Feinleib (1983) found no significant associations of social support networks to morbidity and mortality.

THE ANALYSIS OF AGE IN EPIDEMIOLOGICAL STUDIES

Epidemiological studies are nearly always constrained by sample size, especially those that are prospective and require disease incidence or mortality outcomes. A result is that the effects of age are rarely examined in detail. Instead, age is "adjusted" when examining the results. This may provide a reasonable picture of what would happen in some hypothetical, age-free population, but it fails to account for the fact that many biological effects are age dependent. In other words, the models that explain small, but significant parts of the variations in health of that "adjusted" population might do better if they were specifically tailored to various age groups. In addition, elderly people are more difficult to contact in some settings and, because of their fewer numbers, may require oversampling to define phenomena peculiar to their period in life. Strained budgets often cannot bear the cost of such oversampling, and inappropriate projection of findings from younger age groups onto the geriatric population may result.

Aged people are not the same as younger people, and, yet, age is difficult to define in any way that is biologically consistent (Narang, 1986). Aging is associated with a progressive diminution of the ability to adapt to environmental changes. This, in turn, may be related to a variety of physiological changes strongly associated with chronological age, as has been shown in various studies of animals and humans. A few of these are discussed below; more detailed accounts can be found elsewhere (Birren & Schaie, 1985; Cutler & Narang, 1986).

We adjust for age because we assume it is related to the relationship between our predictor and outcome variables. This implies that different models are appropriate for different age groups. Brody and Schneider (1986) pointed out the difference between age-related and age-dependent diseases. The probability of getting age-related diseases peaks at certain ages, then declines. Multiple sclerosis and amyotrophic lateral sclerosis are examples. There is something, presumably biological, about the unique characteristics of a given chronological age that confers susceptibility to these diseases. Age-dependent diseases, on the other hand, are associated with the process of aging itself, and their probability of incidence rises with age. The appropriate model for relating external stimuli or psychosocial intermediaries to disease may vary, as a result, both by the nature of the disease in question and by the age of the population under consideration.

In a 15-year morbidity and mortality follow-up of persons given a variety of social and psychological measures, various measures of social networks were associated with an increased risk of ischemic heart disease, hypertension, and stroke in younger (under age 45) but not older persons (Vogt et al., 1990). Various measures of control were associated with an increased risk of death and cancer for younger but not older persons. Other measures of mental health state and physical symptoms suggested that low (healthy) scores on such measures are associated with reduced risk of death and functional gastrointestinal diseases in the young, but that low relative to high reporting of physical symptoms was actually associated with an increased risk of mortality among the elderly. Scoring low on a trust scale was associated with a reduced risk of hyperimmune diseases (allergies, arthritis, autoimmune diseases) but with an increased risk for infection among elderly persons only. Biologically, this latter finding makes sense, suggesting that low trust is associated with reduced or impaired immune function, thus lowering risk of diseases associated with excess immune reactions but increasing risk of those associated with impaired immune function.

AGING AND PSYCHOSOCIAL RISK FACTORS

At least eight studies have shown a prospective relationship between social supports/networks and mortality risk (Berkman & Syme, 1979; House, Robbins, & Metzner, 1982; Kaplan, Salonen, Cohen, Brand, & Syme, 1988; Maxwell, 1985; Orth-Gomer & Johnson, 1987; Schoenbach, Kaplan, Fredman, & Kleinbaum, 1986; Tibblin, Svardsudd, Welin, & Larson, 1986; Welin et al., 1985). The influence of social support on morbidity has been little examined. It is presumed that the relationship reflects an association of social connection to disease incidence, but this remains to be shown. Support systems might equally well affect probability of dying after disease had already occurred.

Vogt et al. (1990) examined the relative ability of social network measures to predict death and incidence of various morbid events. They found that social network measures were powerful predictors of death but only moderately good predictors of IHD incidence. Why is this? How can a putatively causal/buffering agent be related to mortality more powerfully than to incidence of the diseases that are the primary causes of mortality? At least two possible explanations can be suggested. The first is that social networks (and perhaps other psychosocial measures as well) may not be related to the incidence of serious disease but to the probability of survival once the disease has occurred. Type A behavior is a similar example, because the behavior that predicts incidence (Type A) is also directly related to an improved probability of survival. In the Vogt et al. study (1990), the investigators examined the probability of cause-specific and all-cause mortality among persons who suffered an incident case on one of nine conditions or groups of conditions. They found that social networks, particularly a measure of the breadth of the network that they termed *network scope*, were powerful predictors of survival among persons with ischemic heart disease, cancer, and hyperimmune conditions.

Another possibility is that social networks and supports as commonly measured do not address the specific social issues relevant to the incidence of disease at various critical ages but do form a summary, albeit weak, measure of the overall risk of death over time. Susceptibility to various diseases is an age-related phenomenon. The presence of strong social ties is not a yes/no issue but a developmental process that has different manifestations at different ages (Bruhn & Philips, 1987). The ability to bond is developed in childhood and manifested in various ways during different stages of life. Traditional measures of social networks (e.g., marital status, number of friends, frequency of contacts) approximate this bonding more or less accurately, depending on which stage of life is under question. Thus, in early adulthood, those network questions that predict risk of disease might be tied to career identification, relationships with the opposite sex, parenthood choices, and similar issues of relevance for the age. In old age, issues such as numbers of friends (because death is common), the ability to expand and develop relations with other peers, and loss of career contacts might be more important.

Kasl and Berkman (1981) suggested that the impact of social factors on health is not dramatically altered by age, although, if there is an age effect, it is that older persons are less affected by social factors. Although this may seem surprising in light of the lower resistance to stress and disease and reduced adaptability of the aged, it is not unexpected if health is viewed as a cumulative function of prior experience. Any new event represents a diminishing proportion of lifetime total events as the individual ages and thus would be expected to have a proportionally reduced impact, at least for chronic conditions with long incubation periods.

Studies of the impact of social and psychological factors on health deal almost exclusively with mortality or short-term health outcomes and fail to address which end of the disease spectrum is most influenced by them (Kasl & Berkman, 1981). Do they affect risk factors, incidence, duration, case fatality, diagnosis and treatment, or some other aspect of the health-illness-disability-death spectrum? Most cohorts in which these questions have been studied have not controlled for health status at the time of the initial assessment (Kaplan et al., 1988, is a notable exception). Because many psychosocial variables are related to health status, this may seriously confound the results of the studies.

Psychological stimuli strongly influence physiological response. The subjective link between these two phenomena is emotion. Emotional theory attempts to integrate three components: what is expressed, what is felt, and what happens inside the body (Birren & Schaie, 1985, p. 534). Emotional responses change with age. The body also changes with age. The production of neurotransmitters in response to stress declines (Bondareff, 1980), and some have attributed many common physical symptoms of age (depression, shuffling gait, tardive movements, rapid fatiguing, decline in sexual function, and sleep disturbances) to this fact alone (McGeer & McGeer, 1980, p. 26). Further, once the aged system is activated, it is more prone to hyperactivity (Welford, 1980) and is slower to return to baseline physiological levels. This decrease in homeostatic response is a fundamental characteristic of aging (Kaack, Ordy, & Trapp, 1975). Because external events and states produce internal physiological responses, and the nature, extent, and duration of those internal responses change with age, it is very likely that the impact of those external events and states on health varies substantially with age and is quite different for the elderly than for the young.

AGING, BIOLOGICAL RESPONSE TO
STRESS, AND RESISTANCE TO DISEASE

The interactions among stress, immunity, and aging are the subject of a book that summarizes these relationships in more detail than can be accomplished here (Cooper, 1984). As aging progresses, immune function becomes both diminished and aberrant (Effros, 1984). T-lymphocyte function degenerates in parallel with thymic involution and a loss of serum thymic hormone activity. T-cell responses to antigens and mitogens decline. Serum immunoglobins are also altered. IgG and IgA concentrations rise and IgM falls (Buckley & Dorsey, 1970; Radl, Sepers, Skuaril, Morell, & Hijmans, 1975). Natural antibody titers decline (Paul & Bunnell, 1932/1982), and autoantibodies increase (Roberts-Thompson, Whittingham, Youngchaiyud, & Mackay, 1974). All these defects seem to be related to defective T-cell collaboration and/or B-cell function (Effros, 1984). It has been suggested that these functional changes are responsible for aging.

The catalog of changes in physiological function related to aging is large. The various relations of social and psychological stressors to disease across the life span constitute an area that is almost untapped. Plasma noradrenalin (NA) levels rise with age (Ziegler, Lake, & Kopin, 1976), as does the NA response to stress. The ability of beta-adrenergic blocking agents such as propranolol to block NA action, however, declines with age (Conway, Wheeler, & Sannerstedt, 1971; Ziegler et al, 1976). If the sensitivity of such receptors declines with age, then the response to noradrenergic agonist and antagonist drugs may also be expected to diminish with age. An extrapolation of this idea would suggest that stress, which triggers a noradrenaline response (fight/flight), might have a physical impact at earlier ages, when receptivity is higher, and a declining impact at later ages. Because atherosclerosis is a lifelong process, it may be that the timing of life stresses is critical in influencing ischemic heart disease and also in raising the low correlation coefficient between stress and immunofunction that bothered Kiecolt-Glaser and Glaser (1987).

THE PHYSIOLOGY OF STRESS

Adrenal-Medullary Response

External stimuli may produce internal physiological responses that have health consequences. Several systems in the brain are involved in the translation of these stimuli ("stress") into physiological changes that may effect susceptibility to disease. The sympathetic adrenal-medullary axis is tied to the fight-flight response first investigated by Cannon (1929). This response is triggered by an external challenge to control over food, water, mate, shelter, or other important resources if the organism perceives that a successful response is feasible. The response involves a range of behaviors/emotions from fear to alertness to aggression. Though fear and anger both involve catecholamine secretion (Henry, 1982), they arise from different locations in the amygdala, and those regions are associated with differential cardiovascular responses. A defensive posture is characterized by the release of adrenaline, and an attack posture by noradrenaline release (Stock, Schlor, Heidt, & Buss, 1978). Others have suggested that adrenaline is released when there is a question of adequacy (Dimsdale & Moss, 1980), while greater noradrenaline rise occurs during exercise when great effort is directed at mastery (Henry, 1982). As noted, this neurotransmitter secretory response is age related, as is the physiological response of the body to the presence of these substances.

Various relaxation and meditation practices represent the opposite of the fight-flight response. Benson (1975) derived the relaxation response as a secularized form of transcendental meditation. Patel, Marmot, and Terry (1981) used rhythmic breathing, deep muscle relaxation, and a variety of other techniques to achieve similar goals. In 1985, Patel and associates published one of the first studies to suggest that long-term practice of such procedures may reduce morbidity. If stress produces negative health effects, it is quite possible that meditation and relaxation exercises practiced regularly might counteract those effects because they all appear to be a part of a single spectrum of physiological response.

Adrenal-Cortical Response

A second system of the brain involved in response to stress is the pituitary-adrenal-cortical axis first described by Selye (1936). This is the system that becomes activated in a hopeless situation, when the organism cannot foresee a successful response. It involves hippocampal arousal, which, in turn, leads to the production of ACTH from the pituitary and consequent production of adrenal-cortical steroids. These are, of course, immunosuppressive agents. Disturbances involving an individual's expectations of proper position in a social hierarchy may produce hippocampal arousal and thereby lead to depression, avoidance of others, and submissiveness (Henry, 1982; Henry & Stevens, 1977). Ambiguity in the social hierarchy may characterize humans after retirement, and depression and avoidance among the elderly are related to such ambiguity.

Among students, pleasant, easily paced tasks are accompanied by catecholamine production, while demanding, distressing tasks leading to loss of mastery cause an increase in cortisol secretion (Frankenhaeuser, Lundberg, & Forsman, 1980). Figure 8.1 summarizes the interaction of the sympathetic and pituitary-adrenal-cortical axes of response to stress. Under the circumstances in which these systems evolved, all parts were adaptive. "Good" and "bad" parts of the axes represent ways in which civilization interacts with biology to make a formerly adaptive response into a nonadaptive one.

Repeated disturbances of these neurophysiological pathways may produce depression or overactivity of the entire hypothalamic pituitary-adrenal system. Cortisol secretion rises and circadian rhythms are disturbed. Cortisol also depresses immunity, which is also related to age, sex, time of day, and levels of thyroid, insulin, and growth hormones (Rogers, Dubey, & Reich, 1979). Chronic stress produces an initial immune enhancement followed by subsequent depression (Dorian et al., 1985). This issue will be discussed later. Aging is associated with a gradual failure of immunoregulation, but these changes are specific to individuals and to various types of stress.

In other words, these two brain systems are linked to stress response. The first, termed variously the *fight-flight reaction* or the *defense response,* involves situations where a feasible response exists; the second, termed the *conservation-withdrawal syndrome,* involves situations where there is little hope of an adequate response. However, these systems also respond to things other than simply the input of stressful stimuli. Henry (1982) provided an overview of the neurophysiology of these systems. Figure 8.2 summarizes the physiological pathways by which stress is related to myocardial infarction. There are multiple paths, several of which involve input from both sympathetic and pituitary-adrenal axes.

Because these systems function throughout life, there is no simple way to separate the effects of current from past environment when we attempt to relate the response patterns to stressful stimuli or to study the modification of those effects by various other characteristics such as social networks, coping skills, and the like. Does repeated stimulation "reset" homeostatic mechanisms so that, later on, we have unhealthy levels of cortisol or catecholamines even in the absence of continued stimulation?

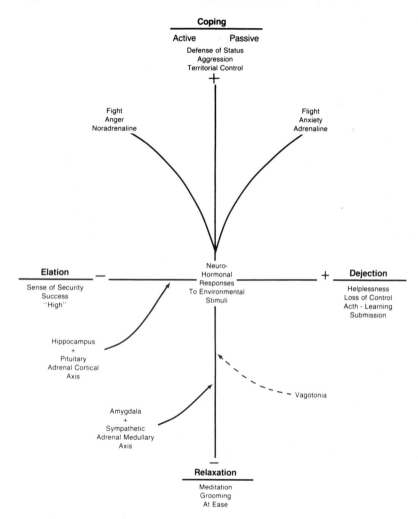

Figure 8.1. Theoretical Vector Diagram Contrasting the Emotion-Related Response Patterns of the Pituitary Adrenal-Cortical and the Sympathetic Adrenal-Medullary Systems

SOURCE: Henry (1982); used by permission.
NOTE: The adrenal-cortical axis activates the high cortisol response of dejection-distress to loss of control and elation-euphoria-attachment to successful control. The sympathetic system is activated by the effort demanded to maintain control. The ensuing active fight-flight response involves release of noradrenaline and fight-rage in association with challenge and an adrenaline-anxiety component or both when there is uncertainty of outcome. The achievement of control normally leads to relaxation, dovetailing with the expression of attachment behavior and low cortisol, serotonin-related changes of the hippocampal, pituitary adrenal-cortical axis.

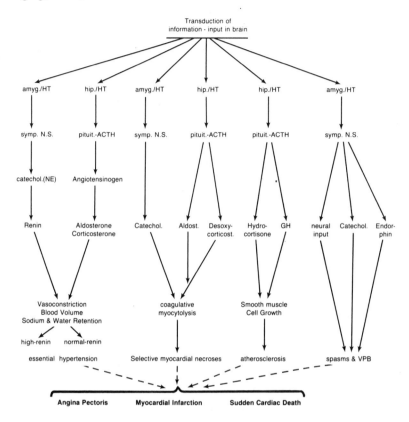

Figure 8.2. Social Factors in the Etiology of Chronic Disease: Selective Relationships Between Neuroendocrine Responses and Cardiovascular Pathology

SOURCE: McQueen and Siegrist (1982); used by permission.
NOTE: Abbreviations—amyg. = amygdala; hip. = hippocampus; symp.N.S. = sympathetic nervous system; pituit. = pituitary; GH = growth hormone; VPB = ventricular premature beats.

Various psychosocial behaviors (Dembroski et al., 1985; Haynes, Feinleib, & Kannel, 1980; Kneier & Temoshok, 1984; MacDougall, Dembroski, Dimsdale, & Hackett, 1985) have been repeatedly related to the risk of disease. Those such as suppression of anger, which are related to chronic sympathetic hyperactivity, are thought to produce an increased risk of cardiovascular disease (Krantz & Manuck, 1984). Indeed, post-myocardial infarction therapy with beta-blocking drugs has been shown to reduce risk of reinfarction, and beta-blocking drugs reduce sympathetic reactivity.

The development of atherosclerotic disease is mediated by complex endocrine interactions (Weinstein & Stemerman, 1981). These interactions involve a variety of hormonal substances with known and unknown relationships to various social and psychological predictors of disease. Some of these are summarized in Figure 8.3. Note the familiar players in that figure—pituitary and adrenal axes, this time operating through a variety of mechanisms not yet discussed. A hormone-free tissue culture of mammalian arterial smooth muscle cells produces normal cells. The addition of hormones to these cultures leads to the spontaneous formation of atherosclerotic plaquelike nodules. In vivo, such cells are exposed to the full complement of serum hormones only after endothelial injury (Goldberg, Stemerman, & Handin, 1980; Ross & Glomset, 1976). It is possible, therefore, that the occurrence of injury, possibly quite minor, is necessary but not sufficient for the initiation of atherosclerotic plaque in the presence of an appropriate hormonal environment. In other words, both the injury and the stress need to be appropriately sequenced. Cortisol has also been tentatively linked to the formation of atherosclerotic plaque and has been suggested as a risk factor for coronary heart disease (Troxler, Sprague, Albanese, Fuchs, & Thompson, 1977).

Similarly, cancer might result from chronic hyperreactivity of the pituitary-adrenal-cortical system (Grossarth-Maticek, Siegrist, & Vetter, 1982). Such hyperreactivity may be associated with submissiveness, lack of aggression, suppression of perceived needs, and adjustment to nonrewarding interpersonal relationships in order to maintain a sense of security and self-esteem. Grossarth-Maticek et al. (1982) categorized the extremes as "emitters of repression" (those at risk of cardiovascular disease and subject to chronic sympathetic adrenal-medullary hyperreactivity) and "receivers of repression" (those at risk of cancer and subject to chronic adrenal-cortical hyperreactivity). An extensive, though inconsistent, literature relates cancer occurrence to these kinds of personal characteristics. Cancer risk has been linked to reduced ability to express emotion (Blumberg, 1954; Greer & Morris, 1975; Grissom, Weiner, & Weiner, 1975), to a reduced insight (Abse et al., 1974; Bahnson & Bahnson, 1966; Pancheri et al., 1979), to hopelessness following the loss of a spouse or other close family member (Greene, 1966; Spence, 1975), to the use of repression and denial as coping mechanisms (Abse et al., 1974; Bahnson, 1966; Bahnson & Bahnson, 1966, Pancheri et al., 1979), and to other similar concepts.

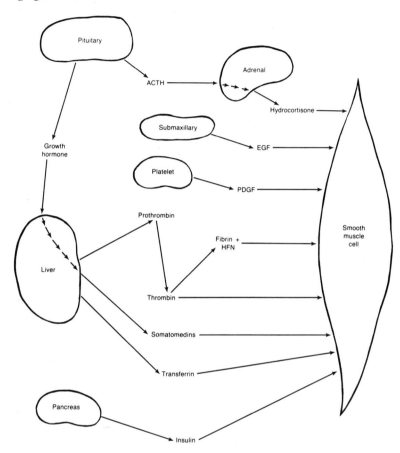

Figure 8.3. Influence of Hormones on Arterial Smooth Muscle Cell
Growth: An Endocrine Approach to Atherosclerosis

SOURCE: Weinstein and Stemerman (1981); used by permission.
NOTE: Depicted are the hormones required for smooth muscle cell growth and their parent
organs, ACTH, adrenocorticotrophic hormone.

A criticism that has been leveled at such studies is that cancer is
not a single disease but a collection of diseases with a similar pathological process. Treating cancer as an outcome is not unlike treating
infection as a single outcome. A way around this is to do studies of
individual cancers. However, it is difficult to find sufficient numbers
of single cancers to conduct such studies. Attempts have been made,
although with conclusions and study designs that leave something to

be desired. Reznikoff (1955) found that women with malignant breast nodules were more likely to report emotional disturbances in infancy and marital discord than those with benign nodules. Schonfield (1975) determined that women with malignant nodules scored higher on the Minnesota Multiphasic Personality Inventory (MMPI) L scale (denial) than those with benign nodules and that they had higher life stress scores. The latter finding was contradicted by Snell and Graham (1971), who found no relation of life stress to breast cancer.

Neuropeptides

Several neuropeptides act as neuromodulators and thus join the brain, glands, and immune system in a network of communication between brain and body, "probably representing the biochemical substrate of emotion" (Pert, Ruff, Weber, & Herkenham, 1985, p. 824S). Opioids have distinct effects on circulatory regulation, and these effects are unique to particular peptides (Faux et al., 1979; Holaday, 1983; Ruth & Eiden, 1984). These range from pressor to depressor effects, and they may serve to buffer the effects of sympathetic stimulation (Belenky & Holady, 1979). Opiates also affect conditioned learning and influence the individual's perception of the degree of aversiveness of a stressor (Riley, Zellner, & Duncan, 1980). Naloxone, a narcotic antagonist, reduces differences in performance between high and low blood pressure groups and results in an increase in the response of blood pressure to stress among those with low pressure but not among those with high blood pressure (McCubbin, Surwit, & Williams, 1985). Thus naturally produced opioids are intimately involved with cardiovascular reactivity, that is, with physiological response of the cardiovascular system to external stimuli. Such reactivity is, in part, genetically determined (Falkner, Onesti, Angelakos, Fernandos, & Langman, 1979; Falkner & Ragonesi, 1986) and may be a risk factor for coronary heart disease (Corse, Manuck, Cantwell, Giordani, & Matthews, 1982; Dembroski, MacDougall, & Lushene, 1979; Keys et al., 1971).

STRESS AND IMMUNITY

We have already discussed how the feasibility of an effective response affects physiological response to stress. The same phenomenon has been observed for immune response. Both animal and human studies have demonstrated abundant and varied effects of stress on immune response (Chang & Rasmussen, 1965; Davis & Read, 1958; Dorian & Garfinkle, 1987; Friedman, Ader, & Grota, 1973; Friedman, Glasgow, & Ader, 1969; Jensen & Rasmussen, 1963; Johnson, Lavender, & Marsh, 1959; Laudenslauger, Ryan, Drugan, Hyson, & Maier, 1983; Levine, Strebel, Wend, & Harman, 1962; Marsh, Lavender, Chang, & Rasmussen, 1963; Plaut, Ader, Friedman, & Ritterson, 1969; Rasmussen, Marsh, & Brill, 1957; Schleifer, Keller, Camerino, Thornton, & Stein, 1983). These effects include immunosuppression, immune stimulation, and a biphasic response to stress. Although often neglected in conceptual models, there is also a reported relationship between stress and susceptibility to arthritis (Amkraut, Solomon, & Kraemer, 1971; Rogers, Trentham, et al., 1979). Tecoma and Huey (1985) and Borysenko (1987) summarized the relation of psychic distress to immune response, and this relationship is further discussed in the chapter by Rodin and Timko in this volume. Immune response can be behaviorally conditioned (Ader & Cohen, 1975, 1982; Bovbjerg, Ader, & Cohen, 1984; Russel et al., 1984), and it may ultimately be possible to develop behavioral training programs that enhance immune response.

RESEARCH PERSPECTIVES: SYNTHESIS VERSUS REDUCTIONISM

Health and disease are, as Cassel (1976) insisted, the end result of genetics and the physical and social environments. Acquiring a disease depends on the interaction of the "dose" of exposure with the degree of susceptibility. The degree of susceptibility is affected by the social and psychological interior and exterior environments and the resulting changes in internal physiological environment. Elderly people undergo major changes in their external environments. Retirement, loss of spouse, separation from children, deteriorating financial conditions, and many other changes mark this period of life and are superimposed on less adaptive internal physiological regulatory mechanisms.

One might divide researchers into two groups: "reductionists" and "synthesizers." Exhaustive reviews of the literature call for models that achieve broader applicability through increased complexity. McQueen and Siegrist (1982) pointed to the problems of general outcomes that suffer from "underspecification." They praised what they termed the "epidemiological approach" because it has tended to focus on disease-specific outcomes rather than on the generalized illness outcomes that are favored by sociologists. Others (Unden & Orth-Gomer, 1989; Weinberger et al., 1990) have emphasized the importance of studying specific social subcomponents and their separate relationships to specific morbid outcomes.

Despite the fact that some epidemiological studies are disease specific, the approach of other epidemiologists and sociologists is more synthetic. The work of Cassel (1976), Kaplan (1985), and Satariano and Syme (1979) is illustrative. Cassel synthesized the results of different types of research into a single conceptual view suggesting that poor social supports and lack of environmental feedback produce declines in health. Satariano and Syme examined common features of Type A behavior, stressful life events, and other social variables to conclude that all had in common an underlying social isolation. Kaplan (1985) examined the direct and indirect effects of a variety of psychosocial predictors of ischemic heart disease. He concluded that the distinction between host and environment is problematic and, because this is true, recognized the importance of a holistic view of the individual's situation. Kaplan examined seven psychosocial predictors of mortality from ischemic heart disease in Alameda County, California. He adjusted each risk factor by the six others and determined which of their relationships were directly linked to mortality from heart disease and which were indirect. Social networks, socioeconomic status, and "helplessness" had direct links to death from heart disease. Depression and life satisfaction were associated with IHD only through their associations with other factors. Health practices were both directly associated with IHD mortality and also indirectly associated via their relationships to social networks and perceived health. Perceived health status was directly linked to IHD and indirectly linked via relationships to SES, helplessness, and health practices.

Kaplan advanced a model (Figure 8.4) that suggests that social networks and health practices both represent day-to-day processes in which the individual acts receive feedback from the external environment. The feedback then modifies behavior. Cassel (1976) emphasized that a key ingredient of adverse outcomes from social and psychological characteristics is the lack of feedback to the individual concerning the consequences of his or her actions. Kaplan suggested that "helplessness" represents a "proactive" orientation to see the world as incoherent and unpredictable and to appraise new situations as stressful and threatening. In other words, the "hopeless" individual assumes from the outset that environmental feedback will be

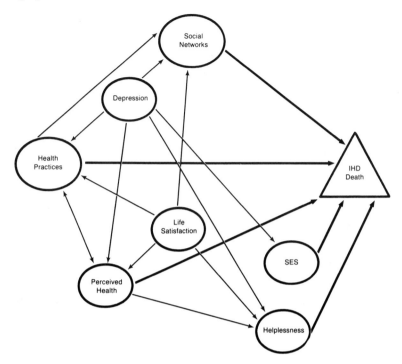

Figure 8.4. Direct and Indirect Associations Between Psychosocial Measures and IHD Death

SOURCE: Kaplan (1985); used by permission.

inadequate to permit appropriate coping responses. Measures of depression and of *helplessness* (Kaplan was not pleased with this term for the scale he used but did not suggest another) do not measure the same thing. Kaplan et al. (1988) confirmed that social connections represent a prospective risk factor for males (but not for females) for death from all causes. The effects of social connection were also modified by the level of blood pressure, a risk factor for stroke and heart disease that is influenced by several of the physiological systems that were described earlier.

Friedman and Booth-Kewley (1987) suggested that, despite weak evidence, there is a generic, disease-prone personality involving depression, anger/hostility, and anxiety. Jacobson (1986) emphasized the limitations of life events models. Stressful life events have been related to morbid events with little attention to the manner in which other social and psychological characteristics might modify that interaction. Consequently, that literature is confusing and highly inconsistent.

MODEL OF PSYCHOSOCIAL DETERMINANTS OF DISEASE

Three synthetic theories relating psychosocial interactions and external stress to illness susceptibility have been presented by Jacobson (1986).

(1) The "needs" model. Each person has specific needs that are met through social interaction. Social structures are established to meet these needs. For example, marriage meets the need for attachment, parenting meets the need for nurturance, friends meet the need for social integration, and experts and professionals meet the need for guidance (Weiss, 1974). Other postulated needs include self-esteem and mastery (Pearlin, Menaghan, Lieberman, & Mullan, 1981; Thoits, 1983, 1985). Disruption of these bonds has a negative impact on health.

(2) The "transactions" model. Stress results when the level of individually perceived demands exceeds the resources available to deal with them (Lazarus & Folkman, 1984; Lazarus & Launier, 1978; McGrath, 1970). These demands may be constant or intermittent. In either case, the nature of the demand is irrelevant; the degree to which it exceeds available resources is crucial.

(3) The "transitions" model. Stress occurs as a result of changes in the persons or environment around us (or within us). Such changes affect our assumptions about the world and our proper place within it. Culture shock is a particularly obvious example. When the world becomes confusing and we do not know how to interpret the meaning of the interactions we have, we suffer stress (Bowlby, 1980).

Other attempts to summarize the data fit generally into these groups. Rowe and Kahn (1987, p. 146) concluded that "the extent to which autonomy and control are encouraged or denied may be a major determinant of whether aging is usual or successful on a number of physiologic and behavioral dimensions." A corollary of their conclusion is that many programs aimed at supporting the elderly are not designed to achieve their goals. Programs that "do for" older people or rely on health warnings may augment helplessness. Teaching, encouraging, and enabling will increase autonomy and, therefore, will lead to an improved sense of support and control.

Jacobson's models are not mutually exclusive. They do suggest that specific items measured in various studies ought to be considered in terms of how they relate to these concepts and that programs designed to support the elderly will not be effective if they are limited simply to prescriptions as to what others ought to do or must do.

Social class is strongly and consistently associated with health-related outcomes. In personal conversation (1987), both Syme and Kaplan have expressed concern that many studies adjust out the effects of this critical variable. Adjustments for all known risk factors fail to abolish this association. What is fundamental to social class that produces such strong associations in the absence of risk-factor differences? That question is fundamental and unanswered. A study by Vogt et al. (1990) of 2,603 adult members of a large health maintenance organization (HMO) offers an interesting clue. Members of the cohort were selected on the basis of two or more years of sustained membership in the HMO. Otherwise, the sample was random and included a diversity of SES groups. The cohort was followed for 15 years, and psychosocial measures taken at baseline were related to subsequent mortality and morbidity rates. Psychosocial and behavioral variables were related to risk in precisely the manner reported in the literature. SES, however, was not related to the assessed outcomes. The selection for stability of HMO membership was the sole characteristic of the population that differentiates it from other samples in which strong associations between SES and morbidity/mortality have been observed, including other studies within the same HMO. However, extremes of wealth and poverty were not common in the sample. Social class is related to more than simply access to food, shelter, and medical care. It is related to the stability of the environment, to options for coping with problems, and to the availability of a network of people who can be called upon to help.

DILEMMAS OF LANGUAGE AND CLASSIFICATION

Confusing Terms

We are inventing the language as we go and may choose the same words to mean different things. Kaplan's *helplessness* is a set of specific questions that should probably have a different name. Berkman (1977) called the same scale "personal uncertainty." The helplessness theorized to be involved in the development of cancer

is entirely different, based as it is on physiological studies of immo-
bilized animals, which, when exposed to stress in the absence of
feasible responses, experience an increase in adrenal-cortical hormone secretion.

The distinction between social support and social network has
become widely accepted; however, the terms that have been used to
describe the subcomponents of social networks are myriad and confusing. Auslander (1988) summarized various questions to describe
the existence, perception, and mobilization of the social network.
Maxwell (1985) discussed the scope, size, frequency, and interaction of the social network. Unden and Orth-Gomer (1989) analyzed
the availability and adequacy of social integration and the availability and adequacy of attachment. This catalog could be much,
much longer. Of course, many of these concepts overlap considerably.
Auslander's mobilization of the network is similar to Maxwell's
frequency, for example. It is time for some collaboration on grouping
these concepts into consistent scales aimed at testing mutually understood concepts.

Different Outcomes

Psychosocial factors are related to both mental and physical pathology. The emphasis in this chapter is on physical health, but the
literature contains models and discussions of the importance of different factors as they relate to both mental and physical pathology.
The appropriate models and the findings of studies may differ across
types of outcomes. Arling (1987) presented a complex set of analyses
in which social contact, social support, life strain, and social resource
availability were used to predict psychological distress among elderly persons. Such findings are not directly comparable to those of
Kaplan (1985), who studied ischemic heart disease.

Disease Classification

If the physiological response to stress is determined to some degree
by the organism's internal (not necessarily conscious) perception of
the feasibility of the response, and if the type of physiological response, when prolonged, enhances susceptibility to a certain complex
of diseases that is determined by the type of physiological response,
then, perhaps, we have been using inappropriate disease classification systems. Most prospective studies that examine social and psychological characteristics as disease predictors use mortality as their

outcome. In most cases, this outcome is chosen because of data limitations. There are few registries of disease incidence, and numbers get very small when one starts to look at specific diseases or even classes of diseases. Traditional disease groups reflect organ system pathology rather than a coherent view of how social and psychological factors affect health. The adrenal-cortical responder to stress, for example, might be expected to have an impaired immune response and to suffer from diseases that occur in weakened immune systems. Cancer and infectious disease might make perfectly acceptable conceptual companions, although they have great differences in incubation periods. But cumulative infection rates should be higher among persons who develop cancer if impaired immune response is involved.

CLASSIFICATION OF STRESS-RELATED ILLNESS

Figure 8.5 presents a system for classifying diseases as they are related to the hypothalamic-pituitary-adrenal response system. There are three groups of stress-related illness. The first includes diseases potentially related to chronic hyperarousal (primarily cardiovascular conditions). The second includes diseases possibly related to adrenal-cortical hyperreactivity, that is, diseases that require a healthy immune response if they are to be resisted.

Finally, diseases of hyperimmune response are grouped together, although we lack a postulated physiological mechanism for the group. These groupings provide larger numbers than would be available from traditional, pathology-based disease groups and also eliminate disease outcomes that may be irrelevant to stress. Much more complex groups could be devised. We are currently comparing this particular system to organ system-based disease classification in a longitudinal study (Vogt et al., 1990).

SUMMARY AND IMPLICATIONS

Mind and body interact constantly. External events produce physiological responses that are dazzling in variety and complexity. Multiple hormonal systems affect, at least in the short term, physical systems that function to protect the body from illness. Similarly, a variety of social and psychological characteristics, which may be viewed as external stressors and/or as stress modifiers, are associated

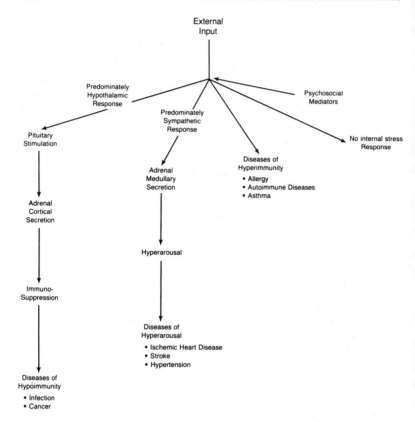

Figure 8.5. Model for Interaction of External Stimuli with Internal
Response for the Hypothalamic/Pituitary and Sympathetic
Systems

NOTE: There is no known mediating system for hyperimmune responses, but they are clearly
related to stressful inputs.

with changes in these hormonal systems. Most psychobiological studies are, for practical reasons, limited to the examination of acute
effects. Most epidemiological studies are limited to short-term, common, or mortal outcomes. It is not clear how age, duration and type
of stress, and behavior interact with one another and with genetic
structure to determine the incidence, type, and severity of disease.
That such interactions occur, and that disease does result from various kinds of life stresses, seems fairly obvious, yet the degree of
specificity of these interaction is not clear. Further, the relation of age

to the interactions of disease susceptibility with psychosocial phenomena has received insufficient attention. Untangling the complexities of these relationships to achieve an understanding of how the modification of the social and psychological environment might affect specific disease outcomes will require both laboratory and large, longitudinal cohort studies. Potential modifications of the social and psychological environment are not value free. Quality of life is a legitimate outcome of such studies, and the aim of extending life must be coupled with the aim of making it more fulfilling. A unique feature of this field of research is that the two goals are so compatible.

REFERENCES

Abse, D. W., Wilkins, M. M., Van de Castle, R. L., Buston, W. D., Demars, J. P., Brown, R. S., & Kirschner, L. G. (1974). Personality and behavioral characteristics of lung cancer patients. *Journal of Psychosomatic Research, 18*, 101-113.

Ader, R., & Cohen, N. (1975). Behaviorally conditioned immunosuppression. *Psychomatic Medicine, 37*, 333-340.

Ader, R., & Cohen, N. (1982). Behaviorally conditioned immunosuppression and murine systemic lupus erythematosus. *Science, 215*, 1534-1536.

Amkraut, A. A., Solomon, G. F., & Kraemer, H. C. (1971). Stress, early experience and adjuvant-induced arthritis in the rat. *Psychosomatic Medicine, 33*, 203-214.

Arling, G. (1987). Strain, social support, and distress in old age. *Journals of Gerontology, 42*, 107-113.

Auslander, G. K. (1988). Social networks and the functional health status of the poor: A secondary analysis of data from the national survey of personal health practices and consequences. *Journal of Community Health, 13*, 197-209.

Bahnson, C. B. (1966). Psychophysiological complementarity in malignancies: Past work and future vistas. *Annals of the New York Academy of Science, 164*, 319-330.

Bahnson, C. B. (1974). Epistemological perspectives of physical disease from the psychodynamic point of view. *American Journal of Public Health, 64*, 1034-1040.

Bahnson, C. B., & Bahnson, M. B. (1966). Role of the ego defenses: Denial and repressions in the etiology of malignant neoplasms. *Annals of the New York Academy of Science, 125*, 827-845.

Belenky, G. L., & Holaday, J. W. (1979). The opiate antagonist naloxone modifies the effects of respiration. *Brain Research, 177*, 414-417.

Benson, H. (1975). *The relaxation response.* New York: William Morrow.

Berkman, L. F. (1977). *Social networks, host resistance, and mortality: A follow-up of Alameda County residents.* Unpublished doctoral dissertation, University of California, Berkeley.

Berkman, L. F., & Syme, S. L. (1979). Social networks, host resistance and mortality: A nine-year follow-up study of Alameda County residents. *American Journal of Epidemiology, 109*, 186-204.

Birren, J. E., & Schaie, K. W. (1985). *Handbook of the psychology of aging.* New York: Van Nostrand Reinhold.

Blumberg, E. M. (1954). Results of the psychological testing of cancer patients. In J. A. Gengerelli & F. J. Kirkner (Eds.), *Psychological variables in human cancer.* Berkeley: University of California Press.

Bondareff, W. (1980). Neurobiology of aging. In J. E. Birren & R. B. Sloane (Eds.), *Handbook of mental health and aging.* Englewood Cliffs, NJ: Prentice-Hall.

Borysenko, M. (1987). The immune system: An overview. *Annals of Behavioral Medicine, 9,* 3-10.

Bovbjerg, D., Ader, R., & Cohen, N. (1984). Acquisition of conditioned suppression of a graft-versus-host response in the rat. *Journal of Immunology, 132,* 111-113.

Bowlby, J. (1980). *Attachment and loss: Vol. 3. Loss, sadness, and depression.* New York: Basic Books.

Brody, J. A., & Schneider, E. L. (1986). Diseases and disorders of aging: An hypothesis. *Journal of Chronic Disease, 39,* 871-876.

Bruhn, J. G., & Philips, B. U. (1987). A developmental basis for social supports. *Journal of Behavioral Medicine, 10,* 213-229.

Buckley, C. E., & Dorsey, F. C. (1970). The effect of aging on human serum immunoglobulin concentrations. *Journal of Immunology, 105,* 964-972.

Cannon, W. B. (1929). *Bodily changes in pain, hunger, fear and rage: An account of recent researches into the function of emotional excitement* (2nd ed.). New York: Appleton.

Cassel, J. (1974a). Psychosocial processes and "stress": Theoretical formulation. *International Journal of Health Services, 4,* 471-482.

Cassel, J. (1974b). An epidemiological perspective of psychosocial factors in disease etiology. *American Journal of Public Health, 64,* 1040-1043.

Cassel, J. (1976). The contribution of the social environment to host resistance. *American Journal of Epidemiology, 104,* 107-123.

Chang, S., & Rasmussen, A. F., Jr. (1965). Stress-induced suppression of interferon production in virus-infected mice. *Nature, 205,* 623-624.

Cohen, S. (1988). Psychological models of the role of social support in the etiology of physical disease. *Health Psychology, 7,* 269-297.

Conway, J., Wheeler, R., & Sannerstedt, R. (1971). Sympathetic nervous activity during exercise in relation to age. *Cardiovascular Research, 5,* 577-581.

Cooper, E. L. (Ed.). (1984). *Stress, immunity, and aging.* New York: Marcel Dekker.

Corse, C. D., Manuck, S. B., Cantwell, J. D., Giordani, B., & Matthews, K. A. (1982). Coronary-prone behavior patterns and cardiovascular response in persons with and without coronary heart disease. *Psychosomatic Medicine, 44,* 449-459.

Cutler, N. R., & Narang, P. K. (Eds.). (1986). *Drug studies in the elderly: Methodological concerns.* New York: Plenum Medical.

Davis, D. E., & Read, C. P. (1958). Effect of behavior on development of resistance in trichinosis. *Proceedings of Social Experimental Biological Medicine, 99,* 269-272.

Dembroski, T. M., MacDougall, J. M., & Lushene, R. (1979). Interpersonal interaction and cardiovascular response in Type A subjects and coronary patients. *Journal of Human Stress, 5,* 28-36.

Dembroski, T. M., MacDougall, J. M., Williams, R. B., Haney, T. L., & Blumenthal, J. A. (1985). Components of Type A, hostility, and anger-in: Relationship to angiographic findings. *Psychosomatic Medicine, 47,* 219-233.

Dimsdale, J. E., & Moss, J. (1980). Plasma catecholamines in stress and exercise. *JAMA, 243,* 340-342.

Dorian, B., & Garfinkel, P. E. (1987). Stress, immunity and illness: A review. *Psychological Medicine, 17*, 393-407.

Dorian, B., Garfinkel, P. E., Keystone, E. C., Gorczynski, R., Garner, D. M., Darby, P., & Shore, A. (1985). Occupational stress and immunity [Abstract]. *Psychosomatic Medicine, 47*, 77.

Effros, R. B. (1984). Aging and immunity. In E. L. Cooper (Ed.), *Stress, immunity, and aging*. New York: Marcel Dekker.

Falkner, B., Onesti, G., Angelakos, E. T., Fernandes, M., & Langman, C. (1979). Cardiovascular response to mental stress in normal adolescents with hypertensive parents. *Hypertension, 1*, 23-30.

Falkner, B., & Ragonesi, S. (1986). Psychosocial stress and reactivity as risk factors of cardiovascular disease. *Journal of American Academy of Child Psychiatry, 25*, 779-784.

Faux, K., Bolme, P., Jonsson, G., Agnati, L. F., Goldstein, M., Hokfelt, T., Schwarcz, R., & Engle, J. (1979). On the cardiovascular role of noradrenalin, adrenalin and peptide containing neuron systems in the brain. In H. Schmitt & P. Meyer (Eds.), *Perspectives in nephrology and hypertension*. Paris: John Wiley.

Frankenhaeuser, M., Lundberg, U., & Forsman, L. (1980). Dissociation between sympathetic-adrenal and pituitary-adrenal responses to an achievement situation characterized by high controllability: Comparison between Type A and Type B males and females. *Biological Psychology, 10*, 79-81.

Friedman, H. S., & Booth-Kewley, S. (1987). The "disease-prone personality": A metanalytic view of the construct. *American Psychologist, 42*, 539-555.

Friedman, S. B., Ader, R., & Grota, L. J. (1973). Protective effect of noxious stimulation in mice infected with rodent malaria. *Psychosomatic Medicine, 35*, 535-537.

Friedman, S. B., Glasgow, L. A., & Ader, R. (1969). Psychosocial factors modifying host resistance to experimental infections. *Annals of the New York Academy of Science, 164*, 381-392.

Goldberg, I. D., Stemerman, M. B., & Handin, R. I. (1980). Vascular permeation of platelet factor 4 after endothelial injury. *Science, 209*, 611-612.

Greene, W. A. (1966). Psychosocial setting of the development of leukemia and lymphoma. *Annals of the New York Academy of Science, 125*, 794-801.

Greer, S., & Morris, T. (1975). Psychological attributes of women who develop breast cancer: A controlled study. *Journal of Psychosomatic Research, 19(2)*, 147-153.

Grissom, J. J., Weiner, B. J., & Weiner, A. (1975). Psychological correlates of cancer. *Journal of Consulting Clinical Psychology, 43*, 119.

Grossarth-Maticek, R., Siegrist, J., & Vetter, H. (1982). Interpersonal repression as a predictor of cancer. *Social Science Medicine, 16*, 493-498.

Haynes, S. G., Feinleib, M., & Kannel, W. B. (1980). The relationship of psychosocial factors to coronary heart disease in the Framingham study: Eight year incidence of coronary heart disease. *American Journal of Epidemiology, 111*, 37-58.

Henry, J. P. (1982). The relation of social to biological processes in disease. *Social Science Medicine, 16*, 369-380.

Henry, J. P., & Stephens, P. M. (1977). *Stress, health, and the social environment: A sociobiologic approach to medicine*. New York: Springer-Verlag.

Hibbard, J. H. (1985). Social ties and health status: An examination of moderating factors. *Health Education Quarterly, 12*, 23-24.

Holaday, J. W. (1983). Cardiovascular effects of endogenous opiate systems. *Annual Review of Pharmacological Toxicology, 23*, 541-594.

House, J. S., Robbins, C., & Metzner, H. L. (1982). The association of social relationships and activities with mortality: Prospective evidence from the Tecumseh Community Health Study. *American Journal of Epidemiology, 116*, 123-140.

Isacsson, S. O., & Janzon, L. (1986). *Social support: Health and disease.* Stockholm: Almqvist and Wiksell International.

Jacobson, D. E. (1986). Types and timing of social support. *Journal of Health and Social Behavior, 27*, 250-264.

Jensen, M. M., & Rasmussen, A. F., Jr. (1963). Stress and susceptibility to viral infections: II Sound stress and susceptibility to vesicular stomatitis virus. *Journal of Immunology, 90*, 21-23.

Johnson, T., Lavender, J. F., & Marsh, J. T. (1959). The influence of avoidance learning stress on resistance to Coxsackie virus in mice. *Federation Proceedings, 18*, 575.

Kaack, B., Ordy, J., & Trapp, B. (1975). Changes in limbic, neuroendocrine and autonomic systems, adaptation, homeostasis during aging. In J. Ordy & K. R. Brizzee (Eds.), *Neurobiology of aging.* New York: Academic Press.

Kaplan, G. A. (1985). Psychosocial aspects of chronic illness: Direct and indirect associations with ischemic heart disease mortality. In G. A. Kaplan & M. H. Criqui (Eds.), *Behavioral epidemiology and disease prevention.* New York: Plenum.

Kaplan, G. A., Salonen, J. T., Cohen, R. D., Brand, R. J., & Syme, S. L. (1988). Social connections and mortality from all causes and from cardiovascular disease: Prospective evidence from Eastern Finland. *American Journal of Epidemiology, 128*, 370-380.

Kaprio, J., & Koskenvuo, M. (1988). A prospective study of psychological and socioeconomic characteristics, health behavior and morbidity in cigarette smokers prior to quitting compared to persistent smokers and non-smokers. *Journal of Clinical Epidemiology, 41*, 139-150.

Kasl, S. V., & Berkman, L. F. (1981). Some psychological influences on the health status of the elderly: The perspective of social epidemiology. In J. L. McGaugh, S. B. Kiesler, & J. G. March (Eds.), *Aging: Biology and behavior.* New York: Academic Press.

Keys, A., Taylor, H. L., Blackburn, H., Brozek, J., Anderson, J. T., & Somonson, E. (1971). Mortality and coronary heart disease among men studied for 23 years. *Archives of Internal Medicine, 128*, 201-214.

Kiecolt-Glaser, J. K., & Glaser, R. (1987). Psychosocial moderators of immune function. *Annals of Behavioral Medicine, 9*, 16-20.

Kneier, A. W., & Temoshok, L. (1984). Repressive coping reactions in patients with malignant melanoma as compared to cardiovascular disease patients. *Journal of Psychosomatic Research, 28*, 145-155.

Krantz, S., & Manuck, S. B. (1984). Acute psychophysiologic reactivity and risk of cardiovascular disease: A review and methodologic critique. *Psychological Bulletin, 96*, 435-464.

Krause, N. (1986). Social support, stress, and well-being among older adults. *Journals of Gerontology, 41*, 512-519.

LaRocco, J. M., House, J. S., & French, J. R. P., Jr. (1980). Social support, occupational stress, and health. *Journal of Health and Social Behavior, 21,* 202-218.

Laudenslager, M. L., Ryan, S. M., Drugan, R. C., Hyson, R. L., & Maier, S. (1983). Coping and immunosuppression: Inescapable but not escapable shock suppresses lymphocyte proliferation. *Science, 221,* 568-570.

Lazarus, R. S., & Folkman, S. (1984). *Stress, appraisal, and coping.* New York: Springer.

Lazarus, R. S., & Launier, R. (1978). Stress-related transactions between person and environment. In L. A. Pervin & M. Lewis (Eds.), *Perspectives in interactional psychology.* New York: Plenum.

Levine, S., Strebel, R., Wend, E. J., & Harman, P. J. (1962). Suppression of experimental allergic encephalomyelitis by stress. *Proceedings of Social Experimental Biological Medicine, 109,* 294-298.

MacDougall, J. M., Dembroski, T. M., Dimsdale, J. E., & Hackett, T. P. (1985). Components of Type A, hostility, and anger-in: Further relationships to angiographic findings. *Health Psychology, 4,* 137-152.

Marsh, J. T., Lavender, J. F., Chang, S., & Rasmussen, A. F., Jr. (1963). Poliomyelitis in monkeys: Decreased susceptibility after avoidance stress. *Science, 140,* 1415-1416.

Maxwell, M. B. (1985). *The impact of social networks on mortality, disease incidence, and disease progression.* Unpublished doctoral dissertation, Portland State University, Portland, OR.

McCubbin, J. A., Surwit, R. S., & Williams, R. B. (1985). Endogenous opiate peptides, stress reactivity, and risk for hypertension. *Hypertension, 7,* 808-811.

McGeer, P. L., & McGeer, E. G. (1980). Chemistry of mood and emotions. *Annual Review of Psychology, 31,* 273-307.

McGrath, J. D. (1970). *Social and psychological factors in stress.* New York: Holt, Rinehart & Winston.

McQueen, D. V., & Celentano, D. D. (1982). Social factors in the etiology of multiple outcomes: The case of blood pressure and alcohol consumption patterns. *Social Science Medicine, 16,* 397-418.

McQueen, D. V., & Siegrist, J. (1982). Social factors in the etiology of chronic diseases: An overview. *Social Science Medicine, 16,* 353-367.

Narang, P. K. (1986). Age: A complex variable. In N. R. Cutler & P. K. Narang (Eds.), *Drug studies in the elderly: Methodological concerns.* New York: Plenum Medical.

O'Reilly, P., & Thomas, H. E. (1989). Role of support networks in maintenance of improved cardiovascular health status. *Social Science Medicine, 28,* 249-260.

Orth-Gomer, K., & Johnson, J. V. (1987). Social network interaction and mortality: A six-year follow-up study of a random sample of the Swedish population. *Journal of Chronic Diseases, 40,* 949-957.

Pancheri, P., et al. (1979). Studio controllato sulle carateristiche di personalita meccanismi di defesa ad eventi stressanti nel carcinoma del collo del' utero. *Rivista di Psichiatria, 114,* 210-221.

Patel, C., Marmot, M. G., & Terry, D. J. (1981). Controlled trial of biofeedback-aided behavioral methods in reducing mild hypertension. *British Medical Journal, 282,* 2005-2008.

Patel, C., Marmot, M. G., Terry, D. J., Carruthers, M., Hunt, B., & Patel, M. (1985). Trial of relaxation in reducing coronary risk: Four year follow-up. *British Medical Journal, 290,* 1103-1106.

Paul, J. R., & Bunnell, W. W. (1982). Classics in infectious diseases: The presence of heterophile antibodies in infectious mononucleosis. *American Journal of Medical Science.* (Reprinted from *Review of Infectious Diseases, 4*, 1062-1068, 1932)

Pearlin, L. I., Menaghan, E. G., Lieberman, M. A., & Mullan, J. T. (1981). The stress process. *Journal of Health and Social Behavior, 22*, 337-356.

Pert, C. B., Ruff, M. R., Weber, R. J., & Herkenham, M. (1985). Neuropeptides and their receptors: A psychosomatic network. *Journal of Immunology, 135*, 820s-826s.

Pinneau, S. R. (1975). *Effects of social support on psychological and physiological stress.* Unpublished doctoral dissertation, University of Michigan, Ann Arbor.

Plaut, S. M., Ader, R., Friedman, S. B., & Ritterson, A. L. (1969). Social factors and resistance to malaria in the mouse: Effects of groups vs. individual housing on resistance to Plasmodium berghei infection. *Psychosomatic Medicine, 31*, 536-552.

Radl, J., Sepers, J. M., Skuaril, F., Morell, A., & Hijmans, W. (1975). Immunoglobin patterns in humans over 95 years of age. *Clinical Experimental Immunology, 22*, 84-90.

Ragland, D. R., & Brand, R. J. (1988). Type A behavior and mortality from coronary heart disease. *The New England Journal of Medicine, 318*, 65-69.

Rasmussen, A. F., Jr., Marsh, J. T., & Brill, N. Q. (1957). Increased susceptibility to herpes simplex in mice subjected to avoidance-learning stress or restraint. *Proceedings of Social Experimental Biological Medicine, 96*, 183-189.

Reed, D., McGee, D., Katsuhiko, Y., & Feinleib, M. (1983). Social networks and coronary heart disease among Japanese men in Hawaii. *American Journal of Epidemiology, 117*, 384-396.

Reker, G. T., Peacock, J., & Wong, P. T. (1987). Meaning and purpose in life and well-being: A life-span perspective. *Journals of Gerontology, 42*, 44-49.

Reznikoff, M. (1955). Psychological factors in breast cancer: A preliminary study of some personality trends in patients with cancer of the breast. *Psychosomatic Medicine, 17*, 96-110.

Riley, A. L., Zellner, D. A., & Duncan, H. J. (1980). The role of endorphins in animal learning and behavior. *Neuroscience Biobehavior Review, 4*, 69-76.

Roberts-Thompson, I. C., Whittingham, S., Youngchaiyud, U., & Mackay, I. R. (1974). Aging, immune response, and mortality. *Lancet, 2*, 368-370.

Rogers, M. P., Dubey, D., & Reich, P. (1979). The influence of the psyche and the brain on immunity and disease susceptibility: A critical review. *Psychosomatic Medicine, 41*, 147-164.

Rogers, M. P., Trentham, D., McCune, J., Ginsberg, B., Reich, P., & David, J. (1979). Abrogation of type II collagen-induced arthritis in rats by psychological stress. *Clinical Research, 27*, 513A.

Ross, R., & Glomset, J. A. (1976). The pathogenesis of atherosclerosis. *The New England Journal of Medicine, 295*, 369-377, 420-425.

Rowe, J. W., & Kahn, R. L. (1987). Human aging: Usual and successful. *Science, 237*, 143-149.

Russel, M., Dark, K. A., Cummins, R. W., Ellman, G., Callaway, E., & Peeke, H. V. (1984). Learned histamine release. *Science, 225*, 733-734.

Ruth, J. A., & Eiden, L. E. (1984). Modulation of peripheral cardiovascular function by enkephalins. In F. Fraioli, A. Isidori, & M. Mazzetti (Eds.), *Opioid peptides in the periphery*. Amsterdam: Elsevier Science.

Satariano, W., & Syme, S. L. (1979, June). *Life change and illness in the elderly: Coping with change*. Paper presented to the National Academy of Sciences Conference on Biology and Behavior, Woods Hole, MA.

Schleifer, S. J., Keller, S. E., Camerino, M., Thornton, J. C., & Stein, M. (1983). Suppression of lymphocyte stimulation following bereavement. *Journal of American Medical Association, 250*, 374-377.

Schoenbach, V. J., Kaplan, B. H., Fredman, L., & Kleinbaum, D. G. (1986). Social ties and mortality in Evans County, Georgia. *American Journal of Epidemiology, 123*, 577-591.

Schonfield, J. (1975). Psychological life experience differences between Israeli women with benign and cancerous breast lesions. *Journal of Psychosomatic Research, 19*, 229-234.

Selye, H. (1936). A syndrome produced by diverse nocuous agents. *Nature, 138*, 32.

Snell, L., & Graham, S. (1971). Social trauma as related to cancer of the breast. *British Journal on Cancer, 25*, 721-734.

Spence, D. P. (1975). Language correlates of cervical cancer. *Psychosomatic Medicine, 37*, 95.

Stock, G., Schlor, K. H., Heidt, H., & Buss, J. (1978). Psychomotor behaviour and cardiovascular patterns during stimulation of the amygdala. *Pfluegers Archives, 376*, 177-184.

Tecoma, E. S., & Huey, L. Y. (1985). Psychic distress and the immune response. *Life Sciences, 36*, 1799-1812.

Thoits, P. A. (1983). Dimensions of life events that influence psychological distress: An evaluation and synthesis of the literature. In B. Kaplan (Ed.), *Psychological stress: Trends in theory and research*. New York: Academic Press.

Thoits, P. A. (1985). Social support and psychological well being: Theoretical possibilities. In I. G. Sarason & B. R. Sarason (Eds.), *Social support: Theory, research, and applications*. Boston: Martinus Nijhoff.

Tibblin, G., Svardsudd, K., Welin, L., & Larson, B. (1986). The theory of general susceptibility. In S. O. Isacsson & L. Janzon (Eds.), *Social support: Health and disease*. Stockholm: Alqvist and Wiksell.

Troxler, R. G., Sprague, E. A., Albanese, R. A., Fuchs, R., & Thompson, A. F. (1977). The association of elevated plasma cortisol and early atherosclerosis as demonstrated by coronary angiography. *Atherosclerosis, 26*, 151-162.

Unden, A. L., & Orth-Gomer, K. (1989). Development of a social support instrument for use in population surveys. *Social Science Medicine, 29*, 1387-1392.

Vogt, T. M., Pope, C. R., Mullooly, J. P., Ernst, D., Hollis, J. F., & Valanis, B. (1990). *Social predictors of morbidity and mortality* (NIA Grant No. 5, R01 AG05682, Final report). Bethesda, MD: National Institute on Aging.

Weinberger, M., Tierney, W. M., Booher, P., & Hiner, S. L. (1990). Social support, stress and functional status in patients with osteoarthritis. *Social Science Medicine, 30*, 503-508.

Weinstein, R., & Stemerman, M. B. (1981). Hormonal requirements for growth of arterial smooth muscle cells in vitro: An endocrine approach to atherosclerosis. *Science, 212*, 818-820.

Weiss, R. S. (1974). The provisions of social relationships. In Z. Rubin (Ed.), *Doing unto others.* Englewood Cliffs, NJ: Prentice-Hall.

Welford, A. (1980). Sensory, perceptual and motor processes in older adults. In J. E. Birren & R. B. Sloane (Eds.), *Handbook of mental health and aging.* Englewood Cliffs, NJ: Prentice-Hall.

Welin, L., Tibblin, G., Svardsudd, K., Tibblin, B., Ander-Peciva, S., Larsson, B., & Wilhelmsen, L. (1985). Prospective study of social influences on mortality: The study of men born in 1913 and 1923. *Lancet, 1,* 915-918.

Wiley, J. A., & Camacho, T. C. (1980). Life-style and future health: Evidence from the Alameda County study. *Preventive Medicine, 9,* 1-21.

Ziegler, M. G., Lake, C. R., & Kopin, I. J. (1976). Plasma noradrenaline increases with age. *Nature, 261,* 333-335.

Zuckerman, D. M., Kasl, S. V., & Ostfeld, A. M. (1984). Psychosocial predictors of mortality among the elderly poor: The role of religion, well-being, and social contacts. *American Journal of Epidemiology, 119,* 410-423.

PART III

Social and Behavioral Interventions

9

Disease Prevention and
Health Promotion with Older Adults

WILLIAM RAKOWSKI

This chapter discusses several considerations underlying the development of disease-prevention and health-promotion (DP/HP) research with older adults. It also addresses the extension of such research to the design of community-based interventions targeted at an older adult audience. *Community-based* denotes interventions with the objective of having large reach or penetration in a designated geographic area, in contrast to behavioral interventions done solely with clinically based samples or persons presenting with a particular symptom. The chapter, therefore, attempts to walk a line between the needs and priorities of research and program implementation— activities that are often quite different but nonetheless have the similar objective of enhancing and maintaining the health of the older population.

When viewed in historical perspective, it is evident that research on preventive health behavior and on interventions to encourage behavior change by older adults is steadily becoming more sophisticated. The questions that can be asked will always outpace and outnumber definitive answers, but so far empirical data argue for continuing to promote life-style change among older persons (e.g., Kaplan & Haan, 1989; Omenn, 1990). The more important issues involve knowing the limitations of our knowledge at any given time and making life-style or even broader public policy recommendations that are firmly grounded in empirical and professional experience.

In the history of developing theories and testing interventions, it would be safe to say that older adults have not been seen as a suitable group for conducting "clean" tests of new constructs, theoretical models, or program delivery strategies. Multiple concurrent illnesses, preexisting pathology in major bodily systems, long-standing habits and attitudes, and any of a variety of sociodemo-graphic factors (e.g., higher poverty rates, less formal education) have been viewed as potential confounds, relative to the ubiquitous college sophomore, the growing child, or the healthy middle-aged volunteer.

It is also important to state at the outset that disease prevention and health promotion are not reserved for the still-well elderly. "Disease prevention" and "health promotion" are objectives that are pursued by any of a variety of intervention strategies. In and of themselves, they specify no target population. Minkler (1984) provided an early call to consider the potential of health promotion even in long-term care settings. Investigations by Perkins, Rapp, Carlson, and Wallace (1986), Fiatarone et al. (1990), Rippey et al. (1987), Lorig, Laurin, and Holman (1984), Glanz, Marger, and Meehan (1986), and Dupree, Broskowski, and Schonfeld (1984) have all been conducted with per-sons with existing health problems.

Moreover, working with an older population presents a compara-bly greater challenge to the comprehensiveness of our theories and interventions. If, on the one hand, it is presumed that results obtained from disease-prevention interventions with nonelderly (and usually volunteer) populations represent the current state of the art, then, by the same token, can the question also be posed as to whether such results also provide inflated standards for the population as a whole? Disease-prevention research and intervention in aging may well be working against a deck that is stacked in some respects. However, any such adversity makes positive results that much more impres-sive. Not that long ago, even working with persons in their sixties and early seventies was novel and a daring step. Now, health-promo-tion programs are being increasingly targeted to include the "old people" aged 75, 80, and older. The significance of this upward shift in the age of our intervention target audiences should not be ignored. It is one of the major developments in aging work over the past 10 to 15 years.

ISSUES FOR STUDYING PREVENTIVE BEHAVIOR AND INTERPRETING RESEARCH

The complexity that accompanies research on preventive behavior and the implementation of behavior change programs becomes evi-dent quickly (Farquhar, 1978; Kirscht, 1983; Salonen, Kottke, Jacobs, & Hannan, 1986; Shumaker & Grunberg, 1986). The objectives of intervention are, at a minimum, to develop a single new health habit and successfully integrate it into an individual's overall behavior profile for a sustained period. However, research on disease prevention and health promotion inevitably interfaces with broader concepts such as "healthy habit patterns," "risk-factor profiles," and more complex objectives such as "life-style modification" and "multiple behavior change." More ambitious, therefore, is the objective (and perhaps the need) of eliminating several undesirable practices, encouraging the learning of other habits more likely to promote health, and maintaining that new life-style over time.

A literature pertinent to designing and implementing community-based disease-prevention/health-promotion (DP/HP) programs with older adults is growing. Some of it is from programs and research actually targeted at behavior change (see the final section). In other instances, the data come from sources such as national surveys of health behavior and epidemiological risk-factor studies and suggest areas where behavior change programs might be productive (e.g., Branch & Jette, 1984; Garland, Barrett-Connor, Suarez, & Criqui, 1983; Harris, Cook, Kannel, & Goldman, 1988; Jajich, Ostfeld, & Freeman, 1984; Kaplan, Seeman, Cohen, Knudsen, & Guralnik, 1987; Rakowski, 1987; Thornberry, Wilson, & Golden, 1986).

Potential target groups that might be at risk of not following desired practices are often identified from responses to behavioral surveys and questionnaires. Secondary analyses are likely to be sources of data for such purposes (e.g., the 1985 and 1987 supplements to the National Health Interview Survey [NHIS]; the 1984 Supplement on Aging to the NHIS, along with the 1986, 1988, and 1990 Longitudinal Study of Aging follow-ups; the 1986 National Mortality Follow-Back Survey). However, secondary data analysis restricts the investigator to the domain of information that was collected and to the specific ways that questions were worded. For this reason and also to benefit the design of future surveys of health habits, three important distinctions should be recognized. They are as important for the conceptual basis of an investigation of health behavior as other concerns such as sampling, data collection procedures, and statistical techniques are for its methodological soundness.

Health Behaviors and Health Practices

The first distinction is the difference between the assessment of a *behavior* and the assessment of a *practice*. It is the usual objective of interventions to encourage practices through skills training and the transfer of behaviors from the teaching/learning situation to daily life settings. For this chapter, a *practice* is defined as the level of analysis of behavior that results from observing or assessing repeated opportunities for a behavioral event or action to occur. At the risk of oversimplification, then, practices represent the longitudinal experience of a behavior. Another perspective might be to say that a *behavior* is taught and adopted, while a *practice* (or habit) is the maintenance of that behavior over time. For example, questions in national surveys about the utilization of health services routinely request the times of the respondent's last medical, dental, and eye exams. Interest is directed at a single visit and whether or not it occurred—essentially a yes/no situation. However, any question about the most recent performance of a target behavior cannot index a habit pattern. We may, of course, infer with some confidence that a nonpreventive style exists when an extended period of time (e.g., four or five years) has elapsed since the individual's last visit.

The interpretation of the frequent finding of only minimal correlation among health-related activities (Harris & Guten, 1979; Langlie, 1979; Rakowski, Julius, Hickey, & Halter, 1987; Stephens, 1986) is one area that might benefit from attention to the distinction between *behaviors* and *practices*. The assessment of behaviors (i.e., performance status as reported at a single time point) may attenuate associations that actually exist among the practices. When constructing survey instruments or interpreting data, therefore, investigators should determine whether the behavioral indicators being used are assessments of a practice pattern or of a behavior. The predictors of adopting a behavior (e.g., most recent breast self-examination) may not be those that predict maintaining the corresponding practice (e.g., regularity of breast self-examination; Sallis et al., 1986).

Health-Related Action Versus Preventive Intention

The second and equally important distinction relates to the difference between activities that are "health related" in a purely statistical sense and activities that we can determine are clearly and specifically intended to be preventive when they are performed. The major element in the latter case, therefore, involves determining the individual's intention that the activity has disease-prevention/health-promotion benefits. Actions may be "health related" whether or not the individual recognizes the fact. Investigations of preventive health behavior can be muddied, however, by not knowing the individual's intentions or purpose.

Questions about the utilization of health services, for example, can be examined from this perspective. Even if surveys ask about a regular practice (e.g., "How many times have you seen your doctor in the past 12 months?"), as opposed to assessing a behavior (i.e., the most recent visit), we might also ask whether the visits were self-initiated or provider-initiated. Also, were the visits for illness care or preventive purposes? Exercise and weight loss are two other examples. As the warmer weather of summer approaches, are efforts in either area pursued for purposes of better health and vigor or because of the desire to look good in the latest summer wear? The hours of sleep question in the classic Alameda health habit index (Belloc & Breslow, 1972; Breslow & Enstrom, 1980; Brock, Haefner, & Noble, 1988) is another example in that survey respondents have no prior knowledge (based on the wording used in most surveys) that the question is being asked as a piece of a larger composite mortality-/morbidity-prevention index.

Point-prevalence studies may not have any objective other than determining the distributions of behaviors and practices in a target population. The extension of the data to intervention planning, however, may be assisted by more complete knowledge of why a behavior/practice is or is not performed. The demographic and psychosocial correlates of health practices observed in a cross-sectional prevalence study (i.e., what behaviors are done and how often) may or may not be replicated if assessments of behavior are reworded to reflect the individual's intention or the objective underlying his or her activity. The basic question is whether the status of having (or not having) a particular health habit results from a conscious decision to be (or not be) preventive in that area. Periodically, individuals may have to review and reconfirm the preventive purposes of their health-related activities, even if they make no changes in those habits. There is a risk that some people will give socially desirable answers when questions are asked that combine intention with performance of the practice. However, unless the wording of a question is clear, there is limited ability to infer that a preventive orientation underlies a given behavior or practice. The issue is not that the individual's definition of what is preventive corresponds with current professional opinion but that the individual has a repertoire of health practices that is consciously consistent with a given purpose (i.e., prevention as self-defined).

Predicting and Understanding Nonevents

The third distinction involves the scope of outcomes that are used to define the behavior or practice in question. Research, analyses, and interpretations are quite understandably designed around observable behaviors and practices. We assess and quantify variables such as visits to health professionals, days of vigorous activity, regularity of self-examination, and types of foods eaten. These represent decisions made and health actions taken that can be checked off on a tally sheet as having actually occurred. Our major concern rests with the reliability and validity of the data collection methods.

Research on disease prevention and health promotion has been less diligent about trying to assess missed opportunities to be preventive or monitoring health-related decision situations where inaction due to a lack of interest was the conscious choice. Because disease prevention and health promotion often involve learning new skills and knowledge, the practice of those skills, and even some risk taking when initiating change in personal behavior, it will be important to understand "nonevents." Events of omission are naturally more difficult to study than events of commission. It is harder to design survey questions to assess when something could have happened but did not. Yet the failure to act preventively in a given situation or to practice an intervention skill can be of great relevance.

Studies of illness behavior often employ nonadherence to treatment and delay of contact after recognizing a symptom as dependent measures, both of which imply inaction. Prevention research with older persons has yet to develop such variables, beyond monitoring dropout and attendance rates in formal, community-based programs (Haber, 1986) or using a single length-of-time report since the desired activity was performed (e.g., time since last medical visit). Studies of the perception of symptoms have the advantage of an anchor point (the symptom experience) around which questions can be structured. To the extent that preventive activities occur in the absence of clear threats to health, it is more difficult to study inaction.

Simply counting the regularity of self-examination or visits to a health professional, for example, gives an incomplete picture if the individual has purposely avoided or delayed an exam because of anxiety over what might be found. Conversely, how often individuals resist opportunities to follow an unhealthful habit, such as when household members or friends have the habits one is trying to eliminate or in some other way work against the new behaviors being implemented, can also be important information (Sallis, Grossman,

Pinski, Patterson, & Nader, 1987). The concept of *resistance* to forces or settings that encourage unhealthy practices may be especially important for understanding personal health psychology.

DIMENSIONS FOR CATEGORIZING INTERVENTIONS AND INTERVENTION RESEARCH

Research on disease prevention/health promotion, like any other area of study, will adopt a wide variety of topics and methods. One of the most fundamental and essential distinctions is the dimension of experimental precision and control, spanning the range from "true" experiment through varying types of quasi-experimental designs to nonexperimental methods (Campbell, 1969; Campbell & Stanley, 1963; Salonen et al., 1986). The growth of an experimental literature relevant to DP/HP intervention lags behind the empirical literature in that few studies have tested research questions and hypotheses using experimental/control designs and random assignment. Of course, initial random selection from a target population, followed by random assignment to experimental and control groups, will always be the desired ideal. However, research investigations have other important distinctions, as discussed below. Although these characteristics are described singly, a multifactorial classification will probably be the most useful. No priority is implied by the order that follows; each is a dimension in its own right.

Disease-Specific Versus Functional Health

The focus and objectives of an intervention may be based upon specified medical diagnostic groups. In such studies, a sample is selected to fit certain categories of illness and/or the investigation is designed around dependent variables for a particular disease (e.g., risk reduction for cancer or heart disease, arthritis self-management). As a result, the literature that develops can be expected to emphasize disease-specific models of health education and health behavior. Intervention techniques (e.g., self-guided learning modules, health-risk appraisals) are developed in conjunction with particular diseases and gradually adapted for others. Eventually, however, meta-analyses are undertaken to identify similarities across the disease-oriented domains.

Another emphasis is on functional health criteria (i.e., activities of daily living [ADLs] and instrumental activities of daily living

[IADLs]; Dawson & Hendershot, 1987; Katz, Downs, Cash, & Grotz, 1970) on the premise that the medical label of a disease conveys less information about its significance for the day-to-day life of an individual than does knowledge about its effects on certain basic self-management competencies. The maintenance of independence and vigor becomes a highlighted feature of these interventions. The intervention itself may then emphasize the management of risk factors and self-care skills that cut across major causes of mortality and morbidity, such as heart disease, osteoporosis, cancer, stroke, and diabetes. Within this context, medical diagnoses or organ-specific pathologies can introduce the need for some disease-specific education, although the overriding theme would be the preservation of functional health. Also of empirical and professional interest is whether an HP/DP intervention is more attractive to an older audience when it is grounded in a single illness or when it highlights systemwide functional health benefits.

High-Risk Versus Communitywide Eligibility

One type of intervention is designed for persons at especially high risk of disease onset, such as those in the top 5% or 10% of a risk-factor distribution (Olson, 1986; Slater, Carlton, Ramirez, & Ashton, 1987). The distribution may, of course, also be based upon multiple risk factors or upon a composite predictive algorithm, such as that derived by the Framingham Study (Truett, Cornfeld, & Kannel, 1967). Another program strategy attempts to reach a communitywide sample, established within purposely broad sociodemographic parameters, to achieve total community "exposure" and participation (Blackburn, 1983; Farquhar, 1978).

High-risk program targeting is represented by the Multiple Risk Factor Intervention Trial, the Hypertension Detection and Follow-Up Program, the Lipids Research Clinics Trial, and the Systolic Hypertension in the Elderly Project (Hypertension Detection and Follow-Up Program, 1979a, 1979b; Lipid Research Clinics Program, 1984a, 1984b; Multiple Risk Factor Intervention Trial, 1982; Siegel et al., 1987). Community-level interventions are represented by projects such as the three National Heart, Lung, and Blood Institute (NHLBI)-supported community demonstrations of cardiovascular risk-factor reduction located at Pawtucket, Rhode Island; Stanford University; and the University of Minnesota; (Farquhar et al., 1985; Lefebvre, Lasater, Carleton, & Peterson, 1987; Maccoby, Farquhar, Wood, & Alexander, 1977; Mittlemark et al., 1986); by the North Karelia Project

(Puska, Salonen, Tuomilehto, Nissenen, & Kottke, 1983; Salonen et al., 1986); and by the Pennsylvania County Health Improvement Program (Cohen, Stunkard, & Felix, 1986; Stunkard, Felix, & Cohen, 1985). To date, many DP/HP programs for older adults have used community-based samples, drawn from any number of well-known sources (e.g., churches, meal sites, housing units). However, we have probably not been as successful (or able, given available resources) in recruiting on a true *communitywide* basis.

Selecting a high-risk population is useful and commonly done when the intervention is being conducted under conditions that are meant to give it an optimal chance of showing an effect, even though generalization to other segments of the population may be difficult. The immediacy of risk to a segment of the population, or even the current state of intervention techniques, may also dictate using a high-risk population. A high-risk strategy is also appropriate when there is a clear-cut point between high and low risk (e.g., when there is a clear demarcation in the dose-response relationship).

In contrast, communitywide interventions are appropriate when the objective is to reduce risk status on a population basis and when risk follows a dose-response continuum. Although rates of morbidity and mortality are greater in the highest-risk groups, the preponderance of cases are observed at moderate levels of the risk factor, where (by definition) the bulk of the population is located (Blackburn, 1983; Farquhar, 1978). Goals of dramatic change, which might be highlighted in a high-risk sample, are sacrificed in favor of more modest improvement but on a broader scale. Interventions that use community-based samples, even without achieving communitywide coverage, make this same choice at least implicitly.

Disease Status Versus Risk-Factor Status

Another distinction relates to a difference between programs based upon disease status in contrast to those that are based on risk-factor status (Safer, 1986). The difference between the two can be important. The former relies upon specifying an illness or pathological state as the basis for recruiting participants (e.g., heart disease, cancer, prevention of repeat falls), where the problems are often in a preclinical or an emergent phase. Persons can be categorized as cases and non-cases, using more of a medical or diagnostic model. Recruitment of participants can be from clinical settings. In contrast, the risk-factor approach is grounded in the concept of susceptibility and in the ascribed probability of developing a target condition. The emphasis in risk-factor reduction programs is, therefore, often on behavioral change, with the objective being to reduce susceptibility. Programs that are attempting to reach a large community audience base their recruitment messages on rationales that are essentially probabilistic, involving a trade-off of current effort for future benefits.

In this context, it is important to remember that susceptibility to illness due to life-style habits is a status ascribed to the individual (e.g., in health-risk appraisal formats) rather than being an observable event, even though the ascribed level of risk may be grounded in empirical findings. One presumed chain of effect might be represented basically as follows:

intervention → change in behavior → change in risk-factor status → lowered susceptibility → improvement on outcome measure(s)

However, lowered susceptibility cannot always be assessed directly, even using a physiological indicator of risk (e.g., blood pressure, saliva cotinine) instead of a behavioral indicator (e.g., physical activity, smoking status). Preclinical physical changes that have already occurred may not be immediately reversed, if they can be at all. In addition, "lower susceptibility" may not be something that can be easily demonstrated to an individual. Therefore, interventions organized around modifying the risk-factor status of asymptomatic older adults (e.g., changing a dietary pattern), as opposed to addressing clear preclinical or emergent disease (e.g., reversing an elevated blood glucose), might consider ways to also incorporate a more concrete indicator with which to demonstrate health benefits.

The Level of Mobilization

Several target audiences for interventions are often highlighted. They include (a) the person (as a unique or individual program participant), so, even in a group setting, messages are targeted and skills are developed on a person-by-person basis; (b) the group (such as families, small clubs, or self-help associations), where the emphasis is on collective or cooperative skill building; (c) organizations (such as the macro-environmental characteristics of a work site, church, or senior center), where the locus of change is the milieu or policies of a given setting; and (d) the community at large (such as item labeling in grocery stores, menu labeling in restaurants, or health-promotion contests), where the objective is to activate one or more sectors of an entire community as the intervention agents or channels.

The ultimate goal in all of these cases is to produce and sustain changes in health practices. The difference among them lies in the level of the community that is activated or mobilized to achieve the change. At the level of the entire community, it becomes possible to consider "sector mobilization"—work sites, senior groups, nutrition sites, medical societies and primary care physicians, housing units, churches, labor unions, health profession organizations, financial institutions, among others that might be listed. Large-scale community interventions often use this strategy (Cohen et al., 1986; Lefebvre, Lasater et al., 1987; Mittlemark et al., 1986), and the sector mobilization approach is implicit in research continua such as Phases IV and V of the five-stage cancer control plan of the National Cancer Institute (Greenwald & Cullen, 1985).

The Phase of Behavior Change

Interventions may be classified by the point of behavior adoption and habit change that they address. Included here might be (a) building awareness and motivation to adopt the health practice; (b) initial skills training; (c) enhancement of a support network to sustain the newly learned skills; (d) prevention of recidivism or relapse during early phases of adoption; and (e) long-term maintenance of the desired practice. Stage-relevant distinctions are commonly found in theories and models of individuals' health-related behaviors (Janz & Becker, 1984; Lefebvre & Flora, 1988; McHugh & Vallis, 1986; Prochaska & DiClemente, 1986; Schiffman, Shumaker, Abrams, & Cohen, 1986). An individual's repertoire of health practices evolves over time. At the level of organizations, sectors, and communities, we might instead focus on health policies and decisions concerning resource allocation.

It should be mentioned that the "support network" cited above is not restricted to a family or friendship model. A single health practice may be strengthened, for example, by skills training in other health practices, to achieve broader life-style change (e.g., combining lower alcohol consumption and smoking cessation would be a possibility or even smoking cessation with weight control; Schoenborn & Benson, 1988). Or an environmental modification may be introduced to reduce the physical energy required to practice and institute a new habit. It may even be possible to mobilize other sectors of a community (e.g., private physicians' offices as a channel for nutrition messages) to reinforce a sector that has been an "early adopter" in the community (e.g., displays in local restaurants and grocery stores).

Such strategies have not been common because of limited funding for DP/HP programs, because of the often substantial task of gaining access to even a single sector, and because of a tendency to address behaviors singly rather than in combination. However, this is a potential avenue for research and program development in aging.

A final point relates to the broader settings to which the newly learned health practices are intended to transfer. When interventions are conducted at the level of individuals and small groups, using didactic teaching strategies and investigating the transfer of skills beyond the program is manageable—if not easy. However, moving intervention to the level of organizations and to sectors of the community, and using techniques such as cable TV and videocassettes, raise issues pertinent to evaluating the practice and reinforcement of new habits. For example, how is "point of purchase" shelf labeling in a grocery store translated into consumers' reading of ingredients on packages and modifying of recipes at home on a day-to-day basis? Or how is the information that is posted on health bulletin boards at union offices, work sites, or churches implemented by the individual employee, union member, or parishioner? Mechanisms will be proposed and investigated, of course, but this represents another new area of health research in aging.

Philosophy of the Intervention

Research and program initiatives in DP/HP have evolved with the view that responsibility for health is shared by individuals, professionals, and all sectors of society (Breslow, 1990). However, it is virtually impossible to address all of these forces in a single project with a realistic budget. Investigators inevitably make choices about what they will emphasize, and it is commonly recognized that broadly different worldviews can influence what an investigator considers to be the appropriate strategies for his or her particular project. One of the classic examples in aging is the dichotomy drawn between "strong" and "weak" theories of human development (Looft, 1973; Overton, 1973; Overton & Reese, 1973; Reese & Overton, 1970). Another is placing the responsibility for change on individuals as opposed to their environments. We are not yet at a point where DP/HP literature in aging can be reviewed to any great extent from the perspective of "dominant philosophies" or "zeitgeists." One project that has made its philosophy clear is the Tenderloin Senior Outreach Project, reported by Minkler and her colleagues (Minkler, 1985;

Wechsler & Minkler, 1986), which has grown in part out of the "critical consciousness" approach of Paulo Friere.

As more programs are implemented and evaluated, attention to implicit or explicit philosophical underpinnings will not be avoided for long. The area of work-site health promotion demonstrates (Sloan, 1987) the debate over whether programs targeted at individual behavior change in fact direct attention away from the employer's responsibility to provide a safe and healthy work environment. It is also likely that the emphasis on personal responsibility and the "culture of character" envisioned in the *Healthy People 2000* objectives for the nation will generate substantial comment (U.S. Department of Health and Human Services, 1990). In fact, the introductory section to the year 2000 objectives is a prime example of trying to designate all sources of responsibility for the public's health, consistent with the ideals of DP/HP, while still directing ultimate attention to individual-level behavioral change.

Currently, it appears that most theories and conceptualizations of personal health behavior have adopted a logical-rational perspective. Individuals are seen as making decisions based upon a review of factors such as health beliefs, symptom experience, causal attribution, cost-benefit estimates, and perceived social norms (Azjen & Fishbein, 1980; Bandura, 1977; Janz & Becker, 1984; McHugh & Vallis, 1986; Prochaska & DiClemente, 1986; Weinstein, 1988). Such approaches readily lend themselves to interventions based upon an educational model, in which information and skills training are expected to lead to the adoption of new habits. Family members, the informal social network, and even a regular source of health care (if there is one) can be viewed as additional sources of information and as potential resources for periodic assistance. In effect, the older person is approached almost exclusively as a decision maker with the luxury of time and resources to draw upon for constructing his or her repertoire of life-style habits.

This perspective on personal health behavior is appropriate but may eventually be expanded by integrating it with models based on a balance between the influences of personal decision making and the influences of contextual/environmental factors. The competence-press model outlined by Lawton and Nahemow (1973) is one example. This integrative type of model implies a dynamic trade-off between what the person and the setting each contribute to a current level of behavior. The model has several key features. It raises the possibility of providing either too much or too little challenge for an individual. The concept of "fit," central to the design of disease-prevention/health-promotion programs, is a primary component. Another explicit element is attention to factors necessary for maintaining any change in behaviors. Balance-type models provide a heuristic for the researcher and the intervention specialist in determining the salient personal and environmental variables and project their course over time to better anticipate when booster contact will be needed.

It is interesting that even traditional experiments and hypothesis testing can represent a particular type of philosophy. The need to follow a standard methodology as closely as possible can limit flexibility in adapting the program to individual participants. As a result, an apparent lack of success in reaching objectives must be interpreted in light of the limits imposed by hypothesis testing and not solely as a failure of the principles guiding the intervention. In contrast is the type of program in which any available resource (e.g., family support, moving to a new program location, trying new procedures in midprogram) can be used on an ad hoc basis if it advances participants' learning. Individualized attention is acceptable, and the package is tailored for each participant. Such flexibility is usually viewed as a barrier to research, because it precludes standardized procedures that would make it possible to identify the effects of separate components and then replicate the effects in other samples. Extreme flexibility allows only for tests of final outcomes (e.g., morbidity/mortality, aggregate cost of health care, personal productivity) as a function of individualized (and, therefore, not readily replicated) intervention.

The line between "adequate standardization" and "loss of rigor" will continue to be a focus of lively debate. Nonetheless, the place of intervention *packages* needs to be addressed, even if it is not always possible to separate the independent effects of each major component. One situation that seems to argue for the acceptability of this approach occurs when the pieces that constitute the package have been individually shown to be useful in prior investigations and when the mix of risk factors (or mediating variables) being addressed is so formidable that no individual component could be expected to have an identifiable impact by itself. Characteristics of one's target group, for example, may make it necessary to have a staged or layered intervention, in which steps of progressive intensity or detail occur in sequence (e.g., muscle strengthening precedes balance training, which precedes training in recovery after a person has fallen, which precedes locomotion inside one's residence, which precedes moving into the general environment). The point at which intervention components are considered valid as a package does in fact represent an important philosophical development in a field of study. Examples are the NHLBI's cardiovascular disease community demonstrations (Farquhar et al., 1985; Lefebvre, Lasater et al., 1987; Maccoby et al., 1977; Mittlemark et al., 1986), and the National Cancer Institute Phase IV and Phase V cancer control investigations (Greenwald & Cullen, 1985).

FACTORS MEDIATING PROGRAM IMPACT AND THE INTERPRETATION OF RESULTS

If judgments about the success of DP/HP intervention depend upon achieving physiologically defined benefits, reduced mortality rates, and/or improvement on morbidity indicators, then research with older adults can be complicated by several factors. Those noted in this section are generic, in that they can apply to any program that uses "hard" biomedical or epidemiologic indices as outcomes. Although not insurmountable barriers, they do require special attention and can make intervention with older adults more difficult. On the positive side, it may be possible to translate some of these concerns into variables that are amenable either to a priori stratification during sample selection or to post hoc statistical control.

Change in Behavior Versus Change in Biological Risk Status

Intervention programs for primary prevention are usually initiated in response to the observation of at-risk status in a segment of the population. However, there can be no guarantee that changes in behavior will be either quickly or isomorphically reflected in changes in risk status. The degree to which risk status that has developed over years (e.g., due to smoking, diabetes, sedentary life-style, or high blood pressure) can be expected to return to "normal" levels, the time span required for this to occur, and the level of intervention required are areas in need of much more study. Moreover, there is no assurance that health-related practices are the major contributors to high-risk status for all persons.

Especially in research with older adult samples, behaviorally and biologically defined risk status may need to be differentiated. A risk factor defined by behavior (e.g., smoking, low calcium in the diet) may be overtly modified or eliminated entirely, while its physical sequelae make a slower reversal, if reversal is possible. Even in a young adult sample, community-level or total-sample changes in morbidity or mortality profiles may take several years to reach statistically detectable levels (e.g., population-level benefits of screening mammography; Andersson et al., 1988; Chu, Smart, & Tarone, 1988). Similarly, individual differences in physiology and genetic predisposition (e.g., nutrient metabolism, endogenous lipid levels) may attenuate the ability to observe effects in smaller samples. Survivorship bias may also complicate the interpretation of risk-factor levels by skewing normative values and creating questions about how we segment the potential target population.

Concomitant Illness

A related consideration is that preexisting and concurrent illness, unrelated to the target condition, may dilute or entirely block the benefits that would otherwise come from a behavior change program. Low visual acuity, for example, may not permit an individual to take outdoor walks for exercise, despite having been in a muscle toning program. This type of confounding may be manifested in practice by the necessity of delivering a greater "dose" or greater "exposure" to intervention to achieve change. Or the effect may be shown by a rapid reversal of gains after an intervention program ends, which is usually accompanied by a withdrawal of staff support and resources. These problems can, of course, occur in samples of all ages. However, the prevalence of chronic impairment in later adulthood carries especially important implications. Existing pathological changes may not be reversible, and possible compensatory mechanisms may themselves be impaired. The intermediate or mediating steps necessary to complete a proposed sequence of behavioral through biological change may be affected by concomitant problems.

Health as a Resource for Behavioral Change

We expect good health status to be associated with a favorable profile of health practices, and, for the most part, epidemiological surveys support this position. What can be overlooked, however, is that health is also a resource that enables individuals to maintain their preventive life-styles and to experiment with modifications. Interventions for disease prevention and health promotion usually involve new skills and knowledge that individuals must make a special effort to learn and then to practice. On a very fundamental and practical level, this translates into expenditure of energy, both physical and mental. Existing illness and functional impairment are almost certain to impose limits on the new tasks a person can take on at any one time.

Even people who are strongly motivated to adopt preventive habits can be severely challenged if they have a limited reserve on which to draw. The effects of reduced stamina and vigor on preventive activities will likely be most evident among population groups such as the aged. The progression of activities in exercise programs are in fact routinely designed to accommodate such needs. This reciprocal influence between health and preventive practices deserves close examination. Although not an optimistic prospect, we may find a "ceiling effect" or point of diminishing returns in the behavior change that certain segments of the older population can be expected to accomplish, short of an unrealistically high infusion of resources. If a ceiling effect is found, it will be important to remember that the societal and human values that underlie providing an intervention are a separate issue from being able to significantly influence (in statistical terms) "hard" outcome indices of health such as morbidity and mortality. The 1990s promise to be an acid test for making such value judgments.

Intervention with the "Oldest Old"

Professionals who work with the aged and issues of aging inherit the results of societal trends in access to health care, personal health behaviors, and changes in medical care technology that affected those age cohorts in their younger years—for better or worse. It is a testimony to past and current efforts that the frontiers of research in aging are continually being pushed toward older and older ages. The period of life between 65 and 75 is becoming a time in which more and more persons can enjoy good functional health. The rapid growth of the population aged 80 and over, our current "old-old" group, reflects the gains in life expectancy that have benefited virtually all age groups. The age boundaries for defining this oldest segment of society are in fact dynamic. In time, age 90 may define the lower boundary of the oldest old.

However, we still live in a world where illnesses eventually catch up with individuals. Almost by definition, those who are the oldest elderly in a given historical period will have more health problems, a more tenuous pool of resources from which to draw support for new endeavors, and statistically fewer years of life expectancy within which life-style changes can develop and show their benefits. To the extent that the potential for change in a target group is limited (e.g., as indexed by higher mortality rates, difficulty in modifying physiological parameters, or shorter duration of success before loss of intervention benefits), larger sample sizes are needed to satisfy power calculations at desired detectable differences. However, the recruitment of samples that are adequate, both in size (considering also any necessary design restrictions) and in requisite background characteristics, may not be feasible. Such a situation has already arisen in the design of a clinical trial to test the effect of diet on mortality from coronary heart disease (Barrett-Connor, 1987); such a study is not considered practical. Similarly, it is possible that certain outcome indicators will not be appropriate with the oldest old. All-cause mortality and morbidity may be sufficiently high to overcome benefits attributable to disease-specific interventions (Mor, Pacala, & Rakowski, 1990). In this situation, quality of life indices, functional health, and behavior change per se (whether or not these factors are associated with decreased morbidity and mortality) may be the areas most amenable to assessment. Especially in this oldest-old age group, we may find that holding the line against decrement, as opposed to achieving clear-cut gains, is a realistic objective at least in initial phases of research and intervention.

THE LARGER CONTEXT OF INTERPRETATION AND APPLICATION OF DATA

Life-style behavior change programs with older adults (and in the field of aging more generally) must deal with other issues that research data per se cannot answer. Some of the questions arise because of the multiplicity and variety of the data themselves. Individual investigators will necessarily make judgments pertinent to the results of their particular studies. Eventually, however, as interpretations are made that influence policymaking and resource allocation at all levels of government, a macro perspective will have to be applied.

Priorities Among Outcome Criteria

Judgment on the effectiveness of an intervention strategy must be based upon clearly defined means for evaluating success. However, the criteria that might be used to judge interventions are numerous and varied. Several of these criteria have been referred to as constituting "courts" of evaluation (Rakowski, 1986), because the reviewer of research data essentially acts as a judge ruling not only on the strength of the evidence but also on whether the type of evidence being presented is appropriate for the type of decision being made. Outcome variables include (a) change in knowledge and attitudes, (b) adoption of a desired health-related activity or the elimination of an undesired habit, (c) change in a physiological indicator associated with the presence of the particular desired behavior or the absence of an undesired one, (d) change in illness or morbidity outcomes, (e) change in functional health parameters, (f) change in indices of personal productivity, (g) change in mortality rates, (h) change at the aggregate level of overall population at-risk status or the quality of life, and (i) change in the cost of health care.

The different types of outcome variables that might be used reflect elements in the chain of effect that is often used as a rationale or framework for DP/HP programs. Behavior change will certainly be a high priority in DP/HP programs, but the hypotheses or research questions for a study are likely to involve outcome measures in more than one of these areas. Epidemiological investigations have traditionally placed a high priority on showing an association between the reputed health-promotive innovation and reduced mortality. Each type of criterion has its attractive points and its drawbacks. None is inherently superior to another, although views on their relative merits are often strongly held. Political and public policy beliefs often influence the type of evidence that is preferred, and the type of outcome criteria for which an affect can be demonstrated will have a major bearing on decisions that are made by policymakers and resource allocation directors.

The Duration of Successful Outcomes

Another significant question has to do with how long an outcome must be maintained after an intervention is withdrawn before success can be claimed (e.g., Emery & Blumenthal, 1990; Perkins et al., 1986; Reich & Zutra, 1989). Success defined in statistical terms as a difference in duration between groups may not translate into time periods that appear long enough to others who must judge results with a practical eye. Initially, even showing short durations of benefit is important and acceptable, simply to demonstrate that an effect can be achieved. As more literature and research become available, standards of comparison are developed and duration criteria may gradually become more strict. Showing progressively longer duration of benefits across successive projects will probably be as important as the duration of effectiveness observed in any one project, particularly in work combating adverse health-related practices that are notoriously resistant to change (e.g., heavy smoking). However, the duration of benefits has no predetermined upper limit, so that an answer to the question of when we have achieved optimal success will always have elements of uncertainty.

Multiple Indicators of Behavior Change

The use of several outcome measures is common and even expected in disease-prevention/health-promotion research. However, multiple indices also introduce the very real possibility that not all of them will equally demonstrate statistical significance. Perhaps the most straightforward example is cause-specific versus total mortality—a distinction often encountered in reviewing the results of large-scale epidemiological clinical trials (e.g., Skrabanek's critique of research on screening mammography, 1988). Traditionally, all-cause mortality is considered to be a difficult variable to affect, and even total mortality in a disease-specific domain (e.g., cardiovascular disease) may not be considered the appropriate outcome measure in a clinical trial (e.g., the initial report of the aspirin/CVD component of the Physicians' Health Study; Steering Committee of Physician's Health Study Research Group, 1988). It is also possible to influence knowledge and attitudes without achieving a comparable influence on behavior.

Distinguishing among causes of mortality is also likely to be important with older persons, where multiple impairments predispose the individual to multiple (or "competing") causes of death. Actually, it is in the domain of psychosocial outcomes that multiple indices are routinely examined, often drawing from different domains (e.g., self-efficacy ratings, knowledge scores, observed behavior, life satisfaction scores, cognitive skills, behavioral intentions). Although showing success along multiple outcome measures can enhance the strength of results, it may also be necessary to resist a temptation to continue upping the ante by prematurely creating an ever larger pool of dependent measures. We have yet to establish a research track record that shows how many or how extensive a set of anticipated outcomes we can expect to achieve, given an intervention of realistic proportions and resources. There may also be a need to decide which outcome indicator(s) should have priority. In initial results from the Stanford Five-City Project (Farquhar et al., 1990), change across the individual cardiovascular risk factors was not as uniform as results on the composite algorithm of cardiovascular disease risk.

Defining the "Preventive" Older Person

The list of desirable health-related activities that a person might incorporate into her or his life-style is extremely lengthy and seems to get longer with each passing year and each new study. The constellation of health practices that should be our highest priority to encourage among older persons remains an open question. Several major focal points can be proposed: control of blood pressure, exercise and activity, smoking cessation, accident and injury prevention, weight management, early-detection cancer screening, diabetes management, self-examination skills, vision care, control of dietary fat and cholesterol, mental health/stress management, safe use of medications, and use of alcohol in moderation. While all of these are reasonable, we are far from being able to specify one or more predictive algorithms for mortality/morbidity that assigns weights to these areas.

Of course, each of the above domains of disease prevention and health promotion are general and subsumes several other behaviors and practices. Achieving and maintaining preventive habits in even one area can involve a significant commitment of time and effort. The task of defining and encouraging a broadly preventive life-style across several areas would seem truly monumental, yet the challenge should not be ignored. The larger network of preventive practices (and preventive attitudes) may provide a kind of supportive matrix within which other practices can be developed. Conversely, trying to introduce a single or isolated preventive habit into an otherwise nonpreventive matrix may doom the effort to failure. Consequently, it may be to our longer-range advantage to work toward identifying (if they exist) groupings of existing health practices that favorably dispose individuals to successfully adopting new practices.

Along these lines, investigators have so far had difficulty identifying factors or clusters of health practices that are statistically strong and that comprise more than only a few questions on a survey (Amir, 1987; Harris & Guten, 1979; Langlie, 1979; Rakowski et al., 1987; Stephens, 1986; Tapp & Goldenthal, 1982). While it does appear that there are different dimensions of personal health behavior (as opposed to a single factor on which all behaviors will load or cluster), these separate factors are not yet well specified. This could be taken as evidence that factors of health behaviors are empirically weak or almost nonexistent. At the same time, it should be remembered that social messages about disease prevention have tended not to highlight clusters or groups of habits. Instead, habits have been addressed individually (e.g., seat belt use, smoking cessation, smoke detectors, exercise, limiting the consumption of red meat). Only recently have state and national public service messages begun pointing to the common objectives or benefits that could be derived from different health habits (e.g., heart disease risk reduction, cancer control).

Because strategies like clustering and factor analyses are *descriptive* in nature, they can find only those associations that exist in the data. However, this can be very specific to a cohort and historical period. If the population as a whole does not practice certain habits as a group at the time of data collection, then factor analysis and strategies like it are bound to show empirically weak and limited associations. This finding should not be surprising. In large part, personal health practices have developed in unique personal, family, and neighborhood contexts, with only the broadest guidance from societal norms. It may not be possible, therefore, for a single cross-sectional survey to identify strong factors based on *inter*individual similarity of health habits. Instead, we may find that clustering of health behavior is an *intra*individual phenomenon, based on personal consistency over time, even though individuals differ in the health habits that they follow. Intervention specialists and researchers might then approach the concept of health behavior factors from an individual-level perspective as well as from a normative, interindividual perspective.

Finally, the prevalence of chronic impairment in an older population introduces another complication into the assessment and definition of the preventive older person. If health is a resource for making changes in behavior, as discussed previously, then the ability to perform a target health practice becomes a consideration. In some instances, it simply may not be possible for an individual to physically perform to a level considered adequate to produce benefits for mortality/morbidity reduction. Yet, the intention or attitudinal commitment to be preventive may be evident in the sheer fact of having made an effort of some magnitude. To ignore this commitment carries the risk of ignoring a potential for change. Perhaps the best example is that of physical activity. Objective indicators of strenuous exercise show lower prevalence among older cohorts (e.g., Thornberry et al., 1986). However, walking does not show such a dramatic age difference, and few people would argue that the modified exercise program that older persons often follow is not worth the effort. Our definition of the preventive older person may well include a dimension for making an effort despite concomitant health problems, regardless of how much change in physiological indicators is actually achieved.

Identifying Major Strategies of Intervention

Because so many health-related activities are suitable targets for DP/HP programs and so many intervention strategies are available, sooner or later a matrix-type approach of Behaviors × Strategies will need to be constructed to review the effectiveness of selected techniques and methodologies. The goal of making this matrix will be to identify whether there are any "optimal" intervention packages based on effectiveness across several health practices so that resources may be allocated accordingly. Presuming that criteria for determining the success of a program have been identified (as discussed previously), attention can be directed at answering questions such as these: Are groups more effective than self-contained kits? Can peer leaders and volunteers be effectively utilized to achieve sustained behavior change? Is cable TV an effective educational medium? What spacing of "booster sessions" is most successful for maintaining behavior change? What are the best ways to encourage high-risk people to utilize several strategies to achieve behavior change? Do group interventions at nutrition sites deserve more funding to promote dietary change or should efforts be directed at communitywide media campaigns? We have yet to tackle such questions using research data from studies in aging, but the time for it is inevitably approaching. However, we should be prepared for answers that are complicated. Evidence is rarely unambiguous, and the inherent differences among health-related practices suggest that any one intervention strategy can hope for no more than partial success.

Overdetermination of Behavior

Research in the behavioral sciences has indicated that a behavior (or habit pattern) can result from or be modified by a number of antecedent factors. In view of the multitude of variables that might be investigated, there is a great deal of validity to the long-standing observation that "everything is important for somebody, but any one thing is not important for everybody." Cross-sectional surveys of health-related practices and their predictors have consistently indicated that neither a single variable nor any set of core variables accounts for a substantial proportion of variance. There is even less indication (especially in aging research) that any one variable or small set of variables is a significant predictor at even a modest level across several health-related activities. The current status of the literature indicates that there is no one "magic bullet" of intervention that can singly reach a communitywide audience.

Self-Selection Bias

Community-based DP/HP programs have a limited capability for carrying out traditional laboratorylike experimental/control procedures. It is rarely possible to mandate attendance at programs, the reading of distributed information, the practice of suggested preventive activities, or other forms of participation. Furthermore, access to delivery points of intervention is usually controlled by gatekeepers such as housing and meal-site directors, work-site managers, physicians, and clergy. The net result is, as commonly observed, that it is difficult for programs to reach many of the people who really need them.

Some compensation for this lack of control may be achieved by randomly assigning individual sites to different experimental conditions (as is often done with work sites and with school classrooms of the same grade level). This may help to "even out" participant characteristics but at the risk of losing substantial degrees of freedom by the use of aggregated data when the site becomes the unit of analysis. In these situations, a multiple time-series strategy may be necessary to increase the number of aggregated points of data collection (Salonen et al., 1986).

We cannot assume, however, that research on disease-prevention/ health-promotion interventions with community-based samples who are, for the most part, voluntary joiners, will produce data that are beyond challenge. Most programs (i.e., local and regional demonstrations conducted with modest resources) will need to give careful attention to the sociodemographic profiles of their participants before proceeding to broad generalizations. The process of recruiting individuals to participate may well evolve into its own specialized area of research, separate from research on how to sustain contact long enough to obtain the desired results. The development of the field of social marketing indicates that this will occur (Lefebvre & Flora, 1988). Researchers and policymakers are in fact well advised to distinguish the process of recruitment (which introduces biases at the outset) from the outcomes of the intervention. The results of intervention are inevitably couched in terms of the characteristics of persons who participated, so that the depth of our data along with our ability to answer questions pertinent to broader issues of aging rely on the nature of our participants.

TRENDS IN COMMUNITY-BASED INTERVENTION WITH OLDER PERSONS

The emphasis in this chapter has been on research and empirical aspects of DP/HP programs. Progress and innovations are being made in many areas, as discussed below. There is also an abundance of ongoing community DP/HP initiatives for older persons. Simply reading local newspapers and community bulletin boards reveals a steady flow of screenings, lectures, support groups, and health fairs. For the most part, these go on without any empirical or evaluative components. To overlook them or to dismiss their contributions, however, is a mistake.

The predominant (and overwhelming) impression one receives is that of the energy, dedication, and creativity of the professionals and the effort that goes into the programs. The energy and commitment of those programs and their participants play a major role in sustaining the much more formal and gradual development of a "scientific knowledge base." Without an already activated clientele to whom results can be disseminated, and who also constitute a visible political lobby, a substantial portion of research on disease prevention and health promotion is of minimal utility. The caveat in writing this section, therefore, is to look toward the future rather than critique past, or even current, efforts. The empirical literature on DP/HP and aging is well on the way to becoming highly diversified. Identifying some key areas where advancements can and will come is of greater benefit.

A Developmental Context

The capability to conduct behaviorally oriented DP/HP interventions depends upon knowing enough about the basic pathology, epidemiology, and physiology of aging to design strategies that have a reasonable chance of success. This requisite knowledge base is itself a somewhat recent phenomenon, and significant areas are still under study (e.g., falls, nutrition). Interventions centered on broadly defined objectives of "wellness" may not need to present a well-documented or biologically plausible chain of effect. However, for investigations intended to test hypotheses based on specific behavioral/biological relationships, the interdependence between the domains of basic science and behavioral research becomes more apparent.

We are also in a process of developing the expertise needed to conduct empirically based disease-prevention/health-promotion interventions. This involves not only applying the principles of DP/HP research design to a "new" area such as older adulthood but also building a collective experience of program implementation and evaluation. This kind of cumulative experience, and the professional networking that accompanies it, will allow better anticipation of the potential pitfalls, hazards, and even fortuitous events that can occur once an intervention is initiated.

Because of where the field began in its process of growth, much of the initially published literature on disease prevention/health promotion with older persons described demonstration-type programs conducted in particular local settings. Senior centers, hospitals, geriatric clinics, churches, schools and other public facilities, and congregate housing were among the most common. Programs were generally of a modest size and implemented with a modest budget. The research elements of programs have often been deemphasized in favor of the service components. Of course, this also reflects the sources of funding for these programs. Only relatively recently has the National Institute on Aging established its various initiatives on maintaining health and functioning in the later years, and other units of the NIH have only gradually introduced aging as a specific component of selected research solicitations. Foundations, hospitals, state and local governments, church groups, and most other possible funding sources have traditionally treated the provision of direct services as the higher priority.

It is safe to say that DP/HP programs have been received favorably by the older population. Participation seems to be adequate (at least for the programs for which there is published information), although this does not mean that participants have been exactly those whom the programs originally hoped to reach (e.g., the severely impaired, those living alone, the poor or less well educated). A report of participation over four years from the Pawtucket Heart Health Program, for example (Lefebvre, Harden, Rakowski, Lasater, & Carleton, 1987), indicated that persons aged 65 and older were better represented than younger age groups in blood pressure and nutrition programs, somewhat less well for weight loss and exercise, and least well in smoking cessation programs.

Areas of Program Development

Many of the reports published to date could probably be described as having objectives of general health promotion or broadly based self-care skills (e.g., Barbaro & Noyes, 1984; Buchner & Pearson, 1989; Emery & Gatz, 1990; Fallcreek & Stam, 1982; Furukawa, 1982; Hopkins, Murrah, Hoeger, & Rhodes, 1990; Leviton & Santa Maria, 1979; Nelson et al., 1984; Selzer, Marshall, & Glazer, 1977; Simmons et al., 1989; Vickery, Golazewski, Wright, & Kalmer, 1988). However, if a trend can be identified, it may be that more disease- or illness-related programs are appearing (Clark et al., 1988; Glanz et al., 1986; Haber, 1986; Lorig et al., 1984; Morisky, Levine, Green, & Smith, 1982; Rimer, Jones, Wilson, Bennett, & Engstrom, 1983; Rimer, Keintz, & Fleisher, 1986; Rippey et al., 1987). There is no reason at the current time to prefer one focus over the other. An interesting area to monitor is the extent to which each type of program stimulates attempts at behavior change beyond the topics covered.

Two characteristics do tend to emerge from the reports to date. The first is that most program delivery has followed a didactic model. For the most part, participants are brought together for presentations and skills training and given the mission of transferring the session content to their daily routines. When conducted in groups, age peers are often trained as coleaders. There has not yet been a great deal of experimentation with different modes of delivery. One report utilized an in-house cable TV system to recruit housing-site residents to health screenings (Selzer et al., 1977); another compared standard class structure with yoga and aerobic formats (Haber, 1986). Vickery et al. (1988) employed a set of mailed materials supplemented with a telephone hot line, and Rook (1986) compared two methods of presenting health-related information. Another recent report examined health education preferences in a sample of employees aged 55 and older (Rakowski, Carl, & Flora, 1988). Overall, though, greater diversity in program techniques is timely for empirical study (e.g., self-contained kits for behavior change, videocassettes, correspondence courses, home monitoring of risk-factor levels). The objective of such work would be to determine the best ways to achieve a "fit" between participant characteristics and the DP/HP strategies that are used.

The second characteristic of programs reported to date has been the preponderance of women as participants. Even with the well-known sex ratio discrepancy in later life, the figures in favor of women seem pronounced. Female participation at rates of 70% to 80% are common (Benson et al., 1989; Emery & Gatz, 1990; Hopkins et al., 1990; Lorig et al., 1984; Morisky et al., 1982; Nelson et al., 1984; Rimer et al., 1986; Rippey et al., 1987). Available survey data on health practices throughout adulthood suggest that women report more favorable health patterns than men, with the exception of vigorous exercise, so this observation on participation should come as no surprise. However, another factor to consider is that a large number of interventions have been done in group settings. Not everyone enjoys learning in situations that might be considered "public" or open for others to watch. Behavior change implies the need for learning new skills, which almost inevitably means that mistakes will be made along the way. Much can be said, and has been, about the traditional male acculturation toward ignoring health threats and appearing tough to maintain sex role stereotypes. We might make some progress on this front by considering the possibility that people often prefer to ease into a new event and even do some practicing in relative privacy. Providing such options may help to increase our representation of men and attract other female audiences also.

Because short follow-ups have been common, outcome measures have focused more on attitude change, knowledge change, and short-term behavior change. However, there are an increasing number of examples of longer-term data collection. Lorig et al. (1984) have up to 20 months of follow-up, while Nelson et al. (1984) report on one-year data, and Morisky et al. (1982) have a five-year follow-up. Vickery et al. (1988) had a follow-up period of 12 months, as did Dupree et al. (1984), who tracked their sample of persons with late-life onset of alcohol abuse. The six-month follow-up of the Staying Healthy After Fifty project (Benson et al., 1989; Simmons et al., 1989) is noteworthy in the number of program implementation sites that had to be managed to achieve data collection. In addition to the project-specific research objectives, one of the most important outcomes of these projects has been to demonstrate that it is possible to collect a comprehensive range of data, across several types of dependent measures, in the context of a disease-prevention program.

Along these lines, improvements in data base management systems and automated data entry will play a major role in the types of projects we can conduct. The California Preventive Health Care for the Aging Program, for example (Luckmann & Weiler, 1988), utilized a record-keeping and tracking system on a statewide level to monitor screening and referral for suspected skin cancer. Disease registries and other data bases may also be linked, with proper precautions for maintaining confidentiality, to augment cross-sectional and even longitudinal data on individuals (e.g., National Death Index, Medicare

A/B records, National Mortality Followback Survey, Longitudinal Survey on Aging).

Some reports have attempted to determine the amount or extent of exposure that program participants have received (Emery & Blumenthal, 1990; Emery & Gatz, 1990). Attendance (largely at group events) is rarely perfect, and record-keeping has often not been done in a way to allow attendance rates to be associated with outcome measures. On a related theme, some process and formative evaluations have been reported (e.g., Glanz et al., 1986; Rimer et al., 1983; Rimer et al., 1986), but there is not yet consensus regarding the variety of information that should be collected from participants and about the intervention setting itself, as a means either to monitor program process or to identify predictors of health behavior change or achievement of program objectives. These observations are probably consistent with the service objectives of most programs, where outcome is more important than experimental/control testing of hypotheses. The most extensive process and formative information about program implementation has been provided for the Staying Healthy After Fifty program, a cooperative effort among the American Association of Retired Persons, the American Red Cross, and the Dartmouth Institute for Better Health, with external support from a major national-level foundation (Simmons et al., 1989). Also conveyed in presentation of the program are many practical factors that can arise in the implementation and evaluation of community-based health-promotion programs.

CLOSING COMMENTS

Many of the points raised in this chapter suggest that empirically verified progress on disease-prevention and health-promotion strategies with older persons will come gradually. This characteristic is not unique to DP/HP initiatives. At the same time, individuals who continue to press and test their limits, in this case, for the maintenance of their health, can reveal aspects of performance and potential not yet evident from research.

The more formidable tasks to be faced will evolve in discussion and debate around areas where there are no "best" choices in an absolute sense. These areas include the definition and measurement of health practices, choice of a strategy from the diverse forms that intervention can take, interpretation of results across investigations, and priority setting among potential outcome indicators. The bigger picture of disease-prevention and health-promotion research with older persons can, by nature, develop only over time. As it does, however, we should be prepared to recognize that prevailing zeitgeists and philosophical perspectives are also a part of the landscape along with empirical data.

The chapter also suggests strongly that the dimension of exposure to an intervention will need close attention and precise definition in the older population. Community-based disease-prevention/health promotion-efforts are almost never simple manipulations of a single abstract variable or learning task. Just as risk-factor status can be graduated according to exposure (e.g., to carcinogenic agents, level of smoking, severity of high blood pressure), individuals can have different exposures even within the same intervention, depending upon such factors as number of programs attended, individual attention from program staff, and practice outside of formal program time. The ability to make even broad distinctions among participants along these lines may yield benefits for understanding intervention effects.

Another implication of this discussion pertains to the search for "risk factors" in aging, which can then be the object of behavioral or environmental intervention. Traditionally, this process has been an epidemiology of identifying statistically independent predictor variables—an attractive and elegant approach made possible by powerful multivariate models. We might, however, consider the usefulness of defining risk by combinations of conditions (e.g., high blood pressure and diabetes; visual impairment and obesity; smoking and sedentary life-style). Such combinations would not be clean by some standards, but they would reflect the problem of concomitant health problems and multiple contributing health practices encountered in later adulthood. Another area of epidemiology from which interventions may benefit relates to information about the progression or sequencing of risk-factor status over time, presuming that at least some typologies can be established. This type of information will make it possible to specify intermediate and long-range outcome objectives and to link them to intervention strategies appropriate to the point in the sequence that is being targeted.

As our efforts continue, we should remember that community-based DP/HP presents us with an open-ended menu and with a tantalizing question: How will we know when the health of the aging population has been optimized? Can there ever be a limit on good health status? We are at an important point in developing this area of investigation, where individual well-designed studies can have a large impact on defining the current state of knowledge and thereby help to set agendas for future investigations. The progress of literature in gerontology supports the potential for benefit; our task is to find the proper keys. Every area of research pursues its horizons, but few have a horizon quite as expansive and elusive as that of disease prevention and health promotion.

REFERENCES

Amir, D. (1987). Preventive behavior and health status among the elderly. *Psychology & Health, 1*, 353-378.

Andersson, I., Aspegren, K., Janzon, L., Landberg, T., Linholm, K., Linell, F., Ljungberg, O., Ranstam, J., & Sigfusson, B. (1988). Mammographic screening and mortality from breast cancer: The Malmo mammographic screening trial. *British Medical Journal, 297*, 943-948.

Azjen, I., & Fishbein, M. (1980). *Understanding attitudes and predicting behavior.* Englewood Cliffs, NJ: Prentice-Hall.

Bandura, A. (1977). Self-efficacy: Toward a unifying theory of behavior. *Psychological Review, 84*, 191-215.

Barbaro, E. L., & Noyes, L. E. (1984). A wellness program for a life care community. *The Gerontologist, 24*, 568-571.

Barrett-Connor, E. (1987). Health promotion: Proof of the pudding. *American Journal of Preventive Medicine, 3*, 2-11.

Belloc, N. B., & Breslow, L. (1972). Relationship of physical health status and health practices. *Preventive Medicine, 1*, 409-421.

Benson, L., Nelson, E. C., Napps, S. E., Roberts, E., Kane-Williams, E., & Salisbury, Z. T. (1989). Evaluation of the Staying Healthy After Fifty educational program: Impact on course participants. *Health Education Quarterly, 4*, 485-508.

Blackburn, H. (1983, December). Research and demonstration projects in community cardiovascular disease prevention. *Journal of Public Health Policy,* pp. 398-421.

Branch, L. G., & Jette, A. M. (1984). Personal health practices and mortality among the elderly. *American Journal of Public Health, 74*, 1126-1129.

Breslow, L. (1990). A health promotion primer for the 1990s. *Health Affairs, 9*, 6-21.

Breslow, L., & Enstrom, J. E. (1980). Persistence of health habits and their relationship to mortality. *Preventive Medicine, 9*, 469-483.

Brock, B. M., Haefner, D. P., & Noble, D. S. (1988). Alameda County redux: Replication in Michigan. *Preventive Medicine, 17*, 483-495.

Buchner, D. M., & Pearson, D. C. (1989). Factors associated with participation in a community senior health promotion program: A pilot study. *American Journal of Public Health, 79*, 775777.

Campbell, D. T. (1969). Reforms as experiments. *American Psychologist, 24*, 409-429.

Campbell, D. T., & Stanley, J. C. (1963). *Experimental and quasi-experimental designs for research.* Chicago: Rand McNally.

Chu, K. C., Smart, C. R., & Tarone, R. E. (1988). Analysis of breast cancer mortality and stage distribution by age for the Health Insurance Plan clinical trial. *Journal of the National Cancer Institute, 80*, 1125-1132

Clark, N. M., Rakowski, W., Wheeler, J. R. C., Ostrander, L. D., Oden, S., & Keteyian, S. (1988). Development of self-management education for elderly heart patients. *The Gerontologist, 28,* 491-494.

Cohen, R. Y., Stunkard, A., & Felix, M. R. J. (1986). Measuring community change in disease prevention and health promotion. *Preventive Medicine, 15,* 411-421.

Dawson, D., & Hendershot, G. (1987, June 10). *Aging in the eighties: Functional limitations of individuals age 65 years and over* (Advance Data No. 133). Hyattsville, MD: National Center for Health Statistics.

Dupree, L. W., Broskowski, H., & Schonfeld, L. (1984). The Gerontology Alcohol Project: A behavioral treatment program for elderly alcohol abusers. *The Gerontologist, 24,* 510-516.

Emery, C. F., & Blumenthal, J. A. (1990). Exercise: Perceived change among participants in an exercise program for older adults. *The Gerontologist, 30,* 516-521.

Emery, C. F., & Gatz, M. (1990). Psychological and cognitive effects of an exercise program for community-residing older adults. *The Gerontologist, 30,* 184-188.

Fallcreek, S., & Stam, S. B. (Eds.). (1982). *The Wallingford Wellness Project: An innovative health promotion program with older adults.* Seattle: University of Washington, School of Social Work, Center for Social Welfare Research.

Farquhar, J. W. (1978). The community-based model of life-style intervention trials. *American Journal of Epidemiology, 108,* 103-111.

Farquhar, J. W., Fortmann, S. P., Flora, J. A., Taylor, C. B., Haskell, W. L., Williams, P. T., Maccoby, N., & Wood, P. D. (1990). Effects of communitywide education on cardiovascular disease risk factors: The Stanford Five-City Project. *JAMA, 264,* 359-365.

Farquhar, J. W., Fortmann, S. P., Maccoby, N., Haskell, W. L., Williams, P., Flora, J. A., Taylor, C. B., Brown, B. W., Solomon, D. S., & Hulley, S. B. (1985). The Stanford Five-City Project: Design and methods. *American Journal of Epidemiology, 122,* 323-334.

Fiatarone, M. A., Marks, E. C., Ryan, N. D., Meredith, C. N., Lipsitz, L. A., & Evans, W. J. (1990). High-intensity strength training in nonagenarians. *JAMA, 263,* 3029-3034.

Furukawa, C. (1982). Adult health conference: Community-oriented health maintenance for the elderly. In T. Wells (Ed.), *Aging and health promotion* (pp. 205-222). Rockville, MD: Aspen.

Garland, C., Barrett-Connor, E., Suarez, L., & Criqui, M. H. (1983). Isolated systolic hypertension and mortality after age 60 years: A prospective population-based study. *American Journal of Epidemiology, 118,* 365-376.

Glanz, K., Marger, S. M., & Meehan, E. F. (1986). Evaluation of a peer educator stroke education program for the elderly. *Health Education Research, 1,* 121-130.

Green, L. W., Wilson, A. L., & Lovato, C. Y. (1986). What changes can health promotion achieve and how long do these changes last? *Preventive Medicine, 15,* 508-521.

Greenwald, P., & Cullen, J. W. (1985). The new emphasis in cancer control. *Journal of the National Cancer Institute, 74,* 543-551.

Haber, D. (1986). Health promotion to reduce blood pressure level among older Blacks. *The Gerontologist, 26,* 119-121.

Harris, D. M., & Guten, S. (1979). Health-protective behavior: An exploratory study. *Journal of Health and Social Behavior, 20,* 17-29.

Harris, T., Cook, E. F., Kannel, W. B., & Goldman, L. (1988). Proportional hazards analysis of risk factors for coronary heart disease in individuals aged 65 or older: The Framingham Heart Study. *Journal of the American Geriatrics Society, 36,* 1023-1028.

Hopkins, D. R., Murrah, B., Hoeger, W. W. K., & Rhodes, R. C. (1990). Effect of low-impact aerobic dance on the functional fitness of elderly women. *The Gerontologist, 30,* 189-192.

Hypertension Detection and Follow-Up Program Cooperative Group. (1979a). Five-year findings of the Hypertension Detection and Follow-Up Program: I. Reduction of mortality of persons with high blood pressure, including mild hypertension. *JAMA, 242,* 2562-2571.

Hypertension Detection and Follow-Up Program Cooperative Group. (1979b). Five-year findings of the Hypertension Detection and Follow-up Program: II. Mortality by race-sex and age. *JAMA, 242,* 2572-2577.

Jajich, C. L., Ostfeld, A. M., & Freeman, D. H. (1984). Coronary heart disease mortality in the elderly. *Journal of the American Medical Association, 252,* 2831-2834.

Janz, N. K., & Becker, M. H. (1984). The Health Belief Model: A decade later. *Health Education Quarterly, 11,* 1-47.

Kaplan, G. A., & Haan, M. N. (1989). Is there a role for prevention among the elderly? Epidemiological evidence from the Alameda County study. In M. G. Ory & K. Bond (Eds.), *Aging and health care: Social science and policy perspectives* (pp. 27-51). London: Routledge.

Kaplan, G. A., Seeman, T. E., Cohen, R. D., Knudsen, L. P., & Guralnik, J. (1987). Mortality among the elderly in Alameda County: Behavioral and demographic risk factors. *American Journal of Public Health, 77,* 307-312.

Katz, S., Downs, T. D., Cash, H. R., & Grotz, R. C. (1970). Progress in the development of the index of ADL. *The Gerontologist, 10,* 20-30.

Kirscht, J. P. (1983). Preventive health behavior: A review of research and issues. *Health Psychology, 2,* 277-301.

Langlie, J. K. (1979). Interrelationships among preventive health behaviors: A test of competing hypotheses. *Public Health Reports, 94,* 216-225.

Lawton, M. P., & Nahemow, L. (1973). Ecology and the aging process. In C. Eisdorfer & M. P. Lawton (Eds.), *The psychology of adult development and aging* (pp. 619-674). Washington, DC: American Psychological Association.

Lefebvre, R. C., & Flora, J. A. (1988). Social marketing and public health education. *Health Education Quarterly, 15,* 299-315.

Lefebvre, R. C., Harden, E. A., Rakowski, W., Lasater, T. M., & Carleton, R. A. (1987). Characteristics of participants in community health promotion programs: Four-year results. *American Journal of Public Health, 77,* 1342-1344.

Lefebvre, R. C., Lasater, T. M., Carleton, R. A., & Peterson, G. (1987). Theory and delivery of health programming in the community: The Pawtucket Heart Health program. *Preventive Medicine, 16,* 80-95.

Leviton, D., & Santa Maria, L. (1979). The Adults Health & Developmental Program: Descriptive and evaluative data. *The Gerontologist, 19,* 534-543.

Lipid Research Clinics Program. (1984a). The Lipid Research Clinics Coronary Primary Prevention Trial Results: I. Reduction in incidence of coronary heart disease. *JAMA, 251,* 351-364.

Lipid Research Clinics Program. (1984b). The Lipid Research Clinics Coronary Primary Prevention Trial Results: II. The relationship of reduction in incidence of coronary heart disease to cholesterol lowering. *JAMA, 251*, 365-374.

Looft, W. R. (1973). Socialization and personality throughout the life span: An examination of contemporary psychological approaches. In P. B. Baltes & K. W. Schaie (Eds.), *Life-span developmental psychology: Personality and socialization* (pp. 26-52). New York: Academic Press.

Lorig, K., Laurin, J., & Holman, H. R. (1984). Arthritis self-management: A study of the effectiveness of patient education for the elderly. *The Gerontologist, 24*, 455-457.

Luckmann, R., & Weiler, P. G. (1988). Screening the elderly for skin disease: A report of the experience of the California Preventive Health Care for the Aging Program. *Family & Community Health, 11*, 53-64.

Maccoby, N., Farquhar, J. W., Wood, P. D., & Alexander, J. (1977). Reducing the risk of cardiovascular disease: Effects of a community-based campaign on knowledge and behavior. *Journal of Community Health, 3*, 100-114.

McHugh, S., & Vallis, T. M. (Eds.). (1986). *Illness behavior: A multidisciplinary model.* New York: Plenum.

Minkler, M. (1984). Health promotion in long-term care: A contradiction in terms? *Health Education Quarterly, 11*, 77-89.

Minkler, M. (1985). Building supportive ties and sense of community among the inner-city elderly: The Tenderloin Senior Outreach Project. *Health Education Quarterly, 12*, 303-314.

Mittlemark, M. B., Leupker, R. V., Jacobs, D. R., Bracht, N. F., Carlaw, R., Crow, R., Finnegan, J., Grimm, R., Jeffery, R. W., Kline, F. G., Murray, D. M., Mullis, R., Perry, C., Pirie, P., Pechacek, T. F., & Blackburn, H. (1986). Community-wide prevention of cardiovascular disease: Education strategies of the Minnesota Heart Health Program. *Preventive Medicine, 15*, 1-17.

Mor, V., Pacala, J., & Rakowski, W. (1990, July). *Universal mammography for older women?* Position paper for NCI/NIA/HCFA-sponsored forum on Breast Cancer Screening in Older Women, Sturbridge, CT.

Morisky, D. E., Levine, D. M., Green, L. W., & Smith, C. R. (1982). Health education program effects on the management of hypertension in the elderly. *Archives of Internal Medicine, 142*, 1835-1838.

Multiple Risk Factor Intervention Trial Research Group. (1982). Multiple Risk Factor Intervention Trial: Risk factor change and mortality results. *JAMA, 248*, 1465-1477.

Nelson, E. C., McHugo, G., Schnurr, P., Devito, C., Roberts, E., Simmons, J., & Zubkoff, W. (1984). Medical self-care education for elders: A controlled trial to evaluate impact. *American Journal of Public Health, 74*, 1357-1363.

Olson, R. E. (1986). Mass intervention vs screening and selective intervention for the prevention of coronary heart disease. *JAMA, 255*, 2204-2207.

Omenn, G. S. (1990). Prevention and the elderly: Appropriate policies. *Health Affairs, 9*, 80-93.

Overton, W. F. (1973). On the assumptive base of the nature-nurture controversy: Additive versus interactive conceptions. *Human Development, 16*, 74-89.

Overton, W. F., & Reese, H. W. (1973). Models of development: Methodological implications. In J. R. Nesselroade & H. W. Reese (Eds.), *Life-span developmental psychology: Methodological issues* (pp. 65-86). New York: Academic Press.

Perkins, K. A., Rapp, S. R., Carlson, C. R., & Wallace, C. E. (1986). A behavioral intervention to increase exercise among nursing home residents. *The Gerontologist, 26,* 479-481.

Prochaska, J. O., & DiClemente, C. C. (1986). Toward a comprehensive model of change. In W. R. Miller & N. Heather (Eds.), *Treating addictive behaviors* (pp. 3-27). New York: Plenum.

Puska, P., Salonen, J. T., Tuomilehto, J., Nissinen, A., & Kottke, T. E. (1983). Evaluating community-based preventive cardiovascular programs: Problems and experiences from the North Karelia Project. *Journal of Community Health, 9,* 49-64.

Rakowski, W. (1986). Research issues in health promotion programs for the elderly. In K. Dychtwald (Ed.), *Wellness and health promotion for the elderly* (pp. 313-326). Rockville, MD: Aspen.

Rakowski, W. (1987). The persistence of personal health practices over a one-year period. *Public Health Reports, 102,* 483-493.

Rakowski, W., Carl, F., & Flora, J. A. (1988). Health education for older workers: Interests and preferences of university employees aged 55 and over. *Family & Community Health, 11,* 65-73.

Rakowski, W., Julius, M., Hickey, T., & Halter, J. (1987). Correlates of personal health behavior in late life. *Research on Aging, 9,* 331-355.

Reese, H. W., & Overton, W. F. (1970). Models of development and theories of development. In L. R. Goulet & P. B. Baltes (Eds.), *Life-span developmental psychology: Research and theory* (pp. 116-145). New York: Academic Press.

Reich, J. W., & Zautra, A. J. (1989). A perceived control intervention for at-risk older adults. *Psychology and Aging, 4,* 415-424.

Rimer, B., Jones, W., Wilson, C., Bennet, D., & Engstrom, P. (1983). Planning a cancer control program for older citizens. *The Gerontologist, 23,* 384-388.

Rimer, B., Keintz, M. K., & Fleisher, L. (1986). Process and impact evaluation of a health communications program. *Health Education Research, 1,* 29-36.

Rippey, R. M., Bill, D., Abeles, M., Day, J., Downing, D. S., Pfeiffer, C. A., Thal, S. E., & Wetstone, S. L. (1987). Computer-based patient education for older persons with osteoarthritis. *Arthritis and Rheumatism, 30,* 932-935.

Rook, K. S. (1986). Encouraging preventive behavior for distant and proximal health threats: Effects of vivid versus abstract information. *Journal of Gerontology, 41,* 526-534.

Safer, M. A. (1986). A comparison of screening for disease detection and screening for risk factors. *Health Education Research, 1,* 131-138.

Sallis, J. F., Grossman, R. M., Pinski, R. B., Patterson, T. L., & Nader, P. R. (1987). The development of scales to measure social support for diet and exercise behaviors. *Preventive Medicine, 16,* 825-836.

Sallis, J. F., Haskell, W. L., Fortmann, S. P., Vranzian, K. M., Taylor, C. B., & Solomon, D. S. (1986). Predictors of adoption and maintenance of physical activity in a community sample. *Preventive Medicine, 15,* 331-341.

Salonen, J. T., Kottke, T. E., Jacobs, D. R., Jr., & Hannan, P. J. (1986). Analysis of community-based cardiovascular disease prevention studies: Evaluation issues in the North Karelia Project and the Minnesota Heart Health Program. *International Journal of Epidemiology, 15*, 176-182.

Schiffman, S., Shumaker, S. A., Abrams, D. B., & Cohen, S. (1986). Models of smoking relapse. *Health Psychology, 5*(Suppl.), 13-27.

Schoenborn, C. A., & Benson, V. (1988, May 27). *Relationship between smoking and other unhealthy habits: United States, 1985* (Advance Data No. 154). Hyattsville, MD: National Center for Health Statistics.

Selzer, J. E., Marshall, C. L., & Glazer, E. R. (1977). The use of cable television as a tool in health education for the elderly: Screening. *Health Education Monographs, 5*, 363-378.

Shumaker, S. A., & Grunberg, N. E. (1986). Proceedings of the National Conference on Smoking Relapse. *Health Psychology, 5*(Suppl.), 3-68.

Sidney, K. H., & Shepard, R. J. (1977). Attitudes toward health and physical activity in the elderly: Effects of a physical training program. *Medicine and Science in Sports, 8*, 246-252.

Siegel, D., Kuller L., Lazarus, N. B., Black, D., Feigal, D., Hughes, G., Schoenberger, J. A., & Hulley, S. B. (1987). Predictors of cardiovascular events and mortality in the Systolic Hypertension in the Elderly Program pilot project. *American Journal of Epidemiology, 126*, 385-399.

Simmons, J. J., Neslon, E. C., Roberts, E., Salisbury, Z. T., Kane-Williams, E., & Benson, L. (1989). A health promotion program: Staying Healthy After Fifty. *Health Education Quarterly, 4*, 461-472.

Skrabanek, P. (1988). The case against. *British Medical Journal, 297*, 971-972.

Slater, C. H., Carlton, B., Ramirez, G., & Ashton, C. (1987). Heart disease: Strategies for prevention. *Evaluation & the Health Professions, 10*, 255-286.

Sloan, R. P. (1987). Workplace health promotion: A commentary on the evolution of a paradigm. *Health Education Quarterly, 14*, 181-194.

Steering Committee of the Physicians' Health Study Research Group. (1988, January 28). Preliminary report: Findings from the aspirin component of the ongoing Physicians' Health Study. *The New England Journal of Medicine, 318*, 262-264 (and related editorial, pp. 245-246).

Stephens, T. (1986). Health practices and health status: Evidence from the Canada Health Survey. *American Journal of Preventive Medicine, 2*, 209-215.

Stunkard, A. J., Felix, M. R. J., & Cohen, R. Y. (1985). Mobilizing a community to promote health: The Pennsylvania County Health Improvement Program (CHIP). In J. C. Rosen & L. J. Solomon (Eds.), *Prevention in health psychology* (pp. 145-190). Hanover: University Press of New England.

Tapp, J. T., & Goldenthal, P. (1982). A factor analytic study of health habits. *Preventive Medicine, 11*, 724-728.

Thornberry, O. T., Wilson, R. W., & Golden, P. M. (1986, September 19). *Health promotion data for the 1990 objectives: Estimates from the National Health Interview Survey of Health Promotion and Disease Prevention: United States, 1985* (Advance Data No. 126). Hyattsville, MD: National Center for Health Statistics.

Truett, J., Cornfeld, J., & Kannel, W. (1967). A multivariate analysis of the risk of coronary heart disease in Framingham. *Journal of Chronic Diseases, 20*, 511-524.

U.S. Department of Health & Human Services. (1990). *Healthy people 2000* (Public Health Service, Office for the Assistant Secretary for Health). Washington, DC: Government Printing Office.

Vickery, D. M., Golazewski, T. J., Wright, E. C., & Kalmer, H. (1988). The effect of self-care interventions on the use of medical service within a medicare population. *Medical Care, 26,* 580-588.

Wechsler, R., & Minkler, M. (1986). A community-oriented approach to health promotion: The Tenderloin Senior Outreach Project. In K. Dychtwald (Ed.), *Wellness and health promotion for the elderly* (pp. 301-311). Rockville, MD: Aspen.

Weinstein, N. D. (1988). The precaution adoption process. *Health Psychology, 7,* 355-386.

10

Intervening in Social
Systems to Promote Health

LENNART LEVI

THE DEFINITION OF
HEALTH AND WELL-BEING

According to the Athenian statesman Pericles (495-429 B.C.), "Health is that state of moral, mental and physical well-being, which enables man to face any crisis in life with utmost facility and grace." This ancient definition highlights two critically important aspects. First, health includes people's interaction with their living conditions. Second, the ability to cope may be lost if the "slings and arrows of outrageous fortune" are sufficiently noxious and if there is no intervention against the resulting breakdown of human adaptation.

Most interventions are focused on the individual, addressing emotional, cognitive, behavioral, and/or physiological reactions to various environmental exposures. The alternative or, better, complementary option of intervening against at least some of the "slings and arrows" is often overlooked. Interventions directed at identifying and ameliorating pathogenic social systems are particularly important for older people, due to increased vulnerabilities associated with advanced age.

Swedish Public Health Service Bill

These new concepts about social determinants of health are reflected in recent Swedish and international initiatives. The Swedish Public Health Service Bill (1985, p. 11) declared that "our health is determined in large measure by our living conditions and lifestyle." The bill enumerates health risks in contemporary society, such as deficient social structures and processes, unemployment and the threat of unemployment, and health-related behaviors and life-styles, "as well as psychological and social strains associated with our relationships—and lack of relationships—with our fellow beings." Such health risks are now a major determinant of our possibilities of living a healthy life and are strongly implicated in today's most common disorders and injuries. Thus "care must start from a holistic approach, [by which is meant] that people's symptoms and illnesses, their causes and consequences, are appraised in both a medical and a psychological and social perspective" (p. 18).

The relationships between the manifestations of ill health and environmental and life-style factors are summarized in Figure 10.1. This environment/life-style/health matrix shows the strength of the relationships without attributing causes. This matrix reveals the range of responses to different life-style or environmental factors (see the discussion in Chapter 8 by Vogt, explaining such inconsistencies in previous literature). Older people are seen as especially vulnerable to the effects of pathogenic environmental influences.

World Health Organization Recommendations

The founders of the World Health Organization (WHO) took a visionary view when they unanimously proposed to define *health* as "not only the absence of disease or infirmity but also a state of physical, mental and social well-being" (WHO, 1946). Drawing on this philosophy in their Health for All (HFA) strategy, the member states of WHO committed themselves to creating the conditions that will enable all people to enjoy a reasonably healthy life by the year A.D. 2000. This strategy reordered the priorities in the health sector and moved from a perspective that was predominantly disease oriented and curative to one focused chiefly on the prevention of ill health, the maintenance and promotion of good health, and the capacity to resist disease.

Interventions in social systems are an essential component in this strategy to promote health. This approach requires broadening the perspective to include intersectorial action among various parts of society. According to the Report of the Technical Discussions of the 39th World Health Assembly (WHO, 1986), health goals defined in these terms cannot be realized through the services delivered by the health sector alone. The achievement of such goals requires the combined effort of several other sectors whose activities have a major impact on health. Improvements in health are perceived as a multisectorial responsibility, in which the main development sectors (e.g.,

Manifestation of ill health

Environment/life-style/health Matrix • indicates some, and ** strong relationships	Cardiovascular diseases	Mental illness	Skeletomuscular disease	Tumours	Injuries	Respiratory diseases
Social upbringing environment	*	**				
Social work environment and unemployment	**	**			*	
Physical work environment		*	**	**	**	**
Social living environment		*				
Physical living environment				*	**	*
Air/water pollutants				*		*
Traffic				*	**	*
Diet	**			**		*
Alcohol and drugs		**		*	**	*
Tobacco	**			**		*

Figure 10.1. Correlation Between Environmental and Behavioral Health Hazards and Ill Health.

food and nutrition, water and sanitation, housing and education, economy and labor) would need to collaborate with the health sector. This report includes a series of recommendations for improving health and the quality of life through intersectoral actions.

The need for a theoretical systems model. Recommendations for a healthy life usually fail to address one essential point. We often do not know how to intervene, when, on whom, under what circumstances, at what cost (in terms of health and well-being but also economy), and at whose expense. This is so because the interactive processes between the physical and social environment—the individual's appraisal of the environmental influences and reactions in terms of emotion, cognition, behavior, and physiology; the modification of these reactions through coping, social support, and other interacting variables; and the resulting changes in health and well-being—are extremely complex and poorly understood. These processes cannot be dealt with effectively in a unifactorial or even multifactorial manner. They must be studied and evaluated interdisciplinarily and intersectorially. All this points to a systems approach, in research, in environmental and health monitoring, in intersectoral health action, and in its interdisciplinary evaluation. A heuristic human ecological model is introduced to describe the interrelated components of the person-environment ecosystem (Kagan & Levi, 1975). Humans modify nature through a variety of social structures and processes (see Box 1 in Figure 10.2). Examples of social structures are a family, a neighborhood, a school, a place of work, a hospital, a city, or a country. A social process is whatever takes place in such a structure—for example, family care, work, or medical care.

These structures and processes are perceived and appraised. Significant, pronounced, or persistent discrepancies between the subject's abilities, needs, and expectations, on the one hand, and environmental stimuli and demands, on the other, can influence health, well-being, and opportunities for human development through a number of pathogenic mechanisms (Box 4). Four types of stress-related mechanisms can be noted: emotional reactions (e.g., anxiety, depression, hypochondriasis), cognitive reactions (e.g., restricted scope of perception), behaviors (e.g., increased consumption of tobacco, alcohol, and certain foods), and physiological reactions (e.g., neuroendocrine "stress" responses). These four types of closely interrelated and potentially pathogenic reactions may in turn lead to transitory disturbances of a number of mental and physical functions (Box 5) and to functional and organic damage (Box 6).

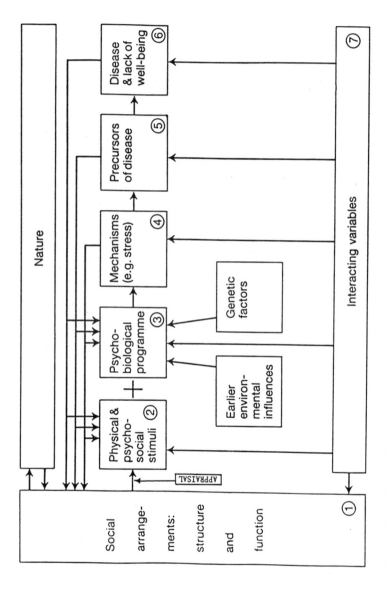

Figure 10.2. Human Ecological System: Human Element Detailed
SOURCE: Kagan and Levi (1975).

The propensity to react with pathogenic processes depends on the individual's psychobiological "programming" (Box 3), which is conditioned not only by genetic factors and previous environmental influences but also by aging and old age. The pathogenic process is modified by interacting variables (Box 7) such as the ability for a needed combination of emotion- and problem-oriented coping and the availability and utilization of social support. The process is cybernetic; that is, a person who sustains a reactive depression or a stress-induced myocardial infarction influences people around him, who in turn influence that person in a different way than previously. The propensity to react and the quality of reactions (i.e., programming) also change. In the worst case, a vicious cycle develops, with successive reinforcement of the pathogenic process.

The conceptual model in Figure 10.2 highlights important research questions. We need to know the content of each "box," which influences are pathogenic, in which individuals, by which mechanisms; which diseases can this lead to; and which interacting variables modify the pathogenic process. Also needed is an understanding of how the various components of the system interact and how we can best describe, analyze, and intervene in this complex system. Additional attention should also be paid to how aging affects, and is affected by, the different structures and processes in this model.

Potentially stressful social structures and processes. Potentially stressful social situations indicated in the model described above include mismatches between person and environment (as appraised by each individual), between individual abilities and environmental demands, between needs and environmental opportunities, and between expectations and the situation as perceived. Such mismatches are threats to survival, health, and well-being; self-esteem; close attachment to significant others; sense of belonging to a valued group; and personal development and self-realization. A common denominator of all these threats is a perceived and/or actual lack of personal control. This, in turn, is a common characteristic of the life of many elderly people all around the world (see Chapter 7 by Rodin & Timko).

Another potential stressor arises in conflicts between competing roles, such as at work and in family life, or in a lack of social role (the latter being increasingly common among the elderly). In general, stress-related ill health can be due to intense or persistent exposure to stressors beyond the coping capacity of the individual.

There is little direct evidence that such social structures and processes and their changes influence the incidence and prevalence of mental and psychosomatic morbidity and mortality. But a substantial body of indirect evidence strongly suggests that such associations exist and emphasizes the need to understand better their role in the etiology of social and health problems as a basis for subsequent preventive action (Levi, 1971, 1975, 1978, 1981, 1987a).

If the interactions among exposure to stressors, vulnerabilities, and lack of protective "buffering" influences are not countered by positive resources, then a number of diseases may develop. These include emotional and personality disorders, suicidal and other self-destructive behaviors, physical functional disorders, and some physical structural disorders such as myocardial infarction and sudden cardiac death (see Elliott & Eisdorfer, 1982; Henry & Stephens, 1977; Levi, 1979). Another large disease group includes virtually all physical functional as well as structural morbidity—in the sense of an emotional overlay, through an influence on health care (compliance) and other behaviors (e.g., tobacco or alcohol abuse) or through psychophysiological mechanisms (Levi, 1971, 1975, 1978, 1981, 1987a).

THE INADEQUACY OF
GOVERNMENTAL RESPONSE

In both developed and developing countries, governmental action against social, environmental, and health problems is often of a troubleshooting and crisis-oriented nature and addresses only one problem or just a few specific problems at a time (e.g., providing meals, or housing, or medical care). Not infrequently, governmental action takes the form of aid for acute disaster in situations where disasters tend to be chronic. In such cases, intervention is usually administered by one of many specialized agencies, with insufficient cooperation with other specialized agencies. A single health problem, such as gastrointestinal infections, may be attacked, while poverty-induced undernourishment, for example, is neglected. More often than not, social and/or behavioral determinants of health problems are left unattended.

This bird's-eye view of social environment and human health—in general and in old age—illustrates that the person-environment ecosystem contains many interacting and probably highly pathogenic factors. Influencing one variable can affect many of the others, with complex interactions and many feedback loops. Consequently, it is usually impossible to cope successfully with current and future environmental, behavioral, and health problems by considering—

in research, therapy, and/or prevention—just one or two of the components of the total ecosystem. Success is more probable if as many as possible of the critical components can be taken into account.

Critical Etiological Factors in the Onset and Course of Disease

Do we really know which environmental exposures are (a) necessary, (b) sufficient, or (c) contributory in causing a certain disease, accelerating its course, and/or triggering its symptoms? Despite many assumptions and suspicions, scientific proof is lacking. Decision makers, often under pressure from the public to act even without evidence that their actions will achieve desired goals, initiate interventions without evaluating the effects and side effects of their actions systematically, interdisciplinarily, and intersectorially. This is why the evaluation of controlled interventions in social systems becomes crucially important. We do not anticipate that all of the policymakers' questions can be answered in this manner. Yet such studies are an important complement to descriptive and analytic approaches.

STEPS IN CONDUCTING STUDIES OF INTERVENTIONS

Answers to Six Key Questions

Research is not an abstraction; it is a tool that can provide better answers to questions about the cause, prevention, and treatment of ill health and suffering. It should provide solid answers to six key questions raised by the President's Commission on Mental Health (1978):

(1) What groups of people are at a high (or low) risk of various types of morbidity and mortality?
(2) What individual and social factors contribute to (or counteract) the risk, and what is the relative importance of each of those factors?
(3) Can the most significant of the risk factors be effectively reduced or eliminated (and health-promoting factors furthered)?
(4) Does eliminating the most significant of the risk factors (or promoting a salutary factor) effectively lower the rate of various types of morbidity and mortality?

(5) If it does, are the costs of intervention justified by the benefits obtained?

(6) Is the program responsive to the principles governing both the rights of individuals and the rights of society?

The answers of these questions may vary considerably over the life span. As emphasized by Ory (1988), there may be critical periods of exposure for any risk factor. People's vulnerability may change with age, or the most susceptible people may not survive to old age. And, even when epidemiological links are found between, for instance, life-style factors and health outcomes, it does not necessarily follow that eliminating or reducing such a factor late in life will improve health and functioning in an elderly person. Consequently, age and aging must be considered in all these and related contexts.

The Application of Knowledge

In developing and evaluating intervention studies, it is necessary to apply existing knowledge and to identify strategies for collecting new data. The three major problem areas in this context—enhancement of health care, prevention of mental and physical ill health, and improvement of well-being—are all complex and affected by a large variety of factors. Although greater understanding is required for each of the three areas, it is highly probable that applying current knowledge would be beneficial. One approach would be to introduce existing knowledge of psychosocial factors, or new ideas where appropriate, into the assessment of health problems and social actions, and to evaluate their impact on health and well-being. The relation of acceptance, availability, and use of health and social actions to the mode of administration, on the one hand, and to health and well-being, on the other, should also be assessed (Kagan & Levi, 1975).

In many instances, our current state of knowledge simply does not allow rational health action even if combined with evaluation. To close such critical gaps, new knowledge must be acquired regarding high-risk situations, high-risk groups, and high-risk reactions. To provide the necessary data, research projects can often be carried out in three complementary steps:

- problem identification, using survey techniques and morbidity data, to find environmental and other correlates of health problems and to describe the size of the problems;

- longitudinal, multidisciplinary, intensive studies of the intersection of high-risk situations and high-risk groups as compared with controls to identify temporal relationships between environmental exposures and pathogenic mechanisms (and among such mechanisms) as modified by interacting factors; and
- controlled intervention, including laboratory experiments as well as therapeutic and/or preventive interventions in real-life settings (for example, natural experiments or interdisciplinary evaluation of health actions).

These approaches could and should include the testing of hypotheses that could increase understanding of the psychosocial factors that affect health in general. Our strategy should be to identify situations and conduct projects by utilizing a combination of applied and basic research. It is often possible and desirable to approach simultaneously the problems of enhancement of health care, prevention of ill health, and increase of well-being—using scarcely more resources for all three than each would require separately (Kagan & Levi, 1975).

Hypothesis Testing and Evaluation of Health Action

Many studies on health and its social and other environmental determinants have been carried out all over the world. Advances have been made at the molecular, cellular, and organ level but very little at the family, neighborhood, or community level (see Markides & Cooper, 1989). Referring to this gap, Kagan (1981) pointed out that, once attention moves from the laboratory to the community, reports on hypothesis-testing studies were hardly ever found. Some notable early exceptions are reviewed by Eisdorfer and Stotsky (1977) and Estes and Freeman (1976).

As soon as one looks beyond clinical trials, it is rare to find an evaluation of community-oriented health action. Numerous studies have shown associations between psychosocial and other environmental factors and health, have speculated on ideas for health or social action, or have put forward hypotheses in relation to the spread and control of disease in the community. In rare, important exceptions, a hypothesis has been tested or action has been evaluated showing that it is possible to carry out controlled, community-oriented social intervention studies (see Kagan, 1981; Levi, Frankenhaeuser, & Gardell, 1982; Markides & Cooper, 1989). Reasons given for not conducting such studies are that they are unethical, technically impossible, too expensive, or too time-consuming. While there is an element of truth in all four objections, the first three can often be addressed adequately, and the fourth can be minimized (Kagan, 1981; Levi, 1987b). Once such research is considered, however, it becomes unethical (and probably more costly) to impose an environmental or health action of unproven value, possible human risk, and high cost without evaluating it or to accept the hypothesis without prior test (Kagan, 1981). For a review of areas for health promotion for the elderly, where intervention is hindered by substantial gaps in information, see Hazzard (1985). It is a philosophical and political question whether controlled intervention studies should await additional fundamental research or provide a way to close these gaps.

Based on descriptive studies, measures that may be presumed to prevent disease and promote health can then be proposed. These measures should be (a) likely to be of greatest causal importance, (b) accessible to change, (c) feasible, and (d) acceptable to all concerned. At a third stage, these measures should be evaluated in an interdisciplinary experimental model study. Fourth, depending on the outcome in terms of benefits, side effects, and costs, a wider application may be implemented, continuously monitored, evaluated, and modified as necessary.

Characteristics of Research Approaches

Briefly, the overall research program should aim at being

- *systems oriented*, analyzing health-related interactions in the human-environment ecosystem (e.g., family, school, work, hospital, and old people's home);
- *interdisciplinary*, covering medical, physiological, emotional, behavioral, social, and economic aspects;
- *oriented to problem solving*, including epidemiological identification of health problems and their environmental and other correlates, followed by longitudinal interdisciplinary field studies of exposures, reactions, and so on, and then by subsequent experimental evaluation under real-life conditions of presumably health-promoting and disease-preventing interventions;
- *health oriented* (not merely disease oriented), trying to identify what constitutes and promotes good health and counteracts ill health;
- *intersectorial*, promoting and evaluating environmental and health actions administered in other sectors (e.g., employment, housing, nutrition, traffic, and education);

- *participatory*, interacting closely with potential caregivers, receivers, planners, and policymakers (see below); and
- *international*, facilitating transcultural, collaborative, and complementary projects with centers in other countries.

Such a research program would be of great benefit in distinguishing among stressful social structures and processes (Figure 10.2, Box 1), reactions to such stressors (Box 4), the consequences of such reactions (Boxes 5 and 6), and the mediators that modify (Box 7) the flow of events. Information is also needed on the determinants that make some events and conditions stressful, on the effects of the resulting stress on a broad range of possible pathogenic mechanisms, and on the health consequences. Information is similarly needed on the components of health-promoting (salutogenic) processes and how they interact (Antonovsky, 1987; Elliott & Eisdorfer, 1982; Lazarus, 1985; Lazarus & Folkman, 1984).

In the past, most studies were unifactorial, in the sense that they focused on a single aspect of the situation (e.g., machine-paced work) or of the individual (e.g., Type A behavior), relating it to a single possibly pathogenic reaction (e.g., catecholamine excretion) and/or morbidity in a specific disease (e.g., myocardial infarction). Since the mid-1970s, studies have become increasingly multifactorial and even interdisciplinary. The next step is to apply a nonlinear, interactional systems approach (see Miller, 1978) to the entire sequence of events, starting with the life situation and its appraisal and ending with the advantages of having a healthy population and including intervening and interacting variables and feedback loops. Although this ecosystem is already admittedly highly complex, attention must also be given to the dynamic influence of the aging processes. Little attention has been paid to stabilities and changes in social structures and processes over an individual's lifetime or to social changes over historical time.

Traditional Versus Participatory Approaches

To be effective and to produce results that are likely to be applied and utilized, the research approaches described above should be participatory. In a traditional approach, the researchers choose the problem to be studied. Usually the choice is based on their own frame of reference. A number of testable hypotheses are formulated from biomedical, social, and/or behavioral theories of human action. Politically or otherwise sensitive and controversial areas, as well as discouragingly complex ones, are usually avoided for reasons of funding and because of problems of winning acceptance from policy-makers or administrators. Even then, motivation for members of the target population to participate in the traditional research study is often low, and dropout rates are accordingly high.

If funded, the traditional research proposal is usually presented to relevant decision makers, and possibly also to those invited to partic-ipate in the study, in attempts to persuade them to agree to the proposal. The study is carried out with subjects, who usually are seen as passive "objects." Data are analyzed in a descriptive statistical fashion and—in the best of cases—presented to the particular "cli-ents," who are often unable to interpret or utilize the findings. When the complete report becomes available, it is usually written in a highly technical language, published in a scientific journal not read by lay people, and available only several years after the collection of the data. By then, the study has usually been completely forgotten by all "clients," and, more often than not, conditions have changed to such an extent that any possible problem-solving proposals—if any evolved from the study—are no longer relevant.

In contrast, the participatory approach starts by formulating the problems to be studied in close collaboration with the "consumers" (e.g., elderly people utilizing home, outpatient, or institutional care or health-promotion or disease-prevention programs). The subjects themselves take an active and creative part in all stages of the research project, including choice of problem areas, formulation of hypothe-ses, choice of methods, review, interpretation, and application of results (see Edgren, 1977). From the perspective of the participants, this approach decreases the attrition rate, increases motivation for and interest in the study, and improves the likelihood that the find-ings will be utilized.

A study of basic and applied problems can often be combined—to the benefit of all concerned. The consumers get information of imme-diate interest to them (e.g., about their health or about which health care alternative to choose), while the researchers are allowed—at very low extra cost for all involved—to study a number of more fundamen-tal scientific problems within the same setting.

Integrated Research Approaches

As already indicated, the complementary research projects—epide-miological, intensive longitudinal, and intervention studies—should be integrated into long-term research programs based on a continuous exchange of data and interpretations with all types of consumers concerned by the study—central and local governments, administrators, caregivers, organizations for retired persons, parties in the labor market, and the general public. Also integrated are, of course, data from other centers as well as results from ethological and animal studies. Such integrated research packages are clearly more desirable than "one-shot" research studies.

Methodological Issues

Several methodological issues impede or limit our ambitious attempts at social intervention. For example, it is impossible to control (or even describe) all relevant variables in a complex and changing social system. Thus our assumptions will become more tenuous and our possibilities for generalizing to other institutions and communities more dubious (see Thorslund, 1986).

Other potential obstacles must also be considered. In some cases, care providers and/or policymakers are not inclined to accept an evaluation of their pet programs, whether innovative or merely established routines based on "agreed standards of good practice." There may also be objections to offering the new treatment only to the experimental (and not the control) group. It is possible that the common denominator of successful treatments may be the availability of a dedicated and enthusiastic program director or the extra attention provided for the experimental group but not the controls.

Additional problems of great importance concern what to monitor, when, how, on whom, and why. As pointed out by Ory (1988), age-related factors can affect both the measurement of health indicators and the design and effectiveness of health-promotion interventions. This has obvious consequences for the design and interpretation of intervention studies on elderly populations (Backer, 1984; Chiriboga, 1989; Evans, 1983; Hendriksen, 1986; Kivelä, 1985; Krause, 1989; Ro, Hendriksen, Kivelä, & Thorslund, 1987; Ro & Hjort, 1985; Thorslund, 1986).

Last but not least, available instruments for measuring interventions and outcomes may lack validity, reliability, and norms with regard to elderly populations. Alternatively, the elderly may find it difficult to provide the participation proposed and the information required (Ory, 1988).

EXPERIMENTAL INTERVENTIONS IN SOCIAL SYSTEMS

Although most health interventions focus on individual variables, a few examine social variables. The following studies, drawn primarily from the Nordic experience, illustrate how persons at different points in the life course can benefit from such social interventions.

Work and Health

Work often plays an important role in structuring and giving meaning to life and in providing personal identity and self-esteem as well as social contacts and material assets. Unemployment deprives people of these opportunities (Jahoda, 1979). In a controlled intervention with 200 unemployed female factory workers in Olofström in the south of Sweden, Arnetz and associates (1988) conducted a multidisciplinary longitudinal evaluation of efforts to prevent negative effects of unemployment. Attempts were made to find or create new jobs or, if this was impossible, to substitute meaningful unpaid collective self-administered activities.

Results from the study demonstrated pronounced mental and physiological stress reactions one month preceding job loss; a diminution of these reactions in the first month of actual unemployment; a subsequent, successive rise in self-rated depression and in cortisol levels over the first year of unemployment, following the initial period of relaxation and relative optimism; and high levels of depression and cortisol and decreased immune function one year after the start of unemployment. The attempt to replace real employment by offering various unpaid collective self-administered activities turned out not to influence significantly the potentially noxious psychosocial and physiological effects of becoming and remaining unemployed. The study illustrates what to expect before and after the onset of unemployment and provides health reasons for promoting gainful employment for all and not forcing the mandatory retirement of older workers.

Counteracting Loneliness Among Pensioners

Elderly, single, female pensioners who rated themselves as lonely and were on a waiting list for service house flats were randomly assigned to an experimental group (n = 35), which was offered group meetings with peers, or to a control group (n = 22), which received no such offer (Andersson, 1984). After six months, the former group displayed significantly less loneliness and alienation, greater self-confidence, more social contacts and interactions, and significantly lower systolic and diastolic blood pressures. These desirable effects of an intervention that was both inexpensive and simple to administer have led to the results being disseminated and these routines being introduced in Stockholm's municipal program for the care of the elderly.

Increased Autonomy and Social Interaction for Institutionalized Pensioners

All 30 pensioners in one section of a senior citizens' apartment building—but not the 30 in another, comparable section—were encouraged to take greater control of their own lives, with the hope that this would lead to an increase in their social activity and, secondarily, to improved mental and physical well-being (Arnetz, 1983). As a result of the intervention, social activities (both planned and spontaneous) tripled, restlessness decreased, various physiological measures improved, and body weight and stature remained steady. This study demonstrates the importance of active participation in care programs and shows that simple measures to this end, in addition to creating social and psychological benefits, favored health and well-being.

For a review of other studies, with particular reference to social interventions to improve health and well-being in the elderly, see Thorslund (1986), Backer (1984), Ro and Hjort (1985), Kivelä (1985), Hendriksen (1986), and Markides and Cooper (1989).

CONCLUSIONS AND RECOMMENDATIONS

In summary, we should strive to identify and modify, where possible, high-risk situations, high-risk groups, and high-risk reactions. This requires close collaboration among decision makers, who formulate political goals, and researchers, who test and evaluate these ideas on a model scale and provide additional knowledge on which to base decisions. If decision makers consider the data and evaluations presented to them by researchers, the entire person-environment system becomes cybernetic and self- corrective.

Figure 10.3 illustrates metaphorically how this could be done. Spanning the river is a bridge—"the road of life"—with many defects and no safety rail. A lot of people fall into the river. Many of them

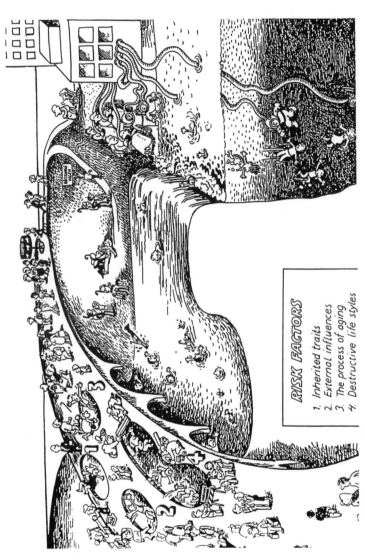

Figure 10.3. Metaphoric Presentation of Therapeutic and Preventive Approaches to Environmental and Behavioral RiskFactors in the Human Ecological System

SOURCE: Gustaf Brynolfsson, Swedish Planning and Rationalization Institute of Health and Social Services (SPRI); used by

cannot swim. To prevent their drowning, the "lifeguards" in primary health care dive into the water, pull them ashore, and begin resuscitation. If the lifeguards do not succeed in reaching the drowning people, the latter will fall over a waterfall and sink to the bottom. The "divers" in our hospitals will then do their best to bring the people to the surface and ashore and subject them to sophisticated and expensive resuscitation.

It is quite clear that both lifeguards and divers, and their institutions and resources, are needed. But we also need resources to

- repair the bridge;
- provide the bridge with a safety rail and warning signs;
- inform people about the dangers of deep water if they cannot swim; and
- teach people to swim and to save other people who cannot swim and need help (Levi, 1985).

Much more knowledge and integration of knowledge is needed to accomplish this effectively. This speaks strongly in favor of interventional research with a participatory and systems approach. It is also important to understand how interventions early in life (i.e., childhood or adolescence) can help people reach old age with more vigor and to understand how interventions directed at older persons can postpone disabilities associated with age-related illness or conditions and compensate for the functional deficits that appear more commonly in later life.

REFERENCES

Andersson, L. (1984). *Aging and loneliness: An interventional study of a group of elderly women*. Stockholm: Karolinska institutet.

Antonovsky, A. (1987). *Unraveling the mystery of health: How people manage stress and stay well*. San Francisco: Jossey-Bass.

Arnetz, B. (1983). *Psychophysiological effects of social understimulation in old age*. Stockholm: Karolinska institutet.

Arnetz, B., Brenner, S., Hjelm, H., Levi, L., Petterson, I., Kallner, A., Eneroth, P., Kvetnansky, R., & Vigas, M. (1988). *Stress reactions in relation to threat of job loss and actual unemployment: Physiological, psychological, and economic effects of job loss and unemployment* (Stress Research Reports No. 206). Stockholm: Karolinska institutet.

Backer, P. (1984). Needs of continuous research into care of the elderly. *Scandinavian Journal of Primary Health Care, 2*, 45-46.

Chiriboga, D. A. (1989). The measurement of stress in later life. In K. S. Markides & C. L. Cooper (Eds.), *Aging, stress and health* (pp. 13-41). Chichester, United Kingdom: John Wiley.

Edgren, B. (1977). *Samarbetsmodellen: En strategi vid tillämpad arbetslivsforskning* [The collaborative model: A strategy in applied work life research] (Stress Research Report No. 56). Stockholm: Karolinska institutet.

Eisdorfer, C., & Stotsky, B. A. (1977). Intervention, treatment, and rehabilitation of psychiatric disorders. In J. E. Birren & K. W. Schaie (Eds.), *Handbook of the psychology of aging*. New York: Van Nostrand Reinhold.

Elliott, G. R., & Eisdorfer, C. (Eds.). (1982). *Research on stress and human health* (National Academy of Sciences, Institute of Medicine, report). New York: Springer.

Estes, C. L., & Freeman, H. E. (1976). Strategies of design and research for intervention. In R. H. Binstock & E. Shanas (Eds.), *Handbook of aging and the social sciences*. New York: Van Nostrand Reinhold.

Evans, J. G. (1983). Evaluation of geriatric services. In W. W. Holland (Ed.), *Evaluation of health care*. Oxford: Oxford University Press.

Hazzard, W. R. (1985). *A state of the art review of preventive strategies and health promotion for the elderly* (Report Submitted by Geriatrics and Gerontology Advisory Committee). Washington, DC: Veterans Administration.

Hendriksen, C. (1986). An intervention study among elderly people. *Scandinavian Journal of Primary Health Care, 4,* 39-42.

Henry, J. P., & Stephens, P. M. (1977). *Stress, health, and the social environment.* New York: Springer.

Jahoda, M. (1979). The impact of unemployment in the 1930s and the 1970s. *Bulletin of the British Psychological Society, 32,* 309-314.

Kagan, A. R. (1981). A community research strategy applicable to psychosocial factors and health. In L. Levi (Ed.), *Society, stress, and disease: Vol. 4. Working life* (pp. 339-342). Oxford: Oxford University Press.

Kagan, A. R., & Levi, L. (1975). Health and environment—psychosocial stimuli: A review. In L. Levi (Ed.), *Society, stress, and disease: Vol. 2. Childhood and adolescence* (pp. 241-260). London: Oxford University Press.

Kivelä, S. L. (1985). Problems in intervention and evaluation. *Scandinavian Journal of Primary Health Care, 3,* 137-140.

Krause, N. (1989). Issues of measurement and analysis in studies of social support, aging and health. In K. S. Markides & C. L. Cooper (Eds.), *Aging, stress and health* (pp. 43-66). Chichester, United Kingdom: John Wiley.

Lazarus, R. S. (1985). Stress: Appraisal and coping capacities. In A. Eichler, M. M. Silverman, & D. M. Pratt (Eds.), *How to define and research stress* (Administrative document; pp. 5-9). Rockville, MD: Department of Health and Human Services, National Institute of Mental Health.

Lazarus, R. S., & Folkman, S. (1984). *Stress, appraisal and coping.* New York: Springer.

Levi, L. (Ed.). (1971). *Society, stress, and disease: Vol. 1. The psychosocial environment and psychosomatic diseases.* London: Oxford University Press.

Levi, L. (Ed.). (1975). *Society, stress, and disease: Vol. 2. Childhood and adolescence.* London: Oxford University Press.

Levi, L. (Ed.). (1978). *Society, stress, and disease: Vol. 3. The productive and reproductive age: Male/female roles and relationships.* Oxford: Oxford University Press.

Levi, L. (Ed.). (1979). Psychosocial factors in preventative medicine. In *Healthy people: The surgeon general's report on health promotion and disease prevention. Background Papers* (pp. 207-252). Washington, DC: U.S. Department of Health, Education, and Welfare.

Levi, L. (Ed.). (1981). *Society, stress, and disease: Vol. 4. Working life.* Oxford: Oxford University Press.

Levi, L. (1985). Stress: Definitions, concepts, and significance. *Cardiovascular Information, 1,* 10-20.

Levi, L. (Ed.). (1987a). *Society, stress, and disease: Vol. 5. Old age.* Oxford: Oxford University Press.

Levi, L. (Ed.). (1987b). Future research. In R. Kalimo et al. (Eds.), *Psychosocial factors at work and their relation to health* (pp. 239-45). Geneva: World Health Organization.

Levi, L., Frankenhaeuser, M., & Gardell, B. (1982). Work stress related to social structures and processes. In G. R. Elliott & C. Eisdorfer (Eds.), *Stress and human health: Analysis and implications of research* (pp. 119-146). New York: Springer.

Markides, K. S., & Cooper, C. L. (Eds.). (1989). *Aging, stress and health.* Chichester, United Kingdom: John Wiley.

Miller, J. (1978). *Living systems.* New York: McGraw-Hill.

Ory, M. (1988). Considerations in the development of age-sensitive indicators for assessing health promotion. *Health Promotion, 3,* 2.

President's Commission on Mental Health. (1978). *Report to the President* (Vol. I.). Washington, DC: Government Printing Office.

Rö, O. C., Hendriksen, C., Kivelä, S., & Thorslund, M. (1987). Intervention studies among elderly people. *Scandinavian Journal of Primary Health Care, 5,* 163-168.

Rö, O. C., & Hjort, P. F. (1985). Interventional research in primary health care for the elderly. *Scandinavian Journal of Primary Health Care, 3,* 133-136.

Swedish Public Health Service Bill No. 1984/85:181. (1985). Stockholm: Ministry of Social Affairs.

Thorslund, M. (1986). Evaluation research in care of the elderly: Some Swedish experiences. *Scandinavian Journal of Primary Health Care, 4,* 33-38.

World Health Organization. (1946). *Definition of health* (Preparatory Committee of the International Health Conference). Geneva: Author.

World Health Organization. (1986). *Report of the technical discussions of the 39th World Health Assembly* (A 39/Technical Discussions/4;15 May 1986). Geneva: Author.

PART IV

Implications for
Public Policy

11

Social Characteristics, Social Structure, and Health in the Aging Population

CARROLL L. ESTES
THOMAS G. RUNDALL

The dominant paradigm used by medicine to understand the etiology of disease focuses on the genetic makeup, biological functioning, and life-style of the individual. This paradigm assumes that physical disorders not genetically determined are caused by individual exposure to infectious organisms, toxic substances, or environmental hazards. The assumptions of this paradigm are clearly evident in our nation's decade-old policy for promoting the health of the aging population. The landmark U.S. health policy document, *Healthy People: The Surgeon General's Report on Health Promotion and Disease Prevention* (U.S. Public Health Service, 1979), established (a) improvement in quality of life and (b) increasing functional independence as the primary health-promotion goals for older adults (age 65 and older). To achieve these goals, *Healthy People* recommended the following eight actions for older adults: (a) maintain an active social life, including work; (b) engage in regular physical activity (appropriate exercise); (c) maintain a nutritious, well-balanced diet; (d) undergo periodic health checkups for specific preventable and diagnosable conditions; (e) review and minimize medications; (f) consult physicians about immunization against pneumococcal pneumonia and influenza; (g) improve home safety to prevent falls and other injuries; and (h) have access to needed community services to maintain independent living.

While much of the attention of researchers and policymakers concentrates on these individual health behaviors and habits that expose people to risks (Omenn, 1990), this view of the causation of personal disease is incomplete. A wealth of data reported by sociologists, epidemiologists, and others suggests that broad social forces also determine the health status of the older population. *Which* older people experience injuries, acute disorders, chronic diseases, and premature death is determined in part by their positions in a society stratified by age, race, sex, and socioeconomic status and organized into residential communities, work organizations, and political and economic structures. Further, *which* older adults regain functional independence once illness and injury have occurred depends to a great extent on the nature of the health care system and the access they have to medical and health care services. Hence, to understand the causes of health and disease in the older population, one must understand not only individual life-style and risk-related behaviors but also the relationships among social characteristics, the structure of the medical care system, and health. This involves the examination of the broad economic, political, and social processes that shape not only the life chances of individuals but also the nation's approach to and definition of public problems such as illness, injury, and premature death.

The purpose of this chapter is to focus attention on the important social structures and health system characteristics that affect the health of the aging population. In each case, the research literature is reviewed and particularly important features of our nation's social structure and medical care system that affect the health of the aging population are identified. The analysis suggests that a broader, more structural approach to enhancing the health of the aging population is required. Finally, a number of suggestions are proposed for changes in the social and medical care systems that hold forth the promise of truly promoting the health of older Americans and of realizing the goals of improving the quality of life and increasing the functional independence of the aging population.

MORTALITY AND MORBIDITY AMONG THE ELDERLY

The decline in mortality and resulting increase in life expectancy of the elderly population during this century are unprecedented in history. While there is still much to learn about the factors contributing to increased longevity as well as the consequences of a longer life span for the elderly population, the development of future social and health policy must acknowledge the reality of an aging population.

Because reductions in mortality rates do not inevitably signal improvements in health, two central questions are raised. First, when longevity increases, what proportion of the additional years of life gained are active functional years versus years of disability and dysfunction? Second, what are the mutable or controllable individual, social, and environmental factors that may modify, maintain, or promote the health of the elderly population, thereby increasing not only the length but also the quality of elders' lives?

With regard to the first question, existing data are limited and do not yet provide a definitive answer. Unfortunately, no data system for assessing morbidity and disability equals the mortality surveillance system. While there are numerous sources for estimating the prevalence of disease and conditions, each has geographic or methodological limitations that restrict its usefulness. Nevertheless, it is important to note that data collected on the health of the elderly consistently show that substantial proportions of them have non-life-threatening but potentially disabling conditions. Moreover, several studies indicate that the proportion of elderly persons with disabling conditions is increasing over time (Colvez & Blanchet, 1981; Kovar, 1977; Manton, 1987; Rice, 1986; Rice & LaPlante, 1988; Verbrugge, 1984). It has even been observed that "trends in the health of middle-aged and older persons since the late 1950s suggest a paradox between longer life and worsening health" (Rice, 1986, p. 164; see also Verbrugge, 1984, 1989).

The data on trends in mortality, morbidity, and disability present a disturbing picture of health and aging. They show increased overall life expectancy for the elderly, but with only a modest addition to the years of active life expectancy, and, on average, a substantial increase in the number of years lived with disabilities. While acknowledging that current data are weak, Brody, Brock, and Williams (1987) estimated that, for each good, active, functional year gained, about 3.5 compromised years are added to the life span. Further, they argue that this phenomenon is likely to persist with its effects magnified, because it is occurring during a period in which family size is shrinking and the usual providers of support, particularly women, will increasingly be in the paid labor force.

The debate about projections of future patterns of mortality, morbidity, and disability has major implications for the future of gerontology and the allocation of societal resources. One theory is that improvements in life-style will delay the onset of disability, reduce the prevalence of disease, and compress the period of morbidity in older ages, resulting in a pattern of "natural" death at the end of a "natural" life span (Fries, 1980). This theory has been contrasted with one suggesting that increased life expectancy will bring an increased prevalence of chronic illness and disability and a pandemic of mental illness and chronic disease (Kramer, 1980). Although a review of the available data lends support to the latter position, the issue is far from settled (Verbrugge, 1989). Indeed, both types of change appear to be unfolding.

With regard to the second question raised above, as a result of decades of empirical research, health and illness are now widely accepted as the products of the interactions among a person's social characteristics and the social and economic structures of the society. In this sense, the social characteristics of older persons (such as income, race, gender, education, and marital status) and the characteristics of the many social institutions that make up society (such as the health care, economic, and political institutions) form a "web of causation" that importantly affects the health of older persons. It must be quickly noted that unraveling the web and identifying causative factors that can be altered with appropriate public policies remain great challenges for social scientists and other researchers. However, there is already a growing body of research to guide policymaking.

SOCIAL AND BEHAVIORAL
FACTORS AND HEALTH

The classic studies of McKeown (1976) underscored the importance of social and economic factors in explaining health. He showed that the decline in mortality over a 150-year span and improvements in health over the past three centuries were predominantly attributable to nutritional, environmental, and behavioral factors. Numerous other studies have linked particular social factors with disease and mortality. Although the conceptual definitions and measurements of the variables in question may vary from one study to another, a growing body of evidence indicates that life-style and exposure to environmental risks are significantly affected by social characteristics such as sex, ethnicity, income, education, marital status, employment, social support, and sense of efficacy and personal control. These social characteristics strongly influence specific life-style factors identified in *Healthy People* and elsewhere as important determinants of health, including smoking, use of alcohol and drugs, dietary habits, exercise, weight, stress control, accident prevention, and use of health providers for early detection and treatment of disorders (Pardini, Passick, Franks, & Rice, 1984; Vogt, 1987).

These specific life-style factors have been discussed at length in a review of the literature on disease prevention and health promotion among the elderly by Kane, Kane, and Arnold (1985). Reports prepared for the Surgeon General's Workshop on Health Promotion and Aging also document the role of social and behavioral factors in eight specific health-promotion areas (U.S. Department of Health and Human Services, 1987). Nevertheless, the complexity of the associations among of these behaviors (e.g., smoking, alcohol, and nutrition) and with a multiplicity of important social (e.g., income) and environmental factors (e.g., availability of health services) calls for carefully designed research to specify the causal chains of relations and cautions policymakers about the great difficulty in designing effective interventions (Ory & Bond, 1989). To clarify these points, we focus the following discussion on three of the most important structural factors affecting the health of the aging population: social class, social support, and access to medical care.

Social Class and Health

A large body of research has substantiated the link between social class and health as measured by mortality, disability, chronic illness (Dutton, 1986; Luft, 1978; Marmot, Kogevinas, & Elston, 1987), and institutionalization (Butler & Newacheck, 1981; Kane & Kane, 1987; see also Kaplan & Haan, 1989). As Butler and Lewis (1982, p. 11) observed, "Demographic data show conclusively that an increasing life expectancy follows in the wake of increasing income and status." The strength of social class as a predictor of health has been underscored in the United States and in virtually all other Western industrialized nations. The famous Black Report in England (Black, Morris, Smith, & Townsend, 1982) provided the classic text on the persistence of class differences in health as well as the difficulties in eradicating these deep inequalities in health, even with universal health coverage such as the British National Health Service:

> While there are a number of quite distinct theoretical approaches to explanation, we wish to stress the importance of differences in material conditions of life. *In our view much of the evidence on social inequalities in health can be adequately understood in terms of specific features of the socioeconomic environment*: Features (such as work accidents, overcrowding, cigarette smoking) which are strongly class related in

Britain and also have clear causal significance. . . . But beyond this there is undoubtedly much which cannot be understood in terms of the impact of so specific factors, but only in terms of the more diffuse consequences of the class structure: Poverty, working conditions, and deprivation in its various forms. (Black et al., 1982, p. 207)

Without doubt, income is one of the most important dimensions of social class in predicting health status. The relation of lower incomes to poorer health outcomes is a consistent finding throughout the life course. Poor elderly people are twice as likely as elderly people with moderate or high incomes to report health problems (44% versus 22%; National Center for Health Statistics [NCHS], 1984). Similarly, data from the 1987 health interview survey show an inverse relationship between family income (age adjusted) and limitations in activity due to chronic conditions (NCHS, 1988). Not only is low income a risk factor in health but reductions in income are also associated with increased risk of mortality (Kaplan & Haan, 1989). The effect of income is also observed on life-style behaviors; Amir (1987) reported data showing a positive relationship between income and preventive health behaviors among elderly persons in Scotland, a finding that is consistent with studies on the North American continent (Norman, 1985).

Although the proportion of the elderly population below poverty has declined (to 12.4% in 1986), nearly one third (28.0%) of the elderly population is poor or "near-poor"—that is, living within 150% of the poverty line. The oldest old (those 85 or older) experience the highest poverty rates of all older groups (17.6%), almost twice the 10.3% rate of those 65 to 74 (U.S. Senate, 1988, pp. 44-45). Poverty among elderly Blacks and Hispanics and among a substantial proportion of older women is pervasive and unrelenting. Minorities experience two to three times the poverty rate of Whites, with 71% of all aged Blacks being poor or "economically vulnerable"—that is, within 200% of the official poverty line (Villers Foundation, 1987, p. 25). Almost one half of old White single women and 80% of old Black single women live at or near the poverty level (Villers Foundation, 1987).

It should not be surprising, then, that life expectancy at age 65 for Black women is 17.0 years, compared with 18.7 years for elderly White women. Overall life expectancy at age 65 is 15.3 years for Blacks and 16.8 years for Whites (NCHS, 1988). It is important to note, however, that, for reasons not well understood, Black/White mortality differentials "cross over" at age 75, with lower Black mortality rates at the oldest ages (Wing, Manton, Stallard, Hames, & Tryoles,

1985). In addition to racial differences in life expectancy, there are racial differences in a variety of chronic conditions and activity limitations (NCHS, 1988). Health status is poorer for older Blacks than for Whites according to both indicators. Further, those with lower incomes and women as well as minorities have the highest rates of activity limitations due to chronic illness (NCHS, 1987a). Women also have a higher prevalence of disability and higher rates of institutionalization at most ages than men (Soldo & Manton, 1985).

Social Support and Health

The often-repeated finding of the importance of social networks and social support in physical and mental health is also striking. The evidence linking stress, illness, and social support dates back 50 years to the work of Cannon (1935) and includes the work of Berkman and Syme (1979; see also Berkman & Breslow, 1983; Lowenthal & Robinson, 1976). More recent treatments of this issue and data that are consistent with earlier work are found in Rowe and Kahn (1987) and Kaplan and Haan (1989).

An important determinant of social support is the marital status of older people. Widows and widowers are five times more likely than married persons to be institutionalized; elderly persons who never married or have been divorced or separated have up to ten times the rate of institutionalization of married individuals. A study by the Commonwealth Fund Commission on Elderly People Living Alone (1988) reported that 8.5 million Americans are over age 65 and live alone. This represents nearly one third of the 27 million Americans in this age group, and their numbers are increasing. Being single (whether widowed, divorced, or never married) is highly associated with low income, particularly for women. Persons experiencing the combination of living alone and having low income have the highest risk of institutionalization (Butler & Newacheck, 1981; Commonwealth Fund Commission, 1988; Kane & Kane, 1987; Wan & Weissert, 1981).

Scientific work has established both a theoretical basis and strong empirical evidence supporting the notion that social relationships affect health. In their review of this issue, House, Landis, and Umberson (1988, p. 241) concluded that

> prospective studies, which control for baseline health status, consistently show increased risk of death among persons with a low quantity, and sometimes low quality, of social relationships. Experimental

and quasi-experimental studies of humans and animals also suggest that social isolation is a major risk factor for mortality from widely varying causes.

The search for a mechanism that might explain why social support exerts so powerful an influence on health has generated a number of hypotheses. Most fall within one of two broad conceptual categories. The first, labeled the direct or *main effect hypothesis*, suggests that social support plays a health-promoting role regardless of stress level. The second, termed the *buffering hypothesis*, argues that social support works by protecting the individual from harmful psychological or physiological effects of stressful events (Coe, Wolinsky, Miller, & Prendergast, 1984; Minkler, 1986a, 1986b; Rundall & Evashwick, 1982).

As researchers have struggled to specify and empirically test these notions, several important issues have arisen. First, what levels of "exposure" to social support (or, conversely, to social isolation) result in a health effect? Second, what are the differential effects, if any, of instrumental and expressive support? Third, which types of social relationships are supportive and which are harmful? Fourth, as Minkler (1986a, p. 36) cautioned,

> Studies on the qualitative dimensions of social support, intervention programs designed to help increase the availability of high quality support, and macro level policies supportive of effectively functioning social networks all may be necessary if we are to help social support reach its potential for promoting health.

Obviously, there is a great deal yet to be learned about social support and its effects on the health of the elderly population. Mechanic (1982) noted that much is unknown about the unique and joint effects of such factors as social class and social support on health. The effects of these social characteristics are interrelated, and rigorous studies are needed to separate confounded effects. In many instances, cause and effect are not clear, and the associations between variables and health status may reflect the fact that people with particular health characteristics systematically select themselves, or are selected, into certain social situations. Nevertheless, there appears to be sufficient evidence, especially with regard to difficulties encountered by elderly persons living alone, to warrant concern over the isolation and the lack of support that characterize the social situations in which many older Americans live.

ACCESS TO MEDICAL CARE

There is debate over the importance of the contribution of medical care to the aggregate health status of the population. In spite of critical analyses (see McKinlay, McKinlay, & Beaglehole, 1989), a number of other researchers (Drake, 1978; Friedman, 1976; Hadley, 1982; NCHS, 1981; Rosenwaike, Yaffe, & Sagi, 1980) have argued that medical care has contributed heavily to the 14% decline in the mortality rate for the entire population between 1970 and 1978. This perspective is based on the observation that declining mortality rates coincided with significant increases in the use of medical care by beneficiaries of federal programs such as Medicaid and Medicare, which were specifically designed to improve access to care. With regard to the aging population in particular, Friedman (1976) showed that morbidity among the aged, as measured by days of restricted activity, was correlated with health expenditures following the establishment of Medicare. The aged "had fewer days of restricted activity and this decline was inversely related to the level of personal health care expenditures by the aged" (Davis, 1984, p. 83; see also Davis & Schoen, 1978).

Interpretation of these findings is difficult in light of the recent review by McKinlay and associates (1989), whose extensive evidence indicates that the nation's unprecedented investment in biomedical research and improvements in medical care contributed little to the changes in patterns of morbidity, mortality, and disability in the United States. Further, as noted earlier, Verbrugge (1989) and a number of other prominent epidemiologists agreed that mortality declines have been accompanied by a real increase in disability and that the net result of medical interventions has been an overall increase in life expectancy, most of which is in years of added disability.

These disparate evaluations of the contribution of medical care to improvements in health status suggest that, although the nation should continue to invest in measures designed to assure and improve access, neither medical care nor biomedical research should constitute the sole, or necessarily even the predominant, thrust of policy interventions to improve the health of the older population. Clearly, a broad approach is necessary, an approach that addresses the matrix of behavioral, social, and demographic as well as biological forces shown throughout this volume to contribute to improving the health of older people. Nevertheless, it is reasonable to assume that the medical care system may play an important role in returning ill and injured older people to functional independence.

Understanding the nature of the medical care system is important to understanding its effectiveness in meeting the needs of older Americans.

THE MEDICAL CARE SYSTEM

Several aspects of the U.S. medical care system merit attention: the public-private character of the system, the medical model orientation of U.S. health policy, the rising cost of care, and the effect of health policy and reimbursement on access to care. Although informal care plays a crucial role in health care delivery, this chapter focuses primarily on the formal medical care system.

The Public-Private Character of the System

The U.S. medical care system is the only one among Western industrialized nations (with the exception of South Africa) that does not provide universal access through some form of national medical care. The mix of private and public financing that underwrites the cost of medical care includes direct out-of-pocket payments by individuals, private health insurance, tax breaks for the purchase of private insurance, and a series of publicly financed sources including Medicare, Medicaid, the Veterans Administration, the armed forces, public employees, state-funded mental health services, and locally funded medical services for the indigent (Lee, 1986). Public financing for medical care is provided primarily through programs for the poor (Medicaid) and for the aged, blind, and disabled (Medicare). In 1987, public funds financed approximately 41% of the national medical expenditures of $500.3 billion, while private health insurance covered about 31%, and U.S. citizens paid approximately 25% directly out of pocket (Levit & Freeland, 1988; Roper, 1988). Medicare provides health insurance protection essentially for hospital and physician services for more than 30 million individuals (90% of whom are 65 and older), and Medicaid covers 21.5 million individuals (young and old) who are extremely poor.

Private insurance affords some protection to approximately 80% of the noninstitutionalized population, including the 72% of the elderly who were covered by some type of supplementary medigap insurance in 1984 (U.S. Senate, 1988, p. 132). The likelihood of purchasing private insurance to defray some of the costs of rapidly rising deductibles and copayments after age 65 is directly linked to income, with only 44% of those with incomes below $5,000 having such insurance compared with 87% of those with incomes greater than $25,000.

The Medical Model of Health and Aging

U.S. health policy for the elderly is predicated on a medical model that finances the treatment of illness and disease rather than public health measures or interventions to redress the economic or social problems known to be associated with at-risk behaviors and the health problems of aging. This acute care bias of Medicare poorly matches the needs of the older population in a society characterized by aging and increasing disability. Meeting the needs of the aging U.S. society clearly calls for the treatment and management of chronic illness as well as disease-prevention and health-promotion efforts targeted early and throughout the life course. Further, health policy should address the array of social and behavioral factors that contribute to health, including underlying environmental and immediate/behavioral causes (Pardini et al., 1984). Unfortunately, the two major public programs designed to provide access to medical care for the aging population—Medicare and Medicaid—have not adopted this broader view of the management and control of disease.

Medicare. Because of its commitment to the coverage of acute care, Medicare coverage excludes virtually all types of long-term care, including nursing home care (except for brief, 150-day periods), in-home services such as personal care and rehabilitation for the chronically ill, dental care, eyeglasses, hearing aids, preventive physical exams, and supportive services (e.g., transportation, meals on wheels, and case management). As a consequence, a significant segment of the population aged 65 and older is underinsured for the mix of medical care and social support services that they will likely need.

New policies affecting the delivery of medical care for older Americans enacted through Medicare have not altered the basic acute care approach of Medicare.[1] We can, for example, examine the effects of the introduction of the prospective payment system (PPS) for hospitals in 1983. This system of hospital payment by patient diagnosis-related groups (DRGs) was designed to contain hospital costs. While the rate of inflation in hospital costs has slowed, the policy has not stemmed the overall rise in the costs of medical care. The high costs of medical care are in line with a health policy that reflects a "medicalization of aging" (Estes & Binney, 1988; Zola, 1986).

Various research studies have identified "ripple effects" throughout the community-based care system as a result of PPS (Estes et al.,

1988). With the immediate two-day reduction in the average length of hospital stay for Medicare patients, under DRGs, a major burden of care was shifted—more than 21 million days of caregiving work were transferred from the hospital to the home, family, and community (Stark, 1987). The DRG policy came into effect at the same time that tight restrictions on Medicare's already limited home health benefits were imposed by the Health Care Financing Administration. The simultaneous implementation of a host of other deregulatory and austerity policies increased competition and reduced already meager funding for social services. The result of these changes in policy is an accumulation of multiple and complex pressures on the beleaguered network of traditionally nonprofit providers of home and community-based health and social services (Estes et al., 1988). Providers are being flooded with very sick and very old clients discharged from the hospital earlier than ever before. The trade-off appears increasingly to be between meeting the needs of postacute care and meeting the needs of chronically ill elders in the community.

Medicaid. Medicaid is the single health policy that finances long-term care, and its primary coverage is for nursing home costs rather than community care. It is available only to those who spend down to poverty levels. The stringent eligibility standards (below poverty level in many states) and the stigma of this welfare program explain why only 36% of the old poor are on Medicaid (Villers Foundation, 1987). As a result, Medicaid has, with some justification, been described as a policy that promotes both impoverishment and dependency. Federal budget tightening aimed at Medicaid from 1981 to now has pressed states to curtail eligibility and utilization, augmenting state-to-state variations in eligibility for and access to Medicaid services (Holahan & Cohen, 1986). As a result, the percentage of poor covered by Medicaid declined from 63% in 1975 to 46% in 1985 (Darling, 1986).

Federal waiver programs have encouraged states to undertake demonstrations of comprehensive and cost-saving approaches (Justice & Etheredge, 1988), but, with the exception of these models, there are few systematic alternatives to institutionalization. Neither are there many integrated and coordinated systems of acute and chronic care (Kane & Kane, 1987; Vogel & Palmer, 1983), again with the exception of selected demonstration models that explicitly marry these separately organized and financed systems of care. Although the fragmentation of service delivery and the limited availability of geriatric assessment and case management services (not automatically reimbursed under Medicare) are particularly problematic for older people who move in and out of acute and long-term care, little is known about the ideal prescriptive formulas that would optimize health outcomes for frail older persons moving between these two sectors of care (Kane & Kane, 1987, p. 304; Ory & Bond, 1989).

The Rising Costs of Medical Care

Overall, national medical care spending in 1990 exceeds $661 billion, reflecting a 10.4% increase over the previous year (U.S. Department of Commerce, 1990) and claiming 11.5% of the nation's GNP. In spite of the medical care reforms of prospective hospital payment, deregulation, and policies designed to promote competition throughout the 1980s, costs of medical care have continued to grow at two to three times the rate of general inflation (Reinhardt, 1986). For example, between 1980 and 1988, these costs grew an average of 14.8% compared with a consumer price index increase of 4.6% annually (Consumer Price Index, 1989). Every component of the aggregate in medical care costs has been increasing: per-capita medical care expenditures, health insurance premiums, costs to employers for health insurance, costs to federal and state governments for Medicare and Medicaid, and individual out-of-pocket costs (Lee, 1986). It is projected that, between 2005 and 2010, annual outlays for Medicare alone will exceed yearly spending for social security (Roper, 1988). It is not surprising that the rising costs of medical care and cost containment have dominated health policy concerns since the late 1970s. Both government and business are pressing for a solution to the high and rising costs of health care. With the population aging, these concerns are understandable, particularly in view of the fact that older people consume nearly one third of national health expenditures while they constitute 12% of the population (NCHS, 1987a).

For the elderly population, the rising cost of medical care has also meant rising copayments and deductibles under Medicare; for example, both the Medicare Part A hospital deductible and the Part B premium each rose 229% between 1980 and 1990, more than five times the rate of inflation (Villers Foundation, 1987). Out-of-pocket medical expenses now exceed 18% of elders' annual incomes and are projected to rise to 20% by 1990 (U.S. House of Representatives, 1987). These medical care costs are rising much faster than social security cost-of-living increases, and the burden of these costs is disproportionately borne by low- and middle-income older people—those who also suffer more illness. Total out-of-pocket health costs constitute more than one fourth of the income (26.6%) of the old who are poor and near-poor. For high-income elders, these costs constitute a mere 2.9% of income (1984 data in Schlesinger & Drumheller, 1988, p. 37). Minorities and women are most likely to fall into these lower-income categories and hence to face high personal medical care costs. In addition, these costs rise with age so that those aged 85 or older spend almost 42% of their income for out-of-pocket medical costs (1985 data in Schlesinger & Drumheller, 1988, p. 38).

As might be expected, nursing home care constitutes the largest single category of these unreimbursed costs, accounting for 81% of out-of-pocket health care expenditures for those who must bear high costs privately (more than $2,000 per year on average; see Rice & Gabel, 1986). The financial catastrophe that nursing home costs can bring is evident in the startling findings of one study in Massachusetts, which showed that, within 13 weeks of nursing home admission, single older persons will be impoverished, while couples will reach poverty before the end of one year (U.S. House of Representatives, 1987).

The Effect of Health Policy and Reimbursement on Access to Care

The goal of Medicare in 1965 was to eliminate financial barriers that discouraged older persons from obtaining needed medical care. Its passage is credited with a major increase in the utilization of hospital services by older persons and the performance of certain types of surgical procedures. Only physician visits per older person remained essentially constant immediately following the passage of Medicare (Davis, 1984, p. 83). Studies of the impact of Medicare on the utilization of services found its early effects to be on subgroups of older persons thought to be most in need of care, such as those living alone, those with low incomes, minorities, and residents of the South and nonmetropolitan areas (Loewenstein, 1971). Later studies identified improvements in access to care for the general population throughout the 1970s, one of the major goals of Medicare and Medicaid (Aday & Anderson, 1975, 1981).

As indicated previously, important changes in patient and hospital behavior occurred when Medicare adopted a prospective payment system for hospitals. Several studies have documented the increased utilization of posthospital care, measured by the percentage of discharged patients using home health and nursing home services, following the implementation of the reimbursement policy (DRGs) that gave hospitals an incentive to shorten lengths of stay (Feder et al., 1988; Gutterman, Eggers, Riley, Greene, & Terrell, 1988; Neu & Harrison, 1988). The average number of home health visits also rose per user for the 1981 to 1984-1985 period, while Medicare-reimbursed skilled nursing facility care (SNF) took on a shorter-term, less "chronic" character (Neu & Harrison, 1988).

Nevertheless, the federal government has attempted to keep the lid on home health costs in spite of the growing need for this type of postacute care service (Estes et al., 1988). Although Medicare outlays for home health services grew rapidly between 1974 and 1983, their annual growth rate was sharply moderated after 1983 (the first year of the implementation of hospital prospective payment). Further, "between FY 1985 and FY 1986, the number of home health care claims filed dropped 5 percent while the number of claims denied increased 73 percent" and a total of 6% of all claims were denied (U.S. Senate, 1988, p. 124; U.S. Health Care Financing Administration, 1987).

Research establishing the import of public and/or private health insurance coverage in explaining the utilization of services (Davis, 1984) is consistent with a number of studies that have identified social and behavioral predictors of health service use by older persons (see Wan, 1989, for a complete review). Income and/or economic dependency have been found in almost all studies to be important "enabling" predictors that, in addition to the variable of "need-for-care" and a variety of "predisposing" variables such as education and marital status, explain different types of service utilization. For example, income and health insurance coverage are strong predictors of physician visits and hospital admissions (Arling, 1985; Eve, 1982; Wan, 1982; Wan & Arling, 1983; Wolinsky & Coe, 1984).

Significant predictors of home health care visits include (a) measures of need such as functional status (activities of daily living [ADL] and instrumental activities of daily living [IADL]), physical condition, and medical needs (Branch et al., 1981; Evashwick, Rowe, Diehr, & Branch, 1984; Soldo, 1985); (b) factors such as eligibility for Medicaid, availability of transportation (Evashwick et al., 1984), receipt of informal services (Soldo, 1985), income, and having a regular physician (Branch et al., 1981); and (c) predisposing variables such as age, race, marital status (Evashwick et al., 1984), and living arrangements (Soldo, 1985). It is important that the mix and balance of care used by older persons are predicted by attributes of the care receiver (age, living arrangements, functional ability, and financial resources) as well as by the perceived burden to the caregiver (Soldo, Agree, & Wolf, 1989).

Because of rapidly rising costs of medical care and the declining proportion of costs covered by Medicare or other forms of private insurance, access to medical care is a growing concern for young and old alike. By the mid-1980s, opinion polls reflected considerable public support for changes in the medical sector (Navarro, 1987); 51% of Americans polled in 1984 indicated that "fundamental changes are needed to make the health care system work better," while 31% in another poll noted that "the American health care system has so much wrong with it that we need to completely rebuild it" (Harris & Associates, 1985; Schneider, 1985; Taylor, 1986). By 1988, Harris poll data revealed the startling finding that only 10% of Americans think their health care system is working well, while 89% see a necessity for fundamental change (Blendon, 1989).

The results of several national opinion polls on long-term care corroborate this dissatisfaction with U.S. health policy. At least four such surveys, including one from younger generation readers of *Rolling Stone* magazine, agreed that "the public not only wants government support for long term care, but is willing to pay for it through higher taxes" (Rovner, 1988, p. 938). These polls and the introduction, for the first time, in the 100th Congress of five long-term care bills indicate the potential for increased foment for health policy changes for older Americans. It is likely as well that advocates for universal health care for citizens of all ages will continue to press for federal solutions to the problems of the uninsured and the rising costs and eroding benefits for those who are insured, including elderly Americans.

OVERRIDING THEMES

Several themes apparent in the preceding review of social class, social support, and medical care issues pertaining to elders in this last decade of the twentieth century deserve particular attention. Six overriding themes are summarized below.

First, the public's perception of older persons often consists of misleading stereotypes. One major stereotype is that to be old is to be sick, frail, dependent, and vulnerable (Estes, 1979). An alternate and equally damaging portrayal is that the elderly are generally wealthy and better off than younger generations. The first view promotes the erroneous idea that acute, high-technology medical care will solve the health problems of the elderly; it justifies Medicare's acute care bias.

The other view fosters the notion that the elderly are so well off that improvements in health care are not needed.

Second, health policy provides public financing and fosters private power in the hands of providers and corporations through services rendered largely in hospitals and physicians' offices. In the resource allocation of U.S. aging policy, medical services receive preferential treatment over the severely underfunded social services, which often are more appropriate for those who are chronically ill.

Third, recent public policy is creating a new "institution" for the elderly—the home (Estes & Wood, 1986). Millions of elders are being discharged from hospitals "sicker and quicker" under prospective payment, and in-home and community-based services cannot adequately respond to increased demands coupled with retrenchment under governmental austerity policies (Estes & Wood, 1986). With virtually no Medicare coverage for rehabilitative and social support services, incarceration in the home is a major unanticipated potential result of hospital cost containment that threatens millions of elders and their caregivers, most of whom are women. This development is in diametric opposition to the goal of promoting a long life span of high quality and active functioning.

Fourth, one of the contradictions in U.S. health policy is that it "pays" to be sick (illness makes one eligible for reimbursed services), yet Medicare does not really insure to keep the elderly well, as evidenced by its historic omission of coverage for regular physical examinations, preventive health care, dental care, and long-term rehabilitative services for the chronically ill.

Fifth, the 1980s version of "blaming the victim" has appeared in the form of a serious national debate on generational equity (Binney & Estes, 1988; Minkler, 1984). Older Americans are blamed by some for a host of the nation's economic woes, including the rise and cost of U.S. health spending. Consistent with the ideology of individualism, blaming the elderly has focused attention on intergenerational conflict rather than on understanding the links between the generations. Yet health in old age can be understood only from a life-course perspective. Inadequate medical care while growing up and other social and behavioral risk factors occurring early in life are likely to be reflected in the health of the aging.

Sixth, because aging is stigmatized and seen primarily in terms of medical need, public policies have promoted a strategy of costly, high-tech medical service instead of adequate redress for other major problem areas such as income, employment, housing, and social support. Far from draining the economy, this strategy of medically oriented service has facilitated the economic growth and expansion of medical technologies, industries, and professions as well as a flourishing biomedical research industry. The effect of U.S. policy has been to transform the multiple needs of the aged into medical and social problems amenable to government-funded and industry-developed interventions via specific economic markets (Estes, 1979; Estes et al., 1984), now called the "medical-industrial complex" (Relman, 1980). This approach has done little to alleviate the existing disparities between rich and poor, men and women, the isolated and socially integrated, and Whites and non-Whites—disparities not taken into account by the current system of service provision.

ANTICIPATING THE FUTURE

Forecasting trends in morbidity and mortality has always proven difficult. Unexpected changes in acute and chronic disease rates and in death rates have surprised demographers and health planners throughout history. Predicting trends in social policy is equally hazardous. Inevitably, there will be an inextricable relationship among trends in the morbidity and mortality of the aging population and trends in health policy as they are played out in the twenty-first century and beyond. The linkages among these trends, however, are not fixed, and a number of alternative scenarios are possible.

Verbrugge (1989) identified three future health scenarios, as follows:

(1) *Tertiary prevention.* Costly medical measures are utilized to save people at death's door "either by maintaining basic life processes (heroic care) or curing/averting fatal complications of disease. Death is deterred without influencing principal illness" (pp. 26-27). Because this approach affects a small number of people, changes in mortality and morbidity curves are slight.

(2) *Secondary prevention.* Attention is given to controlling fatal chronic diseases so that they advance less rapidly and people survive better (i.e., lower case fatality). In this scenario, there is longer life but worsening health as people have disease for more years of their lives. "It has the usual feature that individual gains (less discomfort, lesser disability) are not paralleled in existing population health statistics, which show worsening on many dimensions (rising prevalence of chronic conditions and 'being disabled')" (p. 28).

(3) Primary prevention. Comorbidity diminishes and the chances of acquiring each disease fall, assuming that "striking changes in life-style and medicine have the marvelous outcome of reducing the clinical onset of fatal diseases for most people. Incidence, duration, and prevalence rates of chief killers would fall rapidly. People who did become ill would typically have nonsevere cases" (p. 28).

All three scenarios envision an increase in "population frailty" (Verbrugge, 1989, p. 30). Because "death becomes less selective, . . . intrinsically nonrobust people stay in the living population" (p. 30). Further, as Verbrugge noted, all three scenarios ignore the nonfatal conditions; hence, these conditions, which also cause disability "will remain constant" (p. 30). Verbrugge contended that all three scenarios are correct and that "the decades ahead hold not just one health future, but several futures sequenced in time" (p. 31). The near future will approximate the second scenario, with "gains in mildness (disease progression and impact) but little change in incidence or comorbidity. . . . But the compression of morbidity is not near at hand" (pp. 31-32). We find this perspective persuasive inasmuch as it is generally consistent with the work of Manton (1987), Schneider and Brody (1983), and others (Guralnik, Yanagishita, & Schneider, 1988; Rice, 1986).

Future scenarios for health policy must address formidable obstacles to achieving full access to health care for both young and old. In the past decade, the nation has been moving toward a two-class system of health care—one for those who can pay the accelerating costs and another, increasingly limited system for the poor and near-poor, millions of whom are frozen out of private health insurance. The policies of competition have not slowed the tendency for medical costs to rise much faster than inflation (Fuchs, 1988). In spite of this, competition-based proposals for improving medical care for the elderly abound. Cost sharing and the privatization of Medicare through the purchase of vouchers (a plan by which elders would be given a specified amount of "credit" and sent on their own into the private market to find and purchase their own care), for example, have been touted as the solutions for the health problems of the nation's elders.

One thing is clearly important in any effort to forecast the future of health policy: The aging of the population is a keystone, and the impact of the baby boom (the cohort born between 1945 and 1965) will figure prominently. It is also clear that many of the nation's elders cannot afford to bear the burden of further erosions in Medicare benefits or of increases in out-of-pocket health care expenses. The

Institute for the Future (1987) predicted alternative health policy scenarios for the next century—a "tough choices" scenario and a "health and wealth" scenario.

The tough choices scenario projects a health system driven by cost containment, with managers playing an increasingly important intermediary role between payers and providers. It also anticipates a decline in fee-for-service arrangements, which will be replaced by capitation (a uniform per capita payment or fee) as pressures build for reforms in the system to meet the needs of an aging society. The health and wealth scenario is one in which the desires of an affluent and technologically sophisticated society result in a broad system of services marketed through hybrid financing and delivery mechanisms. Health becomes extremely big business (indeed, the largest identifiable employer group). This scenario shows few controls on the misuse of cost-ineffective technologies and a doubling of real health care spending before the baby boom population reaches eligibility for Medicare.

Regrettably, neither of these health futures is likely to achieve the mainstream integration of preventive health care targeted to risk factors, nor does either incorporate the latest advances in knowledge regarding the contribution of social, behavioral, environmental, and biological factors to health in old age. We remain some distance from implementing policies that are predicated upon the concept of maximizing the active life expectancy of older Americans (Katz et al., 1983).

It has been observed that politics, not demography, determines the definitions of old age in our society and the material conditions of the lives of elders (Myles, 1984). Austerity is among the most important political factors, shaping virtually every facet of the contemporary aging policy landscape. Societal aging compels attention. So also does the growing recognition of the results of the nation's approach to the rationing of health care, which are as follows: more than 37 million Americans under age 65 without health insurance and the more than 27 million elders uninsured for chronic illness and long-term care or for health-promotion, disease-prevention, or social-support services. The views of the public are clear on the issue—health care should be accessible. The aging of the population and the nation's health policy appear to be on a collision course. The situation of millions of un- and underinsured individuals and elders and their families, who are threatened by the financial and psychological exhaustion and devastation of long-term care needs, calls for solution.

The contents of this volume and chapter highlight the need for a number of structural changes to prepare society for the aging population ahead. Social policy must reflect an understanding of health in old age linked to social factors that shape the entire life course. An older person's location in the social structure (e.g., gender, social class, racial/ethnic group) strongly influences individual opportunities to engage in healthful behavior and to receive health care. To know that individual health status at age 65 does not emerge out of nowhere is to understand that an adequate income throughout the life course, an active, integrated social network, and access to health care in every form, including preventive care, are important from birth to death. This perspective highlights the importance of social policy that will assure elders an adequate income and access not only to health services but also to a reasonably healthy living environment (Ball, 1981).

At a minimum, public policy for the aging society must acknowledge and address the inequities of social class, gender, and racial/ethnic origin. The major goals of future policy advances must be (a) income levels in old age adequate to assure that no elderly individuals or families live at or below the poverty level; (b) an integrated strategy of health and social service that assures access, regardless of age, income, or health status, to comprehensive benefits, including preventive and long-term care, with effective cost control; (c) housing policies that meet the needs of a diverse older population yet recognize the need for and value of social networks and supportive living arrangements; and (d) policies that address the growing dearth of caregivers and acknowledge the unpaid work and the financial, psychological, and physical health burdens that women caregivers endure while caring for the old. Indeed, these four goals provide criteria by which alternative public policies may be evaluated.

Concern with the social and behavioral characteristics and social structural factors related to health and health care for the older population is a much needed supplement to the medical perspective that primarily focuses on the health and illness of individual elders. The ability of policymakers to intervene in a planned way to create more healthful social and environmental circumstances for the elderly population is constrained by a number of structural policies and forces: the nature of the current medical care system, the inherent biases and problems in Medicare and Medicaid, and the current social, economic, and political context. Policy reform will no doubt be incremental rather than revolutionary. The most recent statement of federal health-promotion and disease-prevention policy, *Healthy*

People 2000 (U.S. Department of Health and Human Services, 1990), represents just such an incremental advance. In addition to objectives targeting individual habits and risk behaviors, objectives related to social support and regular primary care are also proposed. Still, virtually no attention is given to other socioeconomic factors or characteristics of the medical care system that influence the health of the older adult population.

Clearly, there is much work to be done before health policy promotes the goals of a healthful environment and healthy aging throughout the life course for Americans. The specific goals proposed above are designed to facilitate movement toward this overarching objective. We assert, with a mixture of concern and optimism, that the extent to which policies are consistent with these goals will largely determine the health of the future generations of elders in the twenty-first century.

NOTE

1. The Medicare Catastrophic Coverage Act of 1988, which was repealed in 1990, was criticized for its lack of coverage for long and expensive nursing home stays and other types of long-term care (in home and community) needed by old and chronically ill persons as well as lack of coverage for social support services and for mental health, disease-prevention, and health-promotion programs.

REFERENCES

Aday, L. A., & Anderson, R. (1975). *Access to medical care.* Ann Arbor, MI: Health Administration Press.

Aday, L. A., & Anderson, R. (1981). Equity of access to medical care: A conceptual and empirical overview. *Medical Care, 19*(Suppl.), 4-27.

American Association of Retired Persons (AARP) and the Travelers Companies Foundation. (1988). *National Survey of Caregivers: Summary of findings.* Hartford, CT: Author.

Amir, D. (1987). Preventive behavior and health status among the elderly. *Psychology and Health, 1*(4), 353-378.

Arling, G. (1985). Interactive effects in a multivariate model of physician visits by older people. *Medical Care, 23*(4), 361-371.

Ball, R. M. (1981). Rethinking national policy on health care for the elderly. In A. R. Somers & D. R. Fabian (Eds.), *The geriatric imperative.* New York: Appleton-Century-Crofts.

Berkman, L. F., & Breslow, R. (Eds.). (1983). *Health and ways of living.* New York: Oxford University Press.

Berkman, L. F., & Syme, S. L. (1979). Social networks, host resistance, and mortality: A nine-year follow-up study of Alameda County residents. *American Journal of Epidemiology, 109,* 186-204.

Binney, E. A., & Estes, C. L. (1988). The retreat of the state and its transfer of responsibility: The intergenerational war. *International Journal of Health Services, 18*(1), 83-96.

Black, D., Morris, J. N., Smith, C., & Townsend, P. (1982). The Black Report. In P. Townsend & N. Davidson (Eds.), *Inequalities in health: The Black Report.* Middlesex, United Kingdom: Penguin.

Blendon, R. J. (1989). Three systems: Comparative survey. *Health Management Quarterly, 11*(1), 2-10.

Branch, L., Jette, A., Evashwick, C., Polansky, M., Rowe, G., & Diehr, P. (1981). Toward understanding elders' health services utilization. *Journal of Community Health, 7*(4), 80-91.

Brody, J. A., Brock, D. B., & Williams, T. F. (1987). Trends in the health of the elderly population. In L. Breslow, J. E. Fielding, & L. B. Lave (Eds.), *Annual review of public health* (Vol. 8, pp. 211-234). Palo Alto, CA: Annual Reviews.

Butler, L. H., & Newacheck, P. W. (1981). Health and social factors affecting long term care policy. In J. Meltzer, F. Farrow, & H. Richman (Eds.), *Policy options in long term care.* Chicago: University of Chicago Press.

Butler, R. N., & Lewis, M. L. (1982). *Aging & mental health: Positive psychosocial & biomedical approaches* (3rd ed.). Columbus, OH: Merrill.

Cannon, W. B. (1935). Stresses and strains of homostasis. *American Journal of Medical Sciences, 189,* 1-14.

Coe, R., Wolinsky, F., Miller, D., & Prendergast, J. (1984). Social network relationships and use of physical services: A re-examination. *Research on Aging, 6*(2), 243-256.

Colvez, A., & Blanchet, M. (1981). Disability trends in the United States population 1966-76: Analysis of reported causes. *American Journal of Public Health, 71,* 464-471.

Commonwealth Fund Commission on Elderly People Living Alone. (1988). *Aging alone.* Baltimore, MD: Commonwealth Fund.

Consumer Price Index. (1989). *Statistical abstract of the United States: 1988.* Washington, DC: Government Printing Office.

Darling, H. (1986). The role of the federal government in assuring access to health care. *Inquiry, 23,* 286-295.

Davis, K. (1984). Medicare reconsidered. In *Health care for the poor and elderly: Meeting the challenge* (pp. 77-96). Durham, NC: Duke University Press.

Davis, K., & Rowland, D. (1983). *Long term care.* Baltimore, MD: Johns Hopkins University Press.

Davis, K., & Schoen, C. (1978). *Health and the war on poverty: A ten year approach.* Washington, DC: Brookings Institution.

Drake, D. F. (1978, October 16). Does money spent on health care really improve U.S. health status? *Hospitals.*

Dutton, D. B. (1986). Social class, health & illness. In L. H. Aiken & D. Mechanic (Eds.), *Applications of social science to clinical medicine and health policy* (pp. 31-62). New Brunswick, NJ: Rutgers University Press.

Ehrenreich, J., & Ehrenreich, B. (1971). *The American health empire*. New York: Vintage.

Estes, C. L. (1979). *The aging enterprise*. San Francisco: Jossey-Bass.

Estes, C. L. (1982). Austerity and aging: 1980 and beyond. *International Journal for Health Services, 12*(4), 573-584.

Estes, C. L. (1988). Healthcare policy in the later twentieth century. *Generations: Quarterly Publication of the American Society on Aging, 12*(3), 44-47.

Estes, C. L., & Binney, E. A. (1988). Toward a transformation of health and aging policy. *International Journal for Health Services, 18*(1), 69-82.

Estes, C. L., & Gerard, L. (1983). Governmental responsibility: Issues of reform and federalism. In C. L. Estes & R. J. Newcomer (Eds.), *Fiscal austerity and aging* (pp. 41-58). Beverly Hills, CA: Sage.

Estes, C. L., Gerard, L., Zones, J. S., & Swan, J. H. (1984). *Political economy, health and aging*. Boston: Little, Brown.

Estes, C. L., & Wood, J. B. (1986). The non-profit sector and community-based care for the elderly: A disappearing resource? *Social Science and Medicine, 23*, 1261-1266.

Estes, C. L., Wood, J. B., et al. (1988). *Organizational and community responses to Medicare policy: Consequences for health and social services for the elderly*. San Francisco: University of California, San Francisco, Institute for Health & Aging.

Evashwick, C., Rowe, G., Diehr, P., & Branch, L. (1984). Factors explaining the use of health care services by the elderly. *Health Services Research, 19*(3), 357-382.

Eve, S. (1982). Age strata differences in utilization of health care services among adults in the United States. *Sociological Focus, 17*(2), 105-120.

Feder, J., et al. (1988). *PPS and post-hospital care: Facts and questions*. Paper presented at the Health Services Research Association Fifth Annual Meeting, San Francisco.

Friedman, B. (1976) Mortality, disability, and the normative economics of Medicare. In R. N. Rosett (Ed.), *The role of health insurance in the health services sector*. Washington, DC: National Bureau of Economic Research.

Fries, J. F. (1980). Aging, natural death, and the compression of morbidity. *The New England Journal of Medicine, 303*, 130-135.

Fuchs, V. (1988). The competition revolution in health care. *Health Affairs, 7*(3), 5-24.

Guralnik, J. M., Yanagishita, M., & Schneider, E. L. (1988). Projecting the older population of the U.S.: Lessons from the past and prospects for the future. *Milbank Memorial Fund Quarterly, 66*(2), 283-308.

Gutterman, S., Eggers, P. W., Riley, G., Greene, T. F., & Terrell, S. A. (1988). The first three years of Medicare prospective payment: An overview. *Health Care Financing Review, 9*(3), 59-66.

Hadley, J. (1982). *More medical care: Better health?* Washington, DC: Urban Institute Press.

Harris & Associates. (1985). *1983 Equitable Health Care Survey*. Washington, DC: Author.

Holahan, J. F., & Cohen, J. W. (1986). *Medicaid: The trade-off between cost containment and access to care*. Washington, DC: Urban Institute.

House, J. S., Landis, K. R., & Umberson, D. (1988). Social relationships and health. *Science, 241*, 540-545.

Institute for the Future. (1987). *Looking ahead at American health care: Final report.* Menlo Park, CA: Author.

Justice, D., & Etheredge, L. (1988). *State long term care reform: Development of community care systems in six states.* Washington, DC: National Governors' Association Center for Policy Research.

Kane, R. A., & Kane, R. L. (1987). *Long term care: Principle, programs, and policies.* New York: Springer.

Kane, R. L., Kane, R. A., & Arnold, S. B. (1985). Prevention and the elderly: Risk factors. *Health Services Research, 19*(6), Pt. II, 946-1006.

Kaplan, G. A., & Haan, M. N. (1989). Is there a role for prevention among the elderly? In M. G. Ory & K. Bond (Eds.), *Aging and health care: Social science and policy perspectives.* London: Rutledge.

Katz, S., Branch, L. G., Branson, M. H., Papsidero, J. A., Beck, J. C., & Greer, D. S. (1983). Active life expectancy. *The New England Journal of Medicine, 309,* 1218-1224.

Kovar, M. G. (1977). Elderly people: The population 65 years and over. In *Health, United States, 1976-77* (DHEW Pub. No. [HRA] 77-1232). Hyattsville, MD: National Center for Health Statistics.

Kramer, M. (1980). The rising pandemic of mental disorder and associated chronic diseases and disorders. *Acta Psychiatrica Scandinavica, 62*(Suppl.), 382-396.

Lee, P. R. (1986). *Forecasting the West: Business outlook for the 1990s.* Stanford, CA: Stanford Alumni Association.

Levit, K. R., & Freeland, M. S. (1988). National medical care spending. *Health Affairs, 7*(5), 124-136.

Loewenstein, R. (1971, April). The effects of Medicare on the health care of the aged. *Social Security Bulletin.*

Lowenthal, M. F., & Robinson, B. (1976). Social networks and isolation. In R. H. Binstock & E. Shanas (Eds.), *Handbook of aging and the social sciences* (1st ed., pp. 432-456). New York: Van Nostrand Reinhold.

Luft, H. S. (1978). *Poverty and health: Economic causes and consequences of health problems.* Cambridge, MA: Ballinger.

Manton, K. G. (1987). The interaction of population aging and health transitions at later ages: New evidence and insights. In C. J. Schramm (Ed.), *Health care and its costs* (pp. 185-221). New York: Norton.

Marmot, M. G., Kogevinas, M., & Elston, M. A. (1987). Social/economic status and disease. In L. Breslow, J. E. Fielding, & L. B. Lave (Eds.), *Annual review of public health* (Vol. 8, pp. 111-135). Palo Alto, CA: Annual Reviews.

McKeown, T. (1976). *The role of medicine: Dream, mirage, or nemesis.* London: Nuffield Provincial Hospital Trust.

McKinlay, J. B., McKinlay, S. M., & Beaglehole, R. (1989). Trends in death and disease and the contribution of medical measures. In H. E. Freeman & S. Levine (Eds.), *Handbook of medical sociology* (4th ed.). Englewood Cliffs, NJ: Prentice-Hall.

Mechanic, D. (1982). Disease, mortality, and the promotion of health. *Health Affairs, 1*(3), 28-38.

Minkler, M. (1984). Blaming the aging victim. In M. Minkler & C. L. Estes (Eds.), *Readings in political economy of aging.* Farmingdale, NY: Baywood.

Minkler, M. (1986a, Fall). The social component of health. *American Journal of Health Promotion*, pp. 33-38.

Minkler, M. (1986b). Generational equity and the new victim blaming: An emerging public policy issue. *International Journal of Health Services, 16*(4), 539-551.

Myles, J. F. (1984). *The political economy of public pensions.* Boston: Little, Brown.

National Center for Health Statistics. (1981). *Health US: 1981.* Hyattsville, MD: Government Printing Office.

National Center for Health Statistics. (1984). *National Health Interview Survey, Supplement on Aging* (DHHS Pub. No. [PHS] 87-1323; Public Health Service). Washington, DC: Government Printing Office.

National Center for Health Statistics. (1986a). *Aging in the eighties, age 65 years and over: Use of community services* (Advance Data No. 124). Hyattsville, MD: Author.

National Center for Health Statistics. (1986b). *Current Estimates from the National Health Interview Survey, United States, 1985* (Vital and Health Statistics, 10[160]. DHHS Pub. No. [PHS] 86-1588; Public Health Service). Washington, DC: Government Printing Office.

National Center for Health Statistics. (1987a). *Health statistics on older persons, United States, 1986* (Vital and Health Statistics, 3[25]. DHHS Pub. No. [PHS] 87-1409; Public Health Service). Washington, DC: Government Printing Office.

National Center for Health Statistics. (1987b, December). *Proceedings of the 1987 Public Health Conference on Records and Statistics: Data for an aging population* (DHHS Pub. No. [PHS] 88-1214; Public Health Service). Hyattsville, MD: Government Printing Office.

National Center for Health Statistics. (1988). *Health, United States, 1987* (DHHS Pub. No. [PHS] 88-1232; Public Health Service). Washington, DC: Government Printing Office.

Navarro, V. (1987). Federal health policy in the US: An alternative explanation. *Milbank Memorial Fund Quarterly, 65*(1), 81-111.

Neu, C. R., & Harrison, C. (1988, March). *Posthospital care before and after the Medicare PPS.* Los Angeles: Rand; University of California, Los Angeles, Center for Health Care Financing Policy Research.

Norman, R. (1985). *The nature and correlates of health behavior* (Health Promotion Studies, No. 2). Ottawa, Canada: Health Promotion Directorate.

Omenn, G. S. (1990). Prevention and the elderly: Appropriate policies. *Health Affairs, 9*(2), 80-93.

Ory, M., & Bond, K. (1989). Introduction: Health care for an aging society. In M. Ory & K. Bond (Eds.), *Aging and health care: Social science and policy perspectives.* London: Routledge.

Pardini, A., Passick, R., Franks, P., & Rice, D. (1984). *Health promotion for the elderly: Program and policy.* San Francisco: University of California, San Francisco, Aging Health Policy Center.

Reinhardt, U. E. (1986, October 22). The battle over medical costs isn't over. *The Wall Street Journal.*

Relman, A. (1980). The new medical-industrial complex. *The New England Journal of Medicine, 303,* 963-970.

Rice, D. P. (1986). Living longer in the U.S.: Social and economic implications. *Journal of Medical Practice Management, 1*(3), 162-169.

Rice, T., & Gabel, J. (1986). Protecting the elderly against high health care costs. *Health Affairs, 5.*

Rice, D. P., & LaPlante, M. P. (1988). Chronic illness, disability, and increasing longevity. In S. Sullivan & M. E. Lewin (Eds.), *The economics and ethics of long-term care and disability* (pp. 9-55). Washington, DC: American Enterprise Institute for Public Policy Research.

Roper, W. (1988, November 18). *HHS News* [Press release].

Rose, G. (1985). Sick individuals and sick populations. *International Journal of Epidemiology, 14,* 32-38.

Rosenwaike, I., Yaffe, N., & Sagi, P. C. (1980, October). The recent decline in mortality of the extreme aged: An analysis of statistical data. *American Journal of Public Health.*

Rovner, J. (1988). Lawmakers taking a hard look at problems of long term care. *Congressional Quarterly,* April 9, p. 938.

Rowe, J. W., & Kahn, R. L. (1987). Human aging: Usual and successful. *Science, 237,* 143-149.

Rundall, T. G., & Evashwick, C. (1982). Social networks and help-seeking among the elderly. *Research on Aging, 4*(2), 205-226.

Schlesinger, M., & Drumheller, P. B. (1988). Beneficiary cost sharing in the Medicare program. In D. Blumenthal, M. Schlesinger, & P. B. Drumheller (Eds.), *Renewing the promise: Medicare and its reform.* New York: Oxford University Press.

Schneider, E. L., & Brody, J. A. (1983). Aging, natural death, and the compression of morbidity: Another view. *The New England Journal of Medicine, 309,* 854-856.

Schneider, W. (1985). Public ready for real change in health care. *National Journal, 3*(3), 664-665.

Soldo, B. (1985). In-home services for the dependent elderly: Determinants of current use and implications for future demand. *Research on Aging, 7*(2), 281-304.

Soldo, B., Agree, E., & Wolf, D. A. (1989). The balance between formal and informal care. In M. Ory & K. Bond (Eds.), *Aging and health care: Social science and policy perspectives.* London: Routledge.

Soldo, B., & Manton, K. (1985). Changes in the health status and service needs of the oldest old: Current patterns and future trends. *Milbank Memorial Fund Quarterly, 63*(2), 286-323.

Stark, F. H. (1987, February 26). [Introductory remarks to hearing on Medicare hospital DRG margins] Subcommittee on Health of the Ways and Means Committee, U.S. House of Representatives, Washington, DC.

Taylor, H. (1986, April 8). [Testimony before the U.S. House Select Committee on Aging, Washington, DC].

Tennestedt, S., & McKinlay, J. (1988). Informal care for frail older persons. In M. Ory & K. Bond (Eds.), *Aging and health care: Social science and policy perspectives.* London: Routledge.

U.S. Department of Commerce, International Trade Administration. (1990). *Health and medical services: U.S. industrial outlook 1990.* Washington, DC: Author.

U.S. Department of Health and Human Services. (1987). *Surgeon general's workshops, health promotion and aging: Background papers.* Rockville, MD: Public Health Service.

U.S. Department of Health and Human Services. (1990). *Healthy people 2000* (Conference ed.). Washington, DC: Government Printing Office.

U.S. Health Care Financing Administration. (1987). *Intermediary workload reports: FY 1986*. Baltimore, MD: Author.

U.S. House of Representatives, Committee on Ways and Means. (1987, April 23). *Medicare Quality Protection Act of 1986* (Serial No. 99-75; Hearing).

U.S. Public Health Service. (1979). *Healthy people: The surgeon general's report on health promotion and disease prevention* (DHEW [PHS] Pub. no. 79-55071). Washington, DC: Government Printing Office.

U.S. Senate, Special Committee on Aging. (1985). *Developments in aging: 1984*. Washington, DC: Government Printing Office.

U.S. Senate. (1988). *Aging America: Trends and projections*. Washington, DC: U.S. Department of Health and Human Services.

Verbrugge, L. M. (1984). Longer life but worsening health? Trends in health and mortality of middle-aged and older persons. *Milbank Memorial Fund Quarterly, 62*, 475-519.

Verbrugge, L. M. (1989). Recent, present, and future health of American adults. In J. E. Breslow, J. E. Fielding, & L. B. Lave (Eds.), *Annual review of public health* (Vol. 10). Palo Alto, CA: Annual Reviews.

Villers Foundation. (1987). *On the other side of easy street*. Washington, DC: Author.

Vogel, R. J., & Palmer, H. C. (Eds.). (1983). *Long term care: Perspectives from research and demonstrations*. Baltimore, MD: U.S. Health Care Financing Administration.

Vogt, T. M. (1987). *Psychosocial predictors of morbidity and mortality*. Portland, OR: Kaiser Permanente, Center for Health Research.

Wan, T. (1982). Use of health services by the elderly in low-income communities. *Milbank Memorial Fund Quarterly, 60*(1), 82-107.

Wan, T. (1989). The behavioral model of health care utilization by older people. In M. Ory & K. Bond (Eds.), *Aging and health care: Social science and policy perspectives*. London: Routledge.

Wan, T., & Arling, G. (1983). Differential use of health services among disabled elders. *Research on Aging, 5*(3), 411-431.

Wan, T., & Weissert, W. G. (1981). Social support networks: Patient status and institutionalization. *Research on Aging, 3*(2), 240-256.

Wing, S., Manton, K. G., Stallard, E., Hames, C. G., & Tryoles, H. A. (1985). The Black/White mortality crossover: Investigation in a community-based study. *Journal of Gerontology, 40*(1), 78-84.

Wolinsky, F., & Coe, R. (1984). Physician and hospital utilization among non-institutionalized elderly adults: An analysis of the Health Interview Survey. *Journal of Gerontology, 39*(3), 334-341.

Zola, I. K. (1986). The medicalization of aging and disability: Problems and prospects. In C. W. Mahoney, C. L. Estes, & J. E. Heumann (Eds.), *Toward a unified agenda: Proceedings of a National Conference on Disability and Aging*. San Francisco: University of California, San Francisco, Institute for Health & Aging.

12

Forecasting Health and Functioning in Aging Societies: Implications for Health Care and Staffing Needs

KENNETH G. MANTON

RICHARD SUZMAN

Analyses of current data indicate that the U.S. elderly population will grow rapidly to the year 2020 and beyond, with the most elderly component of that population (i.e., the "oldest old," or those aged 85 and over) projected to be the most rapidly growing component of the entire U.S. population (U.S. Department of Health and Human Services, 1987). Since the elderly and oldest-old populations also have the greatest need for acute, postacute, and long-term care (LTC), the demand for all types of health services and for trained personnel to provide those services can also be expected to grow at a very rapid rate (Manton & Soldo, in press).

To minimize the social and fiscal stress of providing the immense human and financial resources that will be required, it is important to make long-range plans. Long-range planning is demanded not only because of the sheer magnitude of future demands for resources but also because the rate of increase in the demand will fluctuate, influenced by several strategic parameters (e.g., residual life expectancy at later ages). In addition to increasing the capacity to allocate resources flexibly, long-range planning offers opportunities to alter patterns of service, by appropriate adjustments of federal and state mechanisms of reimbursement for health services, in ways that can improve the quality of life and the quality of care. The demand for

AUTHORS' NOTE: Research reported in this chapter was supported by NIA Grant Nos. 1R37 AG07025 and 2R01 AG01159 and HCFA Grant No. 18 C-97710.

certain types of service may also be reduced by targeted health-promotion and disease-prevention activities. Many other developed countries already have such long-range planning. For example, Japan, which is projected to have a quarter of its population over age 65 by 2025, conducted several major multidisciplinary studies of the economic effects of providing necessary social and health services to a rapidly growing elderly population (e.g., Nihon University, 1982).

Unfortunately, no long-range forecasting and planning exercises have been conducted in the United States with the degree of sophistication and breadth of those undertaken in Japan. In this chapter, we present long-term forecasts of the future health and functional status of the elderly population and the implications of those projections for future requirements for health services and manpower. In these forecasts, we attempt to utilize recent scientific data on the mutability of the age trajectory of health and functional changes in the elderly population. Even the sophisticated forecasting efforts conducted by the Japanese do not evaluate the potential of such interventions.

Our forecasts are based on recent scientific research that illustrates heretofore unanticipated potential benefits of long-range interventions for health promotion and disease (and disability) prevention. This scientific evidence shows that much of the prevalence of disease and disability among even very elderly persons is age related but *not* necessarily age determined. That is, the current ill health of many older persons is a result of the cumulative exposure to risk and not simply due to fixed intrinsic processes of biological senescence. It is now realized that many early studies of aging processes were flawed because they did not adequately screen for latent and manifest morbidity in the study population. Because the prevalence of chronic disease and functional impairment in a population tends to increase with age, merely measuring the rate of changes in physiological functioning between two randomly drawn samples of persons of different ages may confound declines in average physiological function due to individual characteristics with age changes in the prevalence of pathology in those populations. To unconfound the measurement of individual rates of physiological change from changes in the population, either detailed statistical controls for health status or careful screening of the population is necessary (e.g., Rowe, 1988; Rowe & Wang, 1988).

Subsequently, studies of selected "healthy" elderly populations have shown that the physiological function of many organ systems can be maintained in certain individuals to quite advanced ages. For example, Lakatta (1985) showed that the cardiac output of healthy 80-year-olds was not unlike that of 30-year-olds. The maintenance of cardiac output resulted from an adaptation—stroke volume increased to offset a lowered ability to increase heart rate—suggesting a large capacity for adaptation to certain physiological consequences of aging. Furthermore, detailed studies have identified some of the biochemical bases for the decreased ability of very elderly persons to maintain high heart rates under physical challenge; such biochemical changes suggest further interventions. Other studies have shown that cognitive performance among many extremely elderly persons was maintained at high levels and that, when these people finally lost cognitive function, they did so rapidly, unlike the slow and regular generalized physiological aging processes (Manton, Siegler, & Woodbury, 1986).

In addition, in contrast to earlier studies, where data mistakenly analyzed suggested age effects (e.g., Kannel & Gordon, 1980), more recent analyses show that many risk factors contribute more strongly to chronic disease at advanced ages than at earlier ages (e.g., Kaplan, Seeman, Cohen, Knudsen, & Guralnik, 1987; Manton, 1986). Other studies suggest that mortality is more changeable, as is the relation of mortality and morbidity, than had been previously thought (e.g., Manton, 1987; Schneider & Guralnik, 1987). All of this evidence supports the concept that we can be effective in shaping the future health of the elderly population and thus modify our delivery of health services to respond in qualitatively positive ways to the large numerical increases in the elderly. However, given the long biological latency of many chronic disease and disability processes, these activities require action considerably in advance. That is, interventions earlier in the life span may prevent disability and disease at later ages and improve the health of the oldest-old population. This is a clear lesson from epidemiological studies of chronic diseases and their functional sequelae. This evidence also suggests that, even when disease and dysfunction are manifested at advanced ages, there is still the potential to improve health and functioning by appropriate rehabilitative action. As the projections below show, we will probably have to implement strategies of both early and late intervention to accommodate the magnitude of the near-term growth of the elderly population—all persons currently alive, many of them middle-aged, currently without the benefits of systematic efforts at health promotion.

To project the health service needs of this nation's elderly population, we need to perform several tasks. First, it is necessary to project the growth of the elderly population. Demographic projections require that we know the size and the structure of both the current elderly population and the population that will become elderly during the interval over which we wish to forecast. These data are available from decennial censuses. The second, more uncertain component of the demographic projections are mortality rates specific to age, sex, race, and relevant health factors, which determine what proportion of those cohorts will survive to age 65 (and 85) at specific future dates. Changes in mortality have been difficult to anticipate (and previously underestimated) because mortality rates at advanced ages were assumed unlikely to decline significantly (Myers, 1981)—an assumption proved false by recent increases in life expectancy at ages 65 and 85 (Manton, 1986). However, even if mortality is modifiable by new technologies, given current budgetary constraints, it is uncertain how rapidly and to what degree these technologies will be implemented.

Second, demographic projections must be made specific to health and functional status. Simply knowing the size of the elderly population (and its age and sex composition) does not tell us directly about the level of need for acute, postacute, and LTC services. It is necessary to know the distribution of functional and health status in that population and within its various components. This is especially important given that recent research on demographic, biomedical, and epidemiological aging makes it clear that the incidence of chronic disease and disability is not absolutely age determined. This observation draws our attention to an additional potential category of health services and personnel that may be increasingly required in the future—physician and ancillary health professional groups providing preventive and health-promotion services.

In projecting the future prevalence of chronic disease and disability, it is important to use measures of the burden of disease and disability that represent the particular health problems of very elderly populations who have a high prevalence of chronic disease. To do this, we employ a model (Figure 12.1) developed by a World Health Organization (WHO) scientific advisory group to describe the burden of disease at advanced ages using measures representing the amount of time people with different types of diseases and disabilities are affected by those problems (WHO, 1984).

Figure 12.1 depicts three types of survival curves describing the probability of surviving to a given age without experiencing one of three types of health event. The vertical axis represents the probability of survival and runs from 100% at the top to 0% at the bottom. The

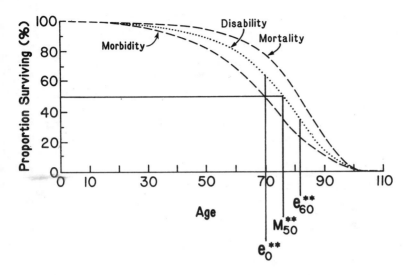

Figure 12.1. The Observed Mortality and Hypothetical Morbidity and Disability Survival Curves for Females in the United States in 1980

SOURCE: World Health Organization (1984).
NOTE: e_0^{**} and e_{60}^{**} are the number of years of autonomous life expected at birth and at age 60, respectively. M_{50}^{**} is the age to which 50% of females could expect to survive without loss of autonomy.

horizontal axis represents age. The outermost curve describes how mortality reduces the proportion surviving to any given age, that is, the survival curve from standard life tables. The innermost curve represents the age-specific probability of surviving to a given age without serious chronic disease. The middle curve describes the probability of surviving to a given age without chronic disability. It is assumed that a chronic disease process must underlie (or precede) the emergence of serious chronic disability—though the disease processes producing most disability may not be the same as those generating mortality.

The areas between the curves have important implications for the use of services in that they represent the average number of years that a person in the cohort spends in a particular health state. Thus the area under the morbidity curve represents the "healthy" life expectancy of the population while the total area under the disability curve represents "active" (functionally intact) life expectancy.

The size of the areas between curves represents the number of years that a person is likely to require various types of service. This is clarified in Figure 12.2, which superimposes the use of different types of LTC service on the survival curves. This illustrates how different types of use of services are distributed over the underlying age-specific risks of functional limitation (Soldo & Manton, 1985). Clearly, more intense types and levels of service use are associated with the higher prevalence of morbidity and disability at later ages. In evaluating the potential effects of various heath-promotion and prevention programs on the demand for services, it is less appropriate to ask whether the need for services is "prevented" than to ask how long the need for acute and LTC services is delayed—with the net effect of reducing the duration that such needs are experienced in a typical life span.

Third, we must translate the numbers of elderly in different health statuses into the aggregate demand for different types of service. The demand for services can be altered either by intervening in the basic disease and disability processes or by altering the types of service used for different types and levels of disability. For example, there has recently been considerable emphasis on substituting community-based services for institutional care. Thus, if community-based services can be designed to respond to the service needs of persons at higher disability levels (i.e., having greater numbers of disabilities), then the "threshold" for institutional care can be raised and more persons successfully managed in community settings (Luce, Liu, & Manton, 1984).

Finally, once the level and types of service that will be required are identified, it is possible to translate that demand into the number and types of medical and ancillary health professional that are required to provide that amount of service. This step is difficult, however, because different types of personnel may be substituted for one another and because different approaches to providing care (and the availability of different levels and types of care) can have an impact on the changes in the health and functional status of the elderly population in future years.

DEMOGRAPHIC PROJECTIONS

Projecting the future growth of the elderly population is difficult because of uncertainty about future trends in mortality. Projections of the U.S. elderly population are produced by the social security

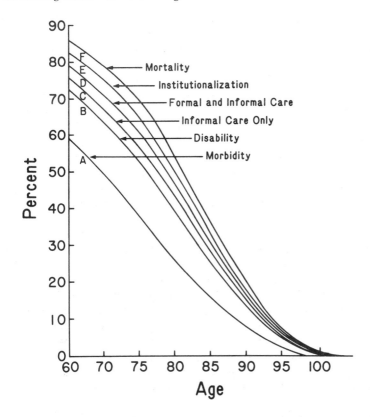

Figure 12.2. The Observed Mortality and Hypothetical Morbidity, Disability, and LTC Service Use Survival Curves for U.S. Females, 1980

SOURCE: Soldo and Manton (1985); used by permission.

actuaries in their preparation of the Social Security Trust Fund report. We will employ these in our analyses because of their importance for the financing of social security and medicare (i.e., all projections are uncertain but the uncertainty of these specific projections has direct programmatic implications for providing services to the elderly). In those projections, future mortality is estimated by extrapolating recent trends in cause and sex-specific mortality. The future life expectancies that are anticipated on the basis of recent changes in mortality are presented in Table 12.1 (U.S. Department of Health and Human Services, 1987). Life expectancy is projected to increase significantly in each of the three scenarios, that is, mortality decreases at half the projected rate (the first alternative, or series I), at the projected rate (the second alternative, or series II), and at twice the projected rate (the third alternative, or series III).

To evaluate the reasonableness of these projections, one may examine countries such as Japan, where life expectancy is higher than in the United States and continues to increase. Japan's male (75.8) and female (81.9) life expectancies in 1988 (WHO, 1989) are much greater than those of series I for U.S. males (75.0) in 2080 and females (80.7) in 2040. Furthermore, the values for age 65 may be compared with the life expectancies observed for males (16.5) and females (21.0) in a large recent study of 460,000 elderly conducted by the American Cancer Society (Lew & Garfinkel, 1984). This population, which was middle class and ostensibly healthy at the start of the study, represents lower bounds to the achievable life expectancy at age 65. From Table 12.1, we see that these levels are not projected to be achieved until 2080 (in series I) or 2020 (in series II). Thus the projected life expectancies clearly encompass the range of what is physiologically possible. Whether such life expectancies will be achieved depends on the behavior of individuals and institutions, but no dramatic changes in medical technology are required.

Regardless of the future rate of improvement in mortality, U.S. elderly and extreme elderly populations will show dramatic growth because life expectancy at advanced ages is already high and because the new cohorts of elderly persons will be much larger. The projected growth of the elderly population under the three mortality scenarios is presented in Table 12.2.

Table 12.2 shows the rate of growth of the U.S. elderly population to be uneven. Under alternative II, the middle variant, the oldest-old population grows rapidly up to the year 2000, increasing to 1.7% of the total U.S. population. From 2000 to 2020, the young-old population grows rapidly as the large post-World War II baby boom cohorts begin to pass age 65. From 2020 to 2080, the oldest-old population increases rapidly as the post-World War II baby boom cohorts pass age 85. By 2060, the oldest-old population is between 2.9% (alternative I, the low life expectancy) and 11.4% (alternative III, the high life expectancy) of the total U.S. population.

Though future increases in the elderly population will necessarily occur because future elderly cohorts are much larger, such projections

Table 12.1

Life Expectancy at Birth and at Age 65, by Sex, Calendar Year, and Alternative (in years)

| | Sex & Alternative | | | | | |
| | I | | II | | III | |
Calendar Year	Male	Female	Male	Female	Male	Female
1987						
at birth	71.5	78.6	71.6	78.7	71.8	78.8
at age 65	14.6	18.8	14.7	18.9	14.7	18.9
1990						
at birth	71.8	78.8	72.3	79.3	72.8	79.7
at age 65	14.7	18.9	14.9	19.2	15.2	19.5
1995						
at birth	72.2	79.2	73.2	80.1	74.2	81.1
at age 65	14.8	19.0	15.3	19.7	15.8	20.3
2000						
at birth	72.6	79.4	73.9	80.8	75.2	82.0
at age 65	14.8	19.2	15.6	20.1	16.3	21.0
2020						
at birth	73.3	80.1	75.1	82.0	77.6	84.5
at age 65	15.2	19.7	16.3	21.0	17.9	22.8
2040						
at birth	73.9	80.7	76.2	83.1	79.8	86.9
at age 65	15.6	20.1	17.0	21.9	19.6	24.6
2060						
at birth	74.5	81.3	77.1	84.2	82.0	89.0
at age 65	16.0	20.6	17.7	22.8	21.2	26.4
2080						
at birth	75.0	81.8	78.1	85.3	84.1	91.1
at age 65	16.4	21.1	18.5	23.7	22.9	28.2

SOURCE: U.S. Department of Health and Human Services, Social Security Administration, Office of the Actuary (1987, pp. 13-14).
NOTE: The life expectancy is the average number of years of life remaining to a person if he were to experience the age-specific mortality rates for the tabulated year throughout the remainder of his life. Series I assumes that mortality rates will decline half as fast as the middle variant, thus producing lower life expectancy. Series II assumes that mortality rates will decline initially as fast as recent trends indicate, tapering to an "ultimate" rate of mortality decline after 25 years. Series III assumes that mortality rates decline twice as fast as the middle variant, thus producing higher life expectancy.

Table 12.2
U.S. Population, Age 65-84, 85 + And 65+, 1985-2080, Under Three Assumptions About the Rate of Mortality Decline (in Thousands)

	Age Group and Mortality Alternative								
	Age 65+			Age 65-84			Age 85+		
Year	I	II	III	I	II	III	I	II	III
1990	31,841	31,911	31,978	28,560	28,598	28,634	3,281	3,314	3,344
2000	34,773	35,626	36,415	30,404	30,895	31,331	4,368	4,731	5,085
2020	50,422	53,099	56,419	44,840	46,361	48,230	5,582	6,738	8,189
2040	64,367	69,051	76,729	54,509	56,617	60,239	9,868	12,433	16,489
2060	65,917	70,381	79,592	54,911	55,751	58,121	11,007	14,629	21,471
2080	74,105	73,484	75,844	61,461	56,700	50,770	12,643	16,784	25,074

SOURCE: U.S. Dept. of Heath & Human Service, Social Security Administration, Office of the Actuary. Social Security Area Population Projections 1987. Actuarial Study No. 99 (by Alice Wade). SSA Pub. No. 11-11546, August, 1987, Table 20. Series I assumes that mortality rates will decline half as fast as the middle variant, thus producing lower life expectancy. Series II assumes that mortality rates will decline initially as fast as recent trends indicate, tapering to an "ultimate" rate of mortality decline after 25 years. Series III assumes that mortality rates decline twice as fast as the middle variant, thus producing higher life expectancy.

are quite sensitive to changes in mortality at later ages. This is because life expectancy has increased to values that are higher than the current age "threshold" of the elderly population. That is, as the life expectancy increases significantly past age 65, we can expect rapid increases in the proportion of survivors to age 65 and rapid increases in the size of the elderly population. Thus we can expect rapid growth in the elderly Black male population in the near future as their life expectancy increases past 65. This is a result of the sharp curvature of the survival function near the life expectancy value for the population. The mean and median life expectancies are similar, so the rate of change in the proportion surviving near the mean can be large (see Figure 12.1). Thus an increase of one year in life expectancy at these ages implies a larger increase in the proportion surviving to older ages than when survival improves at younger ages, where the curve is flatter. White females, in contrast, have life expectancies nearing 80 years. Consequently, future improvements in mortality may cause extremely rapid increases in the size of the oldest-old White female population.

The consequence of such changes in life expectancy are illustrated in Table 12.3. The proportion of the population that is elderly, at a given fertility level (i.e., gross reproductive rate, or GRR), is very

Table 12.3
Simulation II: Proportional Reductions in U.S. Age-Specific Mortality

	Percentage of Reduction in Age Specific Mortality Rates				
	25	75	90	96	99
Life expectancy at birth for White females, 1977 (in years)	81.8	92.0	96.5	98.5	99.6
Proportion of Population 65 and Over Gross Reproduction Rate					
0.57	42.8	55.9	62.7	66.8	69.4
0.86	28.3	38.3	43.9	47.2	49.3
1.14	19.4	26.6	30.6	33.0	34.5
0.5	46.4	59.9	66.9	71.0	73.6
1.0	23.9	32.7	37.5	40.4	42.2
1.5	13.7	18.9	21.7	23.4	24.4

SOURCE: Duke University, Center for Demographic Studies.

sensitive to changes in life expectancy. For example, if life expectancy increases from 78 to 81.8 years as the result of a 25% reduction in mortality, the proportion of the elderly (with replacement-level fertility) jumps from 11% to 23.9%. The degree to which population aging reflects gains in life expectancy is demonstrated in Japanese studies of population aging as the *assumed* upper limit to life expectancy (males at 77.4 years and females at 81.7 by the year 2000; Ogawa, 1982), which is being rapidly approached and exceeded (i.e., 75.8 and 81.9 in 1988; WHO, 1989).

Not only will the size and age composition of the elderly population change dramatically in the United States but also the life experiences of new elderly cohorts will be significantly different. The average number of school years completed, both for current elderly birth cohorts (e.g., those currently aged 70 to 74) and for birth cohorts that will pass age 65 by 2015 (i.e., those now aged 30 to 34), increases from 10.7 years for males and 11.5 years for females to 13.3 and 12.7 years, respectively. The higher educational level of younger cohorts is paralleled by increases in their economic power. With new elderly cohorts having better education, enhanced economic power, and improved life experiences, there may be greater opportunities to provide services to support the disabled elderly in the community and to preserve the functional capacity of the elderly to greater ages with the goal of qualitatively improving the health of the elderly (e.g., Kaplan et al., 1987).

Not all of the changes in the composition of new cohorts of the elderly, however, are beneficial. For example, though the Black population will remain younger than the White population due to higher fertility rates and lower life expectancy, the differences in the median age of the two populations are projected to decrease from 10.1 years for females and 6.2 years for males in 1985 to about 5 years in 2050. The growth of the oldest-old Black population will be extremely rapid. Because of the poorer economic status of the Black population and because long-term structural unemployment has had a strong impact on a number of specific occupational groups (e.g., divesting them of private health insurance coverage), many of the elderly and oldest old will remain in very poor financial circumstances. One compensating mechanism may be that lower socioeconomic groups also tend to have large families—potentially providing more informal care resources. In contrast, the elderly with greater financial resources (but potentially fewer informal care resources due to smaller family sizes) will have greater capacity to purchase acute and LTC insurance coverage and to pay out of pocket for LTC services. Thus planning services for the elderly will require evaluating the very different economic and family situations of different future elderly subpopulations.

Sex and marital status are also important dimensions when discussing the growth of the health and LTC needs of the elderly U.S. population. Life expectancies are higher for women than for men, leading to low sex ratios (i.e., the number of males per 100 females) among the oldest-old population. The sensitivity of these sex ratios to mortality is illustrated in Tables 12.4 and 12.5.

Tables 12.4 and 12.5 depict the median life expectancy at birth, and sex ratios at ages 65-69 and 85-89, for the three sets of mortality assumptions in the social security projections. In 1980, the sex ratios at age 85 were extremely low, suggesting that the problem of delivering care to the oldest old was primarily a problem of caring for elderly females, often without a spouse alive, dependent upon children for informal care, and having few financial resources. Because life expectancy increases faster for females, the sex ratio is projected to become even more unbalanced at age 65 (and 85) up to the year 2000. Beyond 2000, the median life expectancy of both males and females is projected to exceed 85. Consequently, even if life expectancy continues to increase more rapidly for females than for males, the sex ratio for the oldest old could decrease because of relative constraints on the

Table 12.4
Median Life Expectancy at Birth Under Three Alternatives

	1982			2005			2080		
Sex	I	II	III	I	II	III	I	II	III
Males	80.5	80.5	80.5	84.9	83.0	81.7	95.0	90.1	84.0
Females	84.6	84.6	84.6	90.3	88.5	86.3	>95	94.0	89.0

SOURCE: U.S. Department of Health and Human Services, Social Security Administration, Office of the Actuary (1985).

Table 12.5
Sex Ratios* at Ages 65-69, 85-89, and Ages 65+ and 85+ Under Three Alternatives

	1980	1985			2000		
Age		I	II	III	I	II	III
Age 65-69	79.5	82.1	82.1	82.1	84.2	85.3	86.4
Age 85-89	44.5	41.7	41.7	42.0	40.1	41.1	42.3
Age 65+	66.9	66.4	66.4	66.5	65.8	66.4	67.0
Age 85+	42.3	39.0	38.9	39.0	35.6	36.4	37.2

SOURCE: Life expectancy computed from life table survival rates reported in U.S. Bureau of the Census (1984, Table B).
NOTE: Series I assumes that mortality rates will decline half as fast as the middle variant, thus producing lower life expectancy. Series II assumes that mortality rates will decline initially as fast as recent trends indicate, tapering to an "ultimate" rate of mortality decline after 25 years. Series III assumes that mortality rates decline twice as fast as the middle variant, thus producing higher life expectancy.
*Sex ratio represents number of males per 100 females

rate of improvement in female survival to age 85. A continuation of increases in the life expectancy of males does imply an increasing number of intact couples at advanced ages and the possibility of more relatives and siblings in a given family surviving to advanced ages to provide informal care support.

HEALTH AND FUNCTIONAL
STATUS PROJECTIONS

The first factor to consider in projecting health and functional status is medical conditions that cause disability at later ages. The conditions identified in the 1982 and 1984 National Long Term Care

Surveys (NLTCS) as causing most chronic disability among elderly persons are *not* conditions generally viewed as the most lethal; neither are they normally targeted in primary prevention programs. Indeed, for several of the most disabling conditions (e.g., dementia, arthritis), only now are the disease mechanisms being elaborated and major risk factors being identified (Manton, 1989).

Though our understanding of these diseases is in rapid flux, it is clear that their appropriate management can lead to significant rehabilitation and restoration of function. Especially at younger ages, a significant proportion of the disabled elderly manifest significant long-term (i.e., two-year) functional improvement (Manton, 1988). For example, persons aged 65 to 74 in 1982 with five to six impairments in activities of daily living (or ADL) had nearly a 30% chance of showing a long-term (two-year) improvement in functional status.

A wide range of interventions are possible to enhance the health of the elderly and to delay the age at which disability appears (see the chapters by Rakowski & Levi in this volume). For example, one could provide services for primary prevention, with the goal of diminishing risk factors in a population. Such activities generally are delivered at the community level and focus on public action programs rather than on individuals. Primary prevention, to reduce the incidence of disease at younger ages, should, in the elderly, be directed toward delaying the onset of disease. Secondary prevention, to control the progression of the disease process, will also be of considerable importance (e.g., reducing the rate of circulatory degeneration due to diabetes mellitus), while tertiary prevention, directed to limiting the consequences of disease on functioning, is of especial importance for the oldest old. Thus, in addition to the usual efforts to reduce risk factors for chronic disease in individuals, one needs to consider other types of service, including environmental and community interventions to reduce a wide range of unhealthy behaviors, structural environmental changes to reduce the hazard of falls and accidents, and the development of geriatric assessment units to provide services to enhance the functioning of very elderly individuals with multiple disabling conditions and diseases. Some of these activities will require the development of personnel to fill roles that have not traditionally been viewed as primary to the health care of the elderly.

Projections of the effects of efforts to prevent and slow the progression of chronic disease processes must deal with the problem of "dependent" competing risks. Specifically, because the elderly are often subject to multiple diseases, increasing survival by eliminating one disease process may also increase the prevalence of other (nonlethal) disabling conditions (e.g., Feldman, 1983; Manton & Stallard, 1988).

Consider, for example, the projected increases in hip fracture and dementia up to 2050 (Brody, 1984). The increase for both conditions, given projected increases in survival and in the size of future elderly cohorts, is large. Additionally, the incidence of these conditions increases strongly with age. For example, hip fracture increases nearly exponentially with age, doubling about every five years. Thus a delay of five years in the osteoporotic processes generating hip fractures (and resulting disability) might halve the occurrence of hip fracture (Brody, 1984). Increasing life expectancy by five years without reducing the age-specific incidence of hip fractures would double its prevalence.

Predicting changes in disability generated by intervening in chronic disease processes is also difficult, because there is not a simple one-to-one relation of individual disease to disability levels (Manton, 1987). For example, Manton (1986) analyzed the impact of conditions on functional impairment. Three of the ten diseases modeled in the 1982 NLTCS—dementia, stroke, and hip fractures—decreased the level of healthy functioning by 15.4%, 10.4%, and 13.7%, respectively, in the community-dwelling disabled population. Extrapolating the study results to the U.S. population suggests that control of the ten conditions might decrease the number of disabled elderly by 800,000—a reduction of 15.7% in the U.S. disabled community-dwelling elderly population in 1982.

The cumulative effects of the interaction of disability and morbidity among the chronically disabled community-dwelling and institutionalized elderly populations can be projected from disability rates from the 1982 NLTCS and institutionalization rates from the 1977 National Nursing Home Survey (NNHS). These projections show that, consistent with the rapid growth of the extreme elderly population, the number of frail and institutionalized persons would increase from 5.7 million in 1980 to 8.9 million in 2000, to 12.2 million in 2020, and to 17.8 million in 2040. If increases in service were strictly proportional to increases in population, this would imply a need for 197% more providers of services to the community-dwelling disabled elderly and 270% more persons providing care in institutions. Similar projections emerge from more recent data from the 1984 NLTCS and the 1985 NNHS (Manton, 1989).

Modifying the projections to reflect a decrease in morbidity and disability rates paralleling the assumed decrease in mortality rates reduces the projected disabled population to 7.0 million in 2000, 9.0 million in 2020, and 12.1 million in 2040. The reduction for 2020 represents more than 3 million persons who formerly were chronically disabled in the community or in institutions. Assuming that the demand for personnel increased or decreased proportionally with the population size, these proportions suggest large reductions in the amount of personnel potentially required.

To maintain the age- and sex-specific rates that prevailed in 1977, between 1980 and 2040, the number of nursing home beds must grow 2.2% per year on average. Reducing the rate of growth of the construction of nursing home beds by 50% (to 1.1%) curtails the projected number of persons in institutions dramatically, that is, by 1.1 million persons in 2020 and 2.3 million persons in 2040. If these persons were reallocated into the disabled elderly population in the community, according to the proportions that they represented in nursing homes at different health and functional status levels, it would clearly imply a major shift of resources to the home health sector.

PROJECTED CHANGES IN HEALTH SERVICES

In this section, we translate static component projections of the use of health and functional services based on NCHS survey data (Rice & Feldman, 1983) into demand for personnel. Between 1980 and 2040, the consumption of physician visits and acute hospital days by the elderly population is projected to grow rapidly but irregularly. Overall, the growth in the use of acute services roughly doubles for persons aged 65 to 74—from 100 million to 186 million physician visits and from 50 to 93 million acute hospital days—with most of the increase occurring by 2020. In contrast, the use of acute care by persons aged 75 and over quadruples, with a large increase between 2020 and 2040 reflecting differentials in birth cohort size. Physician visits increase from 66 million in 1980 to 115 million in 2000, to 144 million in 2020, and to 241 million in 2040. The same data for acute hospital days are, respectively, 56 million, 102 million, 130 million, and 219 million. Similar patterns are noted for the number of nursing home residents, with the number of residents above age 85—he frailest age group—increasing nearly fivefold, from 563,000 in 1980 to 2.9 million in 2040.

The service needs of the elderly population not only will show large absolute increases but also will become increasingly concentrated among the elderly. Table 12.6 shows the proportion of each of the three classes of service use by the elderly. Use is less concentrated for physician services, which vary less with age. Nursing home residence, being most prevalent among the extreme elderly, is most concentrated. More than 95% of all nursing home use is projected to be among the elderly in 2040 (compared with 87.0% in 1980), with 55.5% of all use among the oldest old (compared with 37.2% in 1980).

An important factor in long-term projections of the use of services is changes in the pattern of services consumed. For example, there have been significant changes in the utilization of medicare. The length of stay for medicare hospital patients dropped from 13.4 days in 1968 to 10.2 days in 1982. By 1984, the first year of the prospective payment system (PPS), it dropped to 8.8 days. In addition, and contrary to expectation, there were also declines in the rate of hospitalization. An important question raised by these changes is what services are being substituted for hospital care and which groups of patients are no longer being admitted to hospitals? This can be answered by examining changes in the case mix of patients. Medicare data show major shifts in the case mix of hospitals pre- and post-PPS, with chronic medical conditions (e.g., diabetes, chronic pulmonary disease) and certain specific procedures (e.g., lens procedures) declining in frequency while acute medical problems and surgical procedures increased. Thus the case mix became more acute and more medically intensive.

What alternative services for chronic care cases are being substituted for acute hospitalization? One substitute is home health care. The number of medicare-certified home health agencies increased from 2,858 in 1979 to 5,247 in 1984. This shift suggests major new demands for geriatric nurse specialists and other rehabilitative and health care specialists providing home services.

In analyzing the demand for LTC services, it is important to consider the private market. Analyses of the 1982 and 1984 NLTCS show that annual out-of-pocket expenditures in 1982 are conservatively estimated at $1.2 billion among 608,000 persons reporting some such payment (average monthly payment $164; Liu et al., 1985). By 1984, these expenditures had increased 60%, to $1.9 billion among 860,000 persons (average monthly payment $184). Out-of-pocket payments for nursing services, though high on a per-capita basis (i.e., from $424 to $529 monthly for 1982 and 1984), are restricted to a relatively small population (58,000 in 1982 and 83,293 in 1984). The projected growth

Table 12.6
Proportion of Physician Visits, Short-Stay Hospital Days and Nursing Home Residents for the Elderly by Age and Sex: United States, 1980-2040

	1980	*2000*	*2020*	*2040*
Physician Visits				
Total				
65-74 years of age	9.0	8.9	12.7	11.5
75 and over	6.0	8.7	9.6	14.9
Male				
65-74 years of age	8.2	8.4	12.2	11.0
75 and over	5.3	7.6	8.5	13.6
Female				
65-74 years of age	9.6	9.2	13.1	11.8
75 and over	6.5	9.5	10.3	15.8
Short-stay hospital days				
Total				
65-74 years of age	17.9	15.6	20.7	16.9
75 and over	20.4	27.5	28.4	40.0
Male				
65-74 years of age	19.7	17.6	23.3	19.4
75 and over	18.1	23.5	24.4	35.7
Female				
65-74 years of age	16.6	14.1	18.7	15.1
75 and over	22.1	30.5	31.5	43.2
Nursing Home Residents				
Total				
65 years and over	87.0	91.1	92.8	95.3
65-74 years of age	15.0	10.4	12.9	8.1
75-84 years of age	35.0	33.4	29.8	31.6
85 and over	37.2	47.3	50.0	55.5
Male				
65 years and over	77.9	83.2	86.7	90.9
65-74 years of age	20.5	16.4	20.2	13.2
75-84 years of age	31.9	35.1	32.4	36.0
85 and over	25.4	31.8	34.1	41.7
Female				
65 years and over	90.5	93.8	94.9	96.7
65-74 years of age	12.8	8.4	10.4	6.4
75-84 years of age	36.0	32.9	29.0	30.1
85 and over	42.0	52.5	55.6	60.1

SOURCE: National Center for Health Statistics, Office of Analysis and Epidemiology; and Rice and Feldman (1983); Used by permission.

of the elderly population implies that, even without the dramatic rate of increase in services between 1982 to 1984, between $5 to $6 billion (in 1984 dollars) will be spent out of pocket in 2040.

Another potential area of substitution of services is that of currently unreimbursed informal care services being replaced by formal care services—a shift promoted by changes in the size and composition of families and the increase of financial resources among new elderly cohorts. In Table 12.7, we present the number of hours per week expended in providing informal services to the community disabled. The annual volume of informal care services (5.8 billion hours in 1980) is tremendous and becoming increasingly concentrated among the older age groups. Even if only 10% of the care in 2020 were shifted to the paid LTC market, this represents a huge new market—that is, 1.3 billion hours per year, or, at $10 per hour as a conservative wage rate, $12.6 billion. Added to the 1984 base level of home health services projected to 2020, this implies a potential home health care market of $16 to $17 billion.

It is also useful to calculate the potential savings if effective health-promotion programs could be instituted. The reductions in use of services, if disease and disability declined as rapidly as mortality, would be large—that is, 3 billion fewer hours of service per year required by 2020. If 10% of this total service use in the future had to be replaced by formal care, this level of health improvement would represent a reduction of 300 million person-hours, requiring 150,000 full-time caregivers, for savings of $3 billion.

Change in acute care services will have an impact on institutional care as well as home health services. In general, it appears that institutional care is becoming more medically intensive—as patients' hospital stays become shorter and as less frail persons increasingly stay in the community.

Other factors may also have fundamental effects on the level and type of acute and LTC services consumed by the elderly. For example, there could be major improvements in the ability to treat and manage chronic diseases. Currently, for instance, a large number of pharmaceutical agents are being developed for the prevention and management of Alzheimer's disease. In addition, advances in genetic engineering (Anderson, 1988) may allow us to respond to the basic age-related cellular mechanisms that underlie much of the pathology now ascribed to "senescent" processes. Any effective treatment for Alzheimer's disease would dramatically reduce the future demand for institutional and home health services (Manton & Stallard, in press).

Table 12.7
Numbers of Hours of Care per Week per Helper Expended Providing Informal Services to Community-Based Disabled Elderly, 1980-2040 (in millions)

Age and Care	1980	2000	2020	2040
Age 65-74:				
IADL Only	12.56	14.70	24.12	23.49
1-2 ADL	13.50	15.86	25.98	25.44
3-4 ADL	7.70	9.11	14.99	14.76
5-6 ADL	12.52	14.64	23.91	23.24
Total	46.28	54.31	89.00	86.92
Age 75-84:				
IADL Only	10.08	16.47	19.71	32.14
1-2 ADL	13.10	21.21	25.26	41.42
3-4 ADL	7.33	12.06	14.37	23.57
5-6 ADL	11.87	19.45	23.28	38.17
Total	42.38	69.19	82.61	135.29
Age 85+:				
IADL Only	3.95	8.19	11.58	20.14
1-2 ADL	7.48	15.94	22.53	32.98
3-4 ADL	4.60	9.73	13.76	24.08
5-6 ADL	7.48	16.15	22.74	39.10
Total	23.50	50.01	70.61	122.30
Age 65+:				
IADL Only	26.59	39.36	55.41	75.76
1-2 ADL	34.08	53.01	73.77	105.83
3-4 ADL	19.63	30.90	43.13	62.40
5-6 ADL	31.87	50.24	69.92	100.51
Total	112.17	173.52	242.23	344.51

SOURCE: Tabulations of the 1982 National Long Term Care Survey, Duke University, Center for Demographic Studies.
NOTE: IADL is instrumental activity of daily living; ADL is activity of daily living.

Future changes in patterns of disease may not be all beneficial. The recent emergence of HIV infection and AIDS reminds us that new epidemics and diseases may put new demands on the requirements for care. Indeed, the elderly, who lose immunological capacity with age, may be at particular risk of AIDS infection (Manton & Singer, 1989). This risk has been recently confirmed in empirical studies, which show the latency time between exposure and manifestation of AIDS declining with age. As more persons live to more advanced ages, there may be created a population at special risk for new disease entities and certainly prone to the especially difficult care problems engendered by multiple chronic diseases.

In addition to possible future changes in disease risks, there is also the possibility of developing new service delivery systems. Several studies have evaluated the costs and benefits of geriatric evaluation units and subacute care centers. Specialized centers for health promotion targeted to preserving function and reducing the risks of disease at advanced ages may emerge. In addition, LTC has tended to emphasize the management of severely physically impaired persons through personal assistance. It is interesting, however, that a large amount of current LTC needs are being met through the provision of specialized equipment and housing modifications (Manton, 1989). It may be that, in the future, low-cost technological developments could fill more of the demand for LTC services.

Thus, in long-range projections, major changes in health status and in the organization of service delivery systems could have a significant impact on the level and types of demand for care. These qualitative factors engender considerable uncertainty about the direction of long-term trends. Consequently, we did not systematically consider their effects in our projections. Nonetheless, one must remain aware of the possibility of such changes.

PROJECTED CHANGES IN
REQUIREMENTS FOR PERSONNEL

The demographic, epidemiological, and health service projections described above have many qualitative and quantitative implications for the requirements for geriatric health personnel. In considering these implications, we must assess, first, whether the current level of personnel is adequate and, second, how demographic and epidemiological factors interact with changes in patterns of service delivery to change the demand for services.

Personnel for Meeting Current Service Needs:
Improving the Current Quality of Care

In assessing the adequacy of current levels of personnel, we again examine three different types of service—hospital, nursing home, and home health. The introduction of PPS for medicare reimbursement of acute hospital stays brought significant declines in both the length of stay and the hospitalization rate of elderly medicare beneficiaries.

These declines have, however, tended to be concentrated in the lighter care cases. As a consequence, the level of care for hospital admissions among medicare beneficiaries has tended to increase. Thus, while some hospitals, especially smaller and rural facilities, have experienced declining occupancy rates (and consequent fiscal problems), major medical centers (partly because of increased reimbursement per case because of the "teaching" hospital adjustments in PPS) have fared much better. Thus, though the number of hospital episodes declined, the demand per case for nursing and physician services increased. This has created a particularly complex situation in nursing, because the increasing intensity of care has increased the demands on the nurses' skill and technological capacity. This has created serious problems with nurses—because of factors such as occupational "burnout," rapid obsolescence of skills, and improved alternative labor markets for women—in the pattern of compensation as hospitals compete for nurses. However, studies of the impact of PPS on the quality of care suggest that, at least through 1985, no serious problems with the quality of care had yet arisen (Liu & Manton, in submission; Manton & Liu, 1990).

A second sector of care consists of nursing homes, which can be crudely described in terms of skilled nursing facilities (SNF), delivering a high level of postacute medical care, and intermediate-care facilities (ICF), delivering less intense medical care. An Institute of Medicine report (1986) raised questions about the quality of care in nursing facilities—a concern focused heavily on staffing. That report suggested that a large proportion of facilities lacked adequate numbers of nurses. Most facilities (12,609 of 13,823) did not achieve a 10-bed per R.N. staffing level. Among SNFs, more than three quarters of facilities (1,840 of 2,370) did not attain this level. Even if one counts both R.N.s and L.P.N.s, only a little more than half of the facilities (i.e., 7501 of 13,823) attained this level of staffing. To reduce the bed/nurse (R.N.) ratio to 10:1 nationally would require 87,000 additional nurses. In SNFs alone, meeting the bed/nurse ratio would require nearly 11,000 R.N.s. To reach this staffing level in all facilities using both R.N.s and L.P.N.s would require 24,000 nurses. These figures suggest that, to meet the lowest estimate of the shortfall of current nursing staff (i.e., 24,000 more nurses needed with 164,000 on staff in 1984), our projections should increase the forecast need for nurses by about 14%. This staff shortage may be underestimated, because it appears that the case mix for nursing facilities may become increasingly medically intensive as patients are discharged earlier, and in a more medically intense state, from hospitals into nursing homes because of PPS. These shortages will also be aggravated as compensation levels in hospitals rise relatively more rapidly than in nursing homes. Moreover, the potentially greater challenges offered by providing hospital care may give hospitals an advantage in the competition for the available pool of nurses.

The third major area of care, home health, is currently the most rapidly expanding type of care. To assess the adequacy of current levels of care, estimates can be made (from the 1982 NLTC survey) of the number of people who have unmet care needs due to chronic ADL or IADL limitations. In those data, approximately 1.5 million chronically disabled elderly persons living in the community reported that they have some chronic IADL limitation that is unmet; more than 190,000 persons reported some chronic ADL limitation unmet. In projecting the future need for medical services, we only consider persons with unmet ADL needs. This suggests that our current estimates of home care needs should be increased by 4.1%. It must also be remembered that unmet need for ADLS and IADLS increases the risk of institutionalization. Consequently, these figures do not tell us how many persons could be managed in the community if adequate home health services were available.

Future Needs for Geriatric Personnel

The projections in Table 12.8 represent increases in the need for physicians, nurses, and home health workers to maintain current levels and patterns of service. These projections required certain assumptions about the current patterns of service. For example, in 1983, there were 424,000 active physicians in the United States (Ginzberg, 1986), of whom 114,000 were hospital based (including 74,000 physicians in training). The effort of the non-hospital-based physicians must be allocated between "office" visits and hospital-based care. With that allocation, we can use the proportion of each type of care delivered to persons aged 65+ in the Rice and Feldman (1983) projections to get physician full-time equivalents (FTEs), which can then be multiplied by the projected demographic growth to determine future levels of personnel needs.

Studies suggest that, of an average 56.8-hour physician week, 25 hours are spent in the office, with the remainder spent on a variety of other activities (e.g., 8.4 hours in hospital rounds and 5.8 hours in surgery). If we assume that half of a physician's effort on patient care is spent in the hospital (this estimate involves averaging in the full-time effort of the 114,000 hospital-based physicians), because 15%

Table 12.8
Projection of Number of Physicians, Nurses, and Home Health Workers
Required to Maintain Current Levels of Service for the Elderly Population,
Under Mortality and Health and Service Variables

Variables	1985	2000	2020	2040
1. Physicians				
A. mortality variables				
a. intermediate	110,000	137,830	206,030	267,760
b. low	110,000	142,067	220,597	299,645
c. high	110,000	129,540	190,906	249,079
B. health and service variables				
a. improved	110,000	109,299	150,196	181,809
b. preserved functional status	110,000	137,830	206,030	267,760
c. increases in number of				
persons switching services	110,000	137,830	206,030	267,760
2. Nurses				
A. mortality variables				
a. intermediate	390,000	488,740	730,650	949,333
b. low	390,000	503,694	782,118	1,062,379
c. high	390,000	493,277	691,029	883,098
B. health and service variables				
a. improved	390,000	387,571	532,644	644,597
b. preserved functional status	390,000	488,740	730,650	949,333
c. increases in number of				
persons switching services	390,000	488,740	730,650	949,333
3. Home Health Workers				
aides				
A. mortality variables				
a. intermediate	198,900	249,258	372,640	484,059
b. low	198,900	256,884	398,880	541,813
c. high	198,900	234,231	352,425	450,380
B. health and services variables				
a. improved	198,900	197,661	271,655	328,676
b. preserved functional status	198,900	223,833	322,334	406,610
c. increases in number of				
persons switching services	198,900	466,158	978,169	1,345,309
nurses				
A. mortality variables				
a. intermediate	22,100	27,695	41,404	53,797
b. low	22,100	28,543	44,320	60,202
c. high	22,100	26,026	39,158	50,042
B. health and services variables				
a. improved	22,100	21,962	30,184	36,528
b. preserved functional status	22,100	24,870	35,815	45,189
c. increases in number of				
persons switching services	22,100	27,695	41,404	53,797

SOURCE: Duke University, Center for Demographic Studies.

of physician office visits are spent on the elderly (i.e., 0.15 × 210,000) and 38.3% on hospital visits (i.e., 0.383 × 210,000)—about 110,000 of the 424,000 total physician FTEs will be required by the elderly. With a projected growth of the elderly of 84% by 2020, 200,000 physician FTEs will be needed.

The projections for nurses are more complex because a larger proportion of care is delivered in nursing homes. (This was assumed to be negligible for physicians—falling into an "other" category.) Furthermore, a number of factors operate to change current patterns of service, such as the rapid turnover of nurses in specific care settings and the withdrawal of many nurses from active practice. These forces are, to a degree, being balanced by rapid increases in nursing salaries and by changes in the profession and practice itself. Depending on how these different forces balance, the future pool of practicing nurses may constrain growth so that the projected need for nurses cannot be met and alternate care strategies will be required. Our projections of the required number of nurses assume that the current level and patterns of care are preserved.

To make these projections, we allocated nurses' service delivery between hospitals, "other places of care," and nursing homes. Nursing home care is likely to require rapid increases of nursing personnel due to the rapid growth of the oldest-old population. In 1984, there were about 1.4 million active registered nurses (U.S. Bureau of Labor Statistics, 1987). There are about 700,000 persons in nursing facilities providing some level of nursing care, with about three fourths being nurses aides and the rest divided between R.N.s and L.P.N.s. In medicare-certified facilities, there are 68,000 R.N. FTEs and almost 100,000 L.P.N. FTEs. These can be projected directly as a function of the earlier projections of the growth of nursing home beds. If we subtract about 100,000 R.N.s (to increase the 68,000 FTEs to account for the 50% who work part-time), then we have 1.3 million active R.N.s not involved in nursing home care. Removing the 53,000 R.N.s involved in community nursing (1980 estimate; National Institute on Aging, 1984) leaves 1.25 million nurses, of whom we will allocate 900,000 into hospital care and 350,000 into direct patient care (the allocation into direct patient care simply assumes that there are as many nurses involved in such care as there are physicians). We can then develop estimates of FTEs using the proportion of care delivered to the elderly projected by Rice and Feldman. This yields about 350,000 nurses (900,000 × 0.38) devoted to delivering care to the elderly in hospitals and about 40,000 nurses (0.15 × 350,000) delivering care in physicians' offices and other places.

With an increase of 84% in the elderly population by 2020, the figure of 390,000 R.N.s in hospitals and in primary care settings will need to increase to about 740,000. We project that the number of nurses required in nursing homes by 2020 will grow by about 150%, or 250,000 R.N.s (400,000 total nurses).

Projecting the need for home health aides and nurses providing home health services is difficult because we do not know the full demand for home health service—the use of home health services has been rapidly expanding and we do not know the point of market saturation. Moreover, there are no clear standards for the staffing of home health services. Nonetheless, we can make crude estimates of the demand for home health aides and nurses using data from the NLTCS and associated Part A medicare files.

The annual average number of medicare home health visits reported in a recent GAO report was 33—an average of 20 visits for persons not chronically disabled and an average of 40 visits for chronically disabled persons. Multiplying these two annual average numbers of visits by the number of nonchronically disabled (694,452) and chronically disabled (785,180) persons reporting medicare home health service use in 1984, we project a total of 45.3 million home health visits.

An additional question is this: How much effort (staff time) will be required for these visits? From the National Opinion Research Center (NORC) caregivers survey for the 1982 NLTCS, the number of hours of care delivered by an individual caregiver to an impaired person (beyond their usual household functions) was estimated as between 3 and 3.5 hours. If a similar amount of care were delivered by a home health agency on a per-visit basis, a home health worker could conduct, on average, two visits per day. This seems consistent with the medicare average reimbursement per visit (in 1982) of $36. Given 250 work days per year (times two visits per day), this implies a need for 90,592 home health workers.

To determine how much of this aid is provided by nurses versus home health aides, we observe, from the 1984 NLTCS, that about 10% of persons paying for informal care (82,293 of 860,504) received nursing services. That suggests that about 81,000 home health aides and 9,000 home health nurses were required in 1985. The calculations do not account, however, for the newness of home health services and the fact that they are not yet available in all areas. Thus we need to estimate the unfulfilled need for home health services. To do this, we refer to estimates from the NLTCS (1982), showing 1,547,964 persons who reported unmet IADL needs and 190,191 persons who reported unmet ADL needs. If these 1,738,155 persons represent the current unmet need for home health services and these persons use 40 home health visits per year (as did the other chronically disabled group), there would be a need for 65.5 million additional home health visits or 131,000 home health aides and nurses.

Combining the two estimates, we project a need for 198,900 home health aides and 22,100 home health nurses in 1985. By 2000, this increases to 249,258 home health aides and 27,695 home health nurses. By 2040, with the rapid growth of the oldest-old population, the demand for home health aides reaches 484,059, and for home health nurses, 53,797.

In Table 12.8, we also present projections illustrating the effect of the different mortality assumptions. The changes due to different mortality conditions by 2020 are modest—on the order of 10% in 2020. This is due to several factors. Much increase is already programmed in, due to increases in birth cohort sizes. Life expectancy at age 65 is already high, so the projected percentage increase in life expectancy past 65 is not large. Additionally, larger fluctuations would be manifest about age 85, with its more uncertain life expectancy.

Table 12.8 also presents the variation of service projections due to improvement in health. The "health improvement only" projection assumes that personnel requirements are reduced proportionately by health-promotion activity. This suggests an overall reduction of 27.1% in 2020. This level of change is much greater than that produced by the variations in the high- and low-mortality assumptions.

Certain types of care may be more sensitive to health-promotion activities. Table 12.8 illustrates the effects if functional status could be preserved—but with only a 50% decline in the demand for acute care. Under these conditions, the projected need would be 223,833 home health aides in 2000. In addition, we combine the impact of increases in the number of persons who switch from relying on informal care services to formal care services with health and acute service uses changing at different rates. In these projections, we assume that 5% will shift in 2000 and 10% will shift in 2020.

A major recent PPS-induced shift in the patterns of care delivered is the consumption of more outpatient services to substitute for the reduction in hospital care. This occurred because hospitalization rates declined for cases that were less care intensive. It is important to note, however, that the more seriously disabled persons in the community tended to consume both informal and formal home care services.

Because the types of care delivered by formal and informal caregivers may be quite different—with formal care being more medically intensive—the two sources of care might not be interchangeable.

CONCLUSIONS

Our projections of the acute and LTC health services and personnel required by the elderly U.S. population are subject to several sources of uncertainty. First, they are subject to uncertainty in projecting the size and health status of the future elderly and oldest-old population. There is uncertainty about future mortality, morbidity, and disability rates, uncertainty about our ability to change these rates, and uncertainty on the resources we will expend to alter these rates.

There is also uncertainty about the types of health services that will be delivered to elderly persons in different health and functional states. To some degree, restrictions on the ability to substitute different types of services are endogenous—the financial, educational, and social resources of the elderly will affect the ability of a person with specific health problems and functional limitations to remain in the community by utilizing home health services. The ability to substitute services will also be constrained by federal and state policies regarding the reimbursement of different types of LTC services.

Underlying both types of uncertainty are potential future changes in the behavior of government, major social institutions (e.g., private markets for acute care, LTC, and housing services), and individuals. Government, with appropriate reimbursement incentives, could promote facilities for health promotion and disease/disability prevention or shift more persons from institutional to home care. Private institutions, in recognition of the increasing economic power of the elderly, could develop new technologies and markets for health and LTC service. Individuals with better education and financial resources could adopt healthier life-styles.

To cope with the future growth in demand for acute and LTC health services, changes will be necessary in all of these areas (i.e., health promotion, organization of the health service delivery systems, the development of new medical and caregiving technologies). The challenge at the federal level is to provide incentives for these changes to occur—but without potentially restrictive overregulation. Efforts to develop such incentives are under way. For example, in the area of reimbursement, it is generally accepted that there will be major roles both for the private acute and LTC insurance market and for publicly reimbursed care (Liu, Manton, & Liu, in press). As a consequence, the government is encouraging efforts to develop better private LTC and medigap insurance policies, though it is also recognized that only a proportion of the elderly population will qualify, either on economic or on medical grounds, for coverage (Rivlin & Wiener, 1988). The Catastrophic Care Legislation enacted in 1988 was designed to eliminate gaps in medicare acute care coverage and to extend benefits, for the first time, to include prescription drugs. The legislation was repealed in 1989, leaving those gaps and raising a new question about the adequacy of supplementary private insurance coverage, which is possessed primarily by the more affluent elderly, and the need for public coverage of LTC services. While considerable effort is being expended on these issues, there seems to be much less activity directed toward facilitating reimbursement for health-promoting medical care activities.

While the challenge in providing adequate levels of care to a rapidly increasing elderly population is clear, the governmental strategies by which we will ensure that such services will be available are not. This area will require considerable future research in the scientific, health services, and public policy arenas. To be effective, such research will require the collection of significant amounts of new population and longitudinal survey data. It is clear that the current level of social and economic data collection and research is woefully inadequate relative to the scope and complexity of the federal programs involved and the magnitude of federal and state expenditures on those programs. This research is needed for all phases of the programs—for identifying the highest-priority areas of need, for the extension or modification of programs, for designing the programs, for monitoring their operation, and for assessing their impact on the health and welfare of the population they service. Large increases in both data collection resources and analyses are thus required to improve and maintain the efficiency and efficacy of the programs.

REFERENCES

Anderson, W. F. (1988). Expectations from recombinant DNA research. In J. B. Wyngaarten & L. H. Smith (Eds.), *Cecil textbook of medicine*. Philadelphia: Harcourt.

Brody, J. A. (1984). The best of times/The worst of times: Aging and dependency in the 21st Century. In S. R. Ingman & I. R. Lawson (Eds.), *Ethical dimensions of geriatric care: Value conflicts of the 21st century* (Philosophy and Medicine Series, No. 25; S. F. Spicker, Ed.; pp. 3-22). Dordrecht, Holland: D. Reidel.

Feldman, J. J. (1983). Workability of the aged under conditions of improving mortality. *Milbank Quarterly, 61,* 430-444.

Ginzberg, E. (Ed.). (1986). *From physician shortage to patient shortage: The uncertain future of medical practice.* Boulder, CO: Westview.

Institute of Medicine. (1986). *Final report of the Subcommittee on Reimbursement and Other Factors Affecting Quality.* Washington, DC: Panel on Nursing Home Regulations, National Academy of Sciences.

Kannel, W. B., & Gordon, T. (1980). Cardiovascular risk factors in the aged: The Framingham Study. In S. G. Haynes & M. Feinleib (Eds.), *Epidemiology of aging* (U.S. DHHS Pub. No. 80-969; pp. 65-90). Washington, DC: Government Printing Office.

Kaplan, G. A., Seeman, T. E., Cohen, R. D., Knudsen, L. P., & Guralnik, J. (1987). Mortality among the elderly in the Alameda County study: Behavioral and demographic risk factors. *American Journal of Public Health, 77,* 307-312.

Lakatta, E. G. (1985). Health, disease, and cardiovascular aging. In *Health in an older society* (Committee on an Aging Society, Institute of Medicine and National Research Council, pp. 73-104)). Washington, DC: National Academy Press.

Lew, E. A., & Garfinkel, L. (1984). Mortality at ages 65 and over in a middle-class population. *Transactions of the Society of Actuaries, 36,* 257-295.

Liu, K., & Manton, K. G. (in submission). *Effects of PPS on hospital readmissions and mortality of disabled medicare beneficiaries.*

Liu, K., Manton, K. G., & Liu, B. (1985). Home health care expenses for noninstitutionalized elderly with ADL and IADL limitations. *HCF Review, 71,* 51-58.

Liu, K., Manton, K. G., & Liu, B. (1990). Morbidity, disability and long-term care: Implications for insurance financing. *Milbank Quarterly, 68,* 445-493.

Luce, B. R., Liu, K., & Manton, K. G. (1984). Estimating the long term care population and its use of services. In *Long term care and social security* (ISSA Studies and Research No. 21, pp. 34-58). Geneva, Switzerland: ISSA.

Manton, K. G. (1986). Past and future life expectancy increases at later ages: Their implications for the linkage of chronic morbidity, disability and mortality. *Journal of Gerontology, 41,* 672-681.

Manton, K. G. (1987). The linkage of health status changes and workability. *Comprehensive Gerontology, 1,* 16-24.

Manton, K. G. (1988). A longitudinal study of functional change and mortality in the U.S. *Journal of Gerontology, 43,* 153-161.

Manton, K. G. (1989). Epidemiological, demographic, and social correlates of disability among the elderly. *Milbank Quarterly, 67,* 13-58.

Manton, K. G., & Liu, K. (1990). Recent changes in service use patterns of disabled medicare beneficiaries. *HCF Review, 11,* 51-66.

Manton, K. G., Siegler, I. C., & Woodbury, M. A. (1986). Patterns of intellectual development in later life. *Journal of Gerontology, 41,* 486-499.

Manton, K. G., & Singer, B. (1989). Forecasting the impact of the AIDS epidemic on elderly populations. In M. W. Riley, M. G. Ory, & D. Zablotsky (Eds.), *AIDS in an aging society* (pp. 169-191). New York: Springer.

Manton, K. G., & Soldo, B. J. (in press). Disability and mortality among the oldest-old: Implications for current and future health and long term care service needs. In R. Suzman, D. Willis, & K. G. Manton (Eds.), *Forecasting the health of the old*. New York: Oxford University Press.

Manton, K. G., & Stallard, E. (1988). *Chronic disease modeling: Measurement and evaluation of the risks of chronic disease processes*. London: Charles Griffin.

Manton, K. G., & Stallard, E. (in press). Cross-sectional estimates of active life expectancy for the U.S. elderly and oldest-old populations. *Journal of Gerontology*.

Myers, G. C. (1981). Future age projections and society. In A. Gilmore et al. (Eds.), *Aging: A challenge and social policy* (pp. 248-261). New York: Oxford University Press.

National Institute on Aging. (1984). *Report on education and training in geriatrics and gerontology, administrative document*. Bethesda, MD: Department of Health and Human Services, Public Health Services.

Nihon University. (1982). *Population aging in Japan: Problems and policy issues in the 21st century*. Tokyo: Nihon University Population Research Institute.

Ogawa, N. (1982). Japan's limit to growth and welfare. In *Population aging in Japan: Problems and policy issues in the 21st century* (pp. 3-1 to 3-28). Tokyo: Nihon University Population Research Institute.

Rice, D. P., & Feldman, J. J. (1983). Living longer in the United States: Demographic changes and health needs of the elderly. *Milbank Quarterly, 61,* 362-396.

Rivlin, A. M., & Wiener, J. M. (1988). *Caring for the disabled elderly: Who will pay?* Washington, DC: Brookings Institution.

Rowe, J. W. (1988). Aging and geriatric medicine. In W. B. Wyngaarten & L. H. Smith (Eds.), *Cecil textbook of medicine*. Philadelphia: Harcourt.

Rowe, J. W., & Wang, S. (1988). The biology and physiology of aging. In J. R. Rowe & R. W. Besdine (Eds.), *Geriatric medicine* (pp. 1-11). Boston: Little, Brown.

Schneider, E. L., & Guralnik, J. M. (1987). The compression of morbidity: A dream which may come true someday! *Gerontologica Perspecta, 1,* 8-13.

Soldo, B. J., & Manton, K. G. (1985). Health status and service needs of the oldest old: Current patterns and future trends. *Milbank Quarterly, 62,* 286-319.

U.S. Bureau of the Census. (1984). Projections of the population of the U.S. by age, sex, and race: 1983-2080. In *Current population reports* (Series P-25, No. 952). Washington, DC: Government Printing Office.

U.S. Bureau of Labor Statistics. (1987). *Employment and earnings, January*. Washington, DC: Government Printing Office.

U.S. Department of Health and Human Services, Social Security Administration, Office of the Actuary. (1985). *Social security area population projections 1985* (Actuarial Study No. 95; SSA Pub. No. 11-11542). Washington, DC: Government Printing Office.

U.S. Department of Health and Human Services, Social Security Administration, Office of the Actuary. (1987). *Social security area population projections 1987* (Actuarial Study No. 99, by Alice Wade; SSA Pub. No. 11-11546). Washington, DC: Government Printing Office.

World Health Organization. (1984). *The uses of epidemiology in the study of the elderly* (Report of a WHO Scientific Group on the Epidemiology of Aging; Technical Report Series 706). Geneva, Switzerland: Author.

World Health Organization. (1989). *World health statistics, Annual, 1989*. Geneva, Switzerland: Author.

Index

About the Authors

Ronald Peter Abeles (Ph.D., Harvard University) is Deputy Associate Director for the National Institute on Aging's Behavioral and Social Research Program. He also serves as Executive Secretary of the National Institutes of Health's Working Group on Health and Behavior. He received his doctorated in social psychology in 1972 and completed a Postdoctoral Fellowship in political science and psychology in 1972 from Yale University. He has conducted research in the areas of life-span development, health and social support, and personal control and efficacy.

Margret M. Baltes (Ph.D.) is Professor of Psychological Gerontology at the Free University of Berlin, Germany, where she holds a joint appointment in the Departments of Gerontopsychiatry and Psychology. She heads the research unit on psychological gerontology. The thrust of her research is in the field of developmental psychology of aging with research projects on dependency in aging; on successful aging, behavioral competence, and everyday activities; and on limits in cognitive plasticity in the very early phase of Alzheimer's disease. She is the author of several books and articles on behavioral gerontology.

Sue Borson (M.D.) obtained her M.D. degree from Stanford University Medical School in 1969. She completed her psychiatric residency and a two-year Geriatric Psychiatry Fellowship at the University of

Washington in 1981. Since 1981, she has been chief of the Geropsychiatry Evaluation and Treatment Unit at the Seattle VAMC. She is the author of 30 publications. She is Associate Professor of Psychiatry and Behavioral Sciences at the University of Washington School of Medicine. Her major research interest has been in psychological disorders associated with medical illness.

Kathryn Dean (Ph.D., M.S.W., R.N.) is Senior Research Scientist with the Institute of Social Medicine, the faculty of Medicine at the University of Copenhagen. She also serves as a Leader of the World Health Organization (WHO) Collaborating Center for Health Promotion Research at the Institute of Social Medicine. She has worked extensively in the areas of health promotion and life-style and life situation influences of health. She has also focused on methodological issues affecting the quality and validity of survey research on health.

Gordon H. DeFriese (Ph.D.) is Professor of Social Medicine, Epidemiology and Health Policy and Administration, and Director of the Health Services Research Center at the University of North Carolina at Chapel Hill. His personal research interests have included studies in the areas of rural health care, child health services, dental care, medical technology assessment, cost-effectiveness and cost-benefit analysis, medical specialization, health promotion and preventive health services, and aging. He was a member of the U.S. Preventive Services Task Force and is a current member of the U.S. Preventive Services Coordinating Committee. A former president of the Association for Health Services Research, he is the editor of *Health Services Research*, the association's official journal.

Carroll L. Estes (Ph.D.) is Chairperson/Professor in the Department of Social and Behavioral Sciences, and Director, Institute for Health & Aging, School of Nursing, University of California, San Francisco. Her Ph.D. is from the University of California, San Diego, and she conducts research and writes on health policy, the sociology of aging, gender, political economy, and medical sociology.

H. Asuman Kiyak (Ph.D.) is a professor in the Department of Oral and Maxillofacial Surgery and an adjunct professor in the Department of Psychology at the University of Washington. She directs the Program in Geriatric Dentistry and is responsible for graduate-level training in geriatric dentistry in the Health Science Schools at the University of Washington. She has conducted research in the fields of health promotion for well and frail elderly, health service utilization among elderly at risk, and health behaviors among minority elderly. She has had grants from the NIH and private foundations on these and other aspects of aging, including person-environment congruence among older persons with Alzheimer's disease and their caregivers. She has published more than 70 articles in gerontology, geriatric dentistry, and health behavior.

Elaine A. Leventhal (M.D., Ph.D.) is Associate Professor in the Department of Medicine and Head of Geriatrics in the Division of General Internal Medicine and Geriatrics, at the University of Medicine and Dentistry of New Jersey, Robert Wood Johnson Medical School. She directs the interdisciplinary and educational, clinical, and research programs and is also an affiliated member of the Institute of Health, Health Care Policy, and Aging Research at Rutgers University. Her research investigates aging and markers of frailty by studying health behaviors in the ambulatory elderly and aging in the institutionalized developmentally disabled elderly. She has also researched the impact of governmental regulations on the most frail—the over 85-year-old nursing home patient before and after DRGs. She is currently studying risk factors for immune competency, morbidity, and mortality and their impact on health and illness (including alcohol abuse) behaviors.

Howard Leventhal (Ph.D.) is Research Professor of Psychology and Chair of the Division of Health of the Institute for Health, Health Care Policy, and Aging Research at Rutgers, the State University of New Jersey. He is director of the interdisciplinary program in health psychology and is responsible for graduate training of students in the Social and Clinical Psychology Programs. He has conducted research in the areas of adolescent health behavior, such as the conditions initiating substance use and techniques for intervening in substance use, illness cognition or lay understanding of health threats, and coping with health threats and has contributed extensively to theoretical writing in psychology of human emotion. He has been a member and is now Chair of the National Institutes of Health Behavioral Medicine Study Section. He has produced more than 175 publications.

Lennart Levi (M.D., Ph.D.) is founder and Chairman of the Department of Stress Reduction/WHO Psychosocial Center of the Karolinska Institutet, Professor of Psychosocial Medicine at the Karolinska Institutet, Director of the National Swedish Institute for Psychosocial Factors and Health (IPM), and a member of the WHO expert panel on mental health.

Paula Darba Lipman (Ph.D.) is a Postdoctoral Fellow in the Laboratory of Socio-Environmental Studies at the National Institute of Mental Health in Bethesda, Maryland. During the development of this volume, she was a Social Science Analyst at the National Institute on Aging. She is interested in the relationship between cognitive functioning in everyday situations and age-related memory changes. Her current research interests are in the area of age differences in macrospatial processing.

Kenneth G. Manton (Ph.D.) is Research Professor and Research Director of Demographic Studies at Duke University and Medical Research Professor at Duke University Medical Center's Department of Community and Family Medicine. He is also a Senior Fellow of the Duke University Medical Center's Center for the Study of Aging and Human Development and Assistant Director of the Duke University Center for Demographic Studies. In 1986, he was named head of the World Health Organization Collaborating Center for Research and Training in the Methods of Assessing Risk and Forecasting Health Status Trends as Related to Multiple Disease Outcomes, based at the Center for Demographic Studies. His current research interests include forecasting morbidity, disability, and mortality among the nation's elderly, reimbursement maintenance of quality of care for both acute and long-term care services consumed by the elderly, mathematical modeling of physiological aging processes of human mortality at advanced ages, and differentials in those processes by sex and race and cross-nationally.

Marcia G. Ory (Ph.D., M.P.H.) is Chief, Social Science Research on Aging, Behavioral and Social Research Program, National Institute on Aging, National Institutes of Health, Bethesda, Maryland. She holds a Ph.D. from Purdue University and a master's of public health from the Johns Hopkins University. She is very active in professional organizations and serves on several national task forces and advisory boards dealing with aging and health issues. Her main areas of interest include aging and health care, health and behavior research, and gender differences in health and longevity. She has published widely on these topics.

William Rakowski (Ph.D.) is Associate Professor of Community Health (Research) in the Center for Gerontology and Health Care Research and the Department of Community Health at Brown University. His research interests are in health behavior and health promotion with middle-aged and older adults and in the relationships among multiple health-related practices.

Judith Rodin (Ph.D.) is Chair of the Department of Psychology and the Philip R. Allen Professor of Psychology at Yale University. She also serves as Professor of Medicine and Psychiatry at Yale University. She received her Ph.D. from Columbia University in 1970 and was a National Science Foundation Post-Doctoral Fellow in Neurobiology. She is currently President of the Society for Behavioral Medicine and is past president of both the Eastern Psychological Association and the Division of Health Psychology (38) of the American Psychological Association. Her work covers a broad spectrum of areas related to psychosocial and biobehavioral determinants of health and disease.

Thomas G. Rundall (Ph.D.) is Professor of Health and Sociology in the School of Public Health at the University of California, Berkeley. He received his Ph.D. in sociology from Stanford University and has served on the faculty of the Sloan Program in Health Services Administration at Cornell University. Since 1987, he has served as Chair of the Department of Social and Administrative Health Sciences and as the editor of *Medical Care Review*. His primary areas of interest include the sociology of health and illness, organizational theory, and evaluation research.

Pamela M. Schaefer is a graduate student in clinical psychology at the University of Wisconsin, Milwaukee. Under the direction of Howard and Elaine Leventhal, she has conducted research on the psychological aspects of health care utilization in middle-aged and elderly adults, examined perceptions of health and aging in similar populations, and studied aging in the developmentally disabled. Currently, she is studying the psychological and physical effects of stress.

Richard Suzman (Ph.D.) is the Chief of Demography and Population Epidemiology, Behavioral and Social Research Program, National Institute on Aging, National Institutes of Health, Bethesda, Maryland.

He is also the staff Director of the Federal Forum on Aging-Related Statistics. His major areas of interest are demography of aging, population epidemiology, and health and retirement economics. He has published widely on these topics.

Christine Timko (Ph.D.) is Associate Director of the Center for Health Care Evaluation at the VA Medical Center in Palo Alto, California. The center is a program of the Health Services Research and Development (HSR&D) Service in the Department of Veterans Affairs. She is also a member of the Social Ecology Lab, which is affiliated with the VA and Stanford University Medical Center in Palo Alto. She is currently conducting research on the quality of care in residential treatment facilities for older people. In addition, she is supported by the HSR&D in the Department of Veterans Affairs to examine the quality of care in inpatient and residential psychiatric and substance abuse treatment programs.

Thomas M. Vogt (M.D., M.P.H.) is Senior Investigator and Director of the Program in Epidemiology and Disease Prevention at the Kaiser Permanente Center for Health Research in Portland, Oregon. He is also Director of the Tobacco Reduction and Cancer Control (TRACC) program, an NCI-funded program project directed at cost-effectively integrating cancer prevention and control activities into the routine delivery of medical care. His other research interests and projects include psychological and social predictors of survival, morbidity, and mortality, cardiovascular disease epidemiology and clinical trials, risk factors for osteoporosis, and hypertension prevention. He is the author of about 50 articles on epidemiological, health behavior, and gerontological issues.

Hans-Werner Wahl (Ph.D.) is a consultant to the Berliner Aging Study of the Berlin Academy of Sciences, Berlin, Germany. His research interests lie in the field of ecological gerontology with a specific emphasis on person-environment fit models with regard to everyday competence of the elderly. He has published a number of articles in gerontological and gerontopsychiatric journals.

Alison Woomert (Ph.D.) is Research Associate at the Health Services Research Center at the University of North Carolina at Chapel Hill. Currently, she is Project Coordinator for a national study of self-care behavior of elderly persons. Her research activities have focused on health promotion and disease prevention, self-care organizations, assessing self-care behavior of community-based elderly persons, home care alternatives to institutionalization for elderly persons, smoking cessation, and asthma care costs. Recently receiving her Ph.D. in sociology, her dissertation examined social support, self-efficacy, and behavior change in a self-help smoking cessation program.

DEMCO